Surfactants and Polymers in Drug Delivery

DRUGS AND THE PHARMACEUTICAL SCIENCES

Executive Editor
James Swarbrick
PharmaceuTech, Inc.
Pinehurst, North Carolina

Advisory Board

Larry L. Augsburger
University of Maryland
Baltimore, Maryland

David E. Nichols
Purdue University
West Lafayette, Indiana

Douwe D. Breimer
Gorlaeus Laboratories
Leiden, The Netherlands

Stephen G. Schulman
University of Florida
Gainesville, Florida

Trevor M. Jones
The Association of the
British Pharmaceutical Industry
London, United Kingdom

Jerome P. Skelly
Alexandria, Virginia

Hans E. Junginger
Leiden/Amsterdam Center
for Drug Research
Leiden, The Netherlands

Felix Theeuwes
Alza Corporation
Palo Alto, California

Vincent H. L. Lee
University of Southern California
Los Angeles, California

Geoffrey T. Tucker
University of Sheffield
Royal Hallamshire Hospital
Sheffield, United Kingdom

Peter G. Welling
Institut de Recherche Jouveinal
Fresnes, France

DRUGS AND THE PHARMACEUTICAL SCIENCES

A Series of Textbooks and Monographs

Surfactants and Polymers in Drug Delivery

Martin Malmsten

*Institute for Surface Chemistry and
Royal Institute of Technology
Stockholm, Sweden*

MARCEL DEKKER, INC.   NEW YORK • BASEL

ISBN: 0-8247-0804-0

This book is printed on acid-free paper.

Headquarters
Marcel Dekker, Inc.
270 Madison Avenue, New York, NY 10016
tel: 212-696-9000; fax: 212-685-4540

Eastern Hemisphere Distribution
Marcel Dekker AG
Hutgasse 4, Postfach 812, CH-4001 Basel, Switzerland
tel: 41-61-261-8482; fax: 41-61-261-8896

World Wide Web
http://www.dekker.com

The publisher offers discounts on this book when ordered in bulk quantities. For more information, write to Special Sales/Professional Marketing at the headquarters address above.

Current printing (last digit):
10 9 8 7 6 5 4 3 2 1

PRINTED IN THE UNITED STATES OF AMERICA

Preface

Surfactant and polymer systems play an important role in modern drug delivery, where they may allow control of the drug release rate, enhance effective drug solubility, minimize drug degradation, contribute to reduced drug toxicity, and facilitate control of drug uptake. In all, they contribute significantly to therapeutic efficiency. However, although understanding of the physicochemical properties and behavior of surfactants and polymers in solution and at interfaces has undergone dramatic development in the past couple of decades, the new findings have generally not been fully implemented in drug delivery, most likely as a result of lack of interdisciplinary communication. Things are gradually changing, however, and scientists and engineers in both academia and industry are paying increasing attention to physicochemical aspects of surfactant and polymer systems and recognizing their importance for the design and controlled use of advanced drug delivery formulations. This is fueled by the development of new biopharmaceuticals in the wake of recent advances in genomics and proteomics. In parallel, a push for advanced drug delivery formulations based on surfactants and polymers has originated from the development of many new synthetic drugs that are sparingly soluble and noncrystallizing compounds, which often are difficult to formulate by traditional means. Here, surfactant and polymer systems of various types offer real potential.

The present book represents an attempt to discuss the basics of surfactant and polymer surface activity and self-assembly, the various types of structures formed by such compounds, and how they may be used in drug delivery. For this purpose, individual chapters are devoted to micelles, liquid crystalline phases, liposomes, microemulsions, emulsions, gels, and solid particles. Because bio-degradation of surfactant and polymer systems has a particularly important effect on their use in drug delivery, a separate chapter is devoted to this topic. Finally, further processing of such formulations, for example, through spray-drying and freeze-drying, is discussed.

I would like to thank Professors Björn Lindman, Thomas Arnebrant, and Per Claesson for fruitful discussions on these topics and for helpful comments on the manuscript. I also express my gratitude to Maud Norberg for her skillful help with the figures and Britt Nyström for help with literature issues.

Martin Malmsten

Contents

Contents

Surfactants and Polymers in Drug Delivery

1

Introduction

Surfactants and polymers are extensively used as excipients in drug delivery. However, although the understanding of the physicochemical properties and behavior of such compounds both in solution and at interfaces has undergone a dramatic development in the last couple of decades, the new findings are frequently not implemented to the full extent possible in various application areas. One reason for this is probably that surface and colloid chemistry is a relatively young scientific discipline, which only during the few last decades has matured into a broad research area, and which commonly is not extensively covered in the curriculum in the training of researchers for adjacent research areas, such as galenic pharmacy. Things are changing, however, and scientists and engineers in both academia and industry are paying increasing attention to surface and colloid chemistry and recognizing its importance, e.g., for the design and controlled use of advanced drug delivery formulations. Such formulations play an important role in modern drug delivery, since the demands on delivery vehicles increase, e.g., regarding drug release rate, drug solubilization capacity, minimization of drug degradation, reduction of drug toxicity, etc., but also since the vehicle as such may be used to control the drug uptake and biological response. This is the case not the least for new biopharmaceuticals being developed based on recent advances in genomics and proteomics. A particular role in this context is taken by surfactants and polymers, which may form various structures which may be

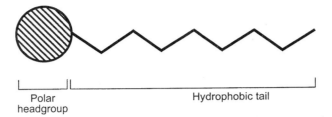

Polar
headgroup

Hydrophobic tail

Figure 1.1   Schematic illustration of a surfactant molecule.

useful for drug delivery applications. The purpose of the present book is therefore to go through the basics of surfactant and polymer surface activity and self-assembly, and the various types of structures formed by such compounds, as well as how such structures may be used in drug delivery.

1.1   INTRODUCTION TO SURFACTANTS

Surfactants are low to moderate molecular weight compounds which contain one hydrophobic part, which is generally readily soluble in oil but sparingly soluble or insoluble in water, and one hydrophilic (or polar) part, which is sparingly soluble or insoluble in oil but readily soluble in water (Figure 1.1). Due to this ''schizophrenic'' nature of surfactant molecules, these experience suboptimal conditions when dissolved molecularly in aqueous solution. If the hydrophobic segment is very large the surfactant will not be water-soluble, whereas for smaller hydrophobic moieties, the surfactant is soluble, but the contact between the hydrophobic block and the aqueous medium nevertheless energetically less favorable than the water-water contacts. Alternatives to a molecular solution, where the

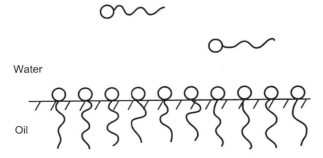

Water

Oil

Figure 1.2   Schematic illustration of the adsorption of surfactants at the oil-water interface.

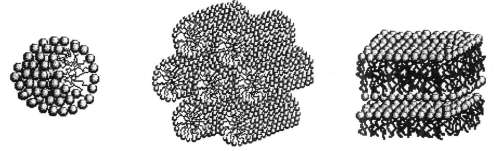

FIGURE 1.3 Schematic illustration of some different self-assembled structures formed in surfactant systems. (Redrawn from Jönsson et al., Surfactants and Polymers in Aqueous Solution, Wiley, 1998.)

contact between the hydrophobic group and the aqueous surrounding is reduced, therefore offer ways for these systems to reduce their free energy. Consequently, surfactants are surface active, and tend to accumulate at various interfaces, where the water contact is reduced (Figure 1.2).

Another way to reduce the oil-water contact is self-assembly, through which the hydrophobic domains of the surfactant molecules can associate to form various structures, which allow a reduced oil-water contact. Various such structures can be formed, including micelles, microemulsions, and a range of liquid crystalline phases (Figure 1.3). The type of structures formed depends on a range of parameters, such as the size of the hydrophobic domain, the nature and size of the polar head group, temperature, salt concentration, pH, etc. Through varying these parameters, one structure may also turn into another, which offers interesting opportunities in triggered drug delivery.

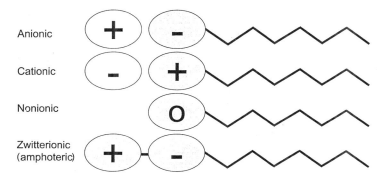

FIGURE 1.4 Schematic illustration of the various types of surfactants.

Surfactants are classified according to their polar headgroup; i.e., surfactants with a negatively charged headgroup are referred to as anionic surfactants, whereas cationic surfactants contain polar headgroups with a positive charge. Uncharged surfactants are generally referred to as nonionic, whereas zwitterionic surfactants contain both a negatively charged and a positively charged group (Figure 1.4).

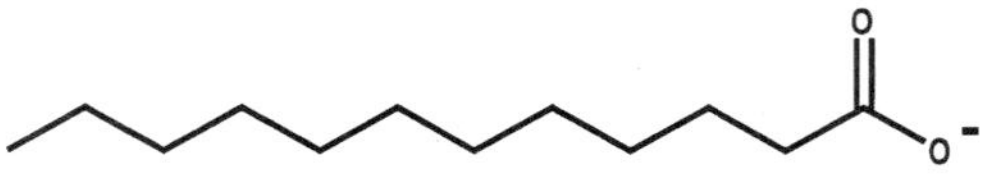

Soap

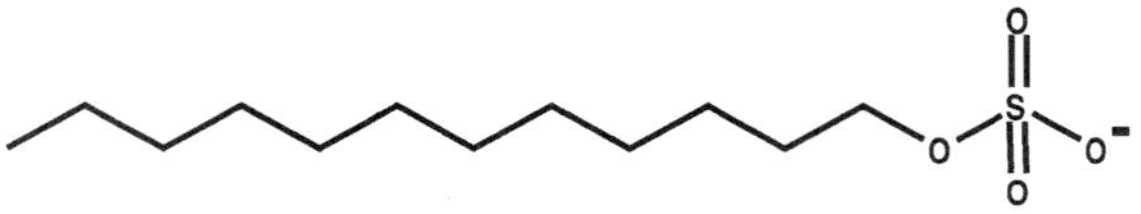

Na lauryl sulphate (SDS)

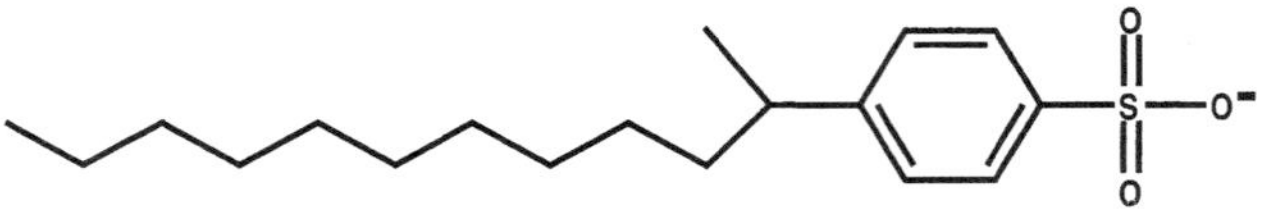

Alkyl benzene sulphonate

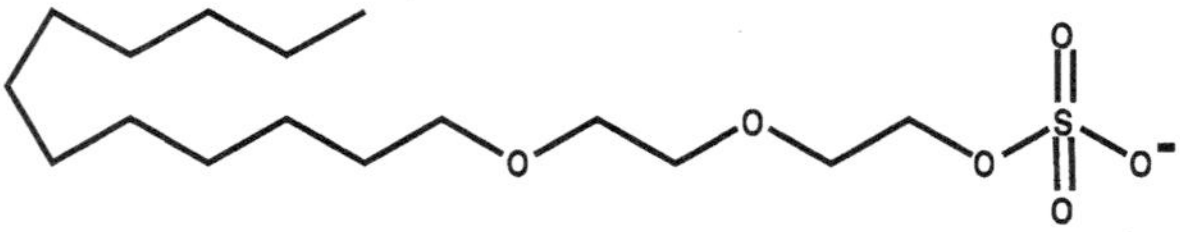

Alkyl ether sulphate

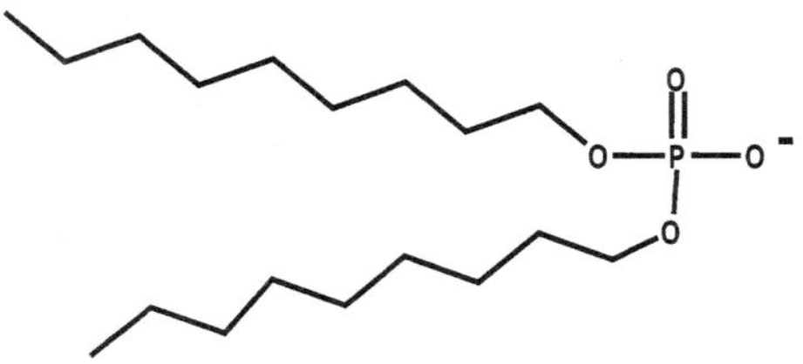

Phosphate ester

FIGURE 1.5 Chemical structure of some commonly used anionic surfactants.

Anionic surfactants (Figure 1.5) constitute the largest group of available surfactants. Examples of such surfactants include,

1. Fatty acid salts (''soaps'')
2. Sulfates
3. Ether sulfates
4. Phosphate esters

A common feature of all anionic surfactants is that their properties, e.g., surface activity and self-assembly, are quite sensitive to salt, and particularly divalent or multivalent cations. A commonly experienced illustration of this is poor solubility, foaming, and cleaning efficiency of alkyl sulfate surfactants in salt or hard water. Naturally, this salt dependence also offers opportunities in drug delivery. Sulfates are also somewhat sensitive toward hydrolysis, particularly at low pH,

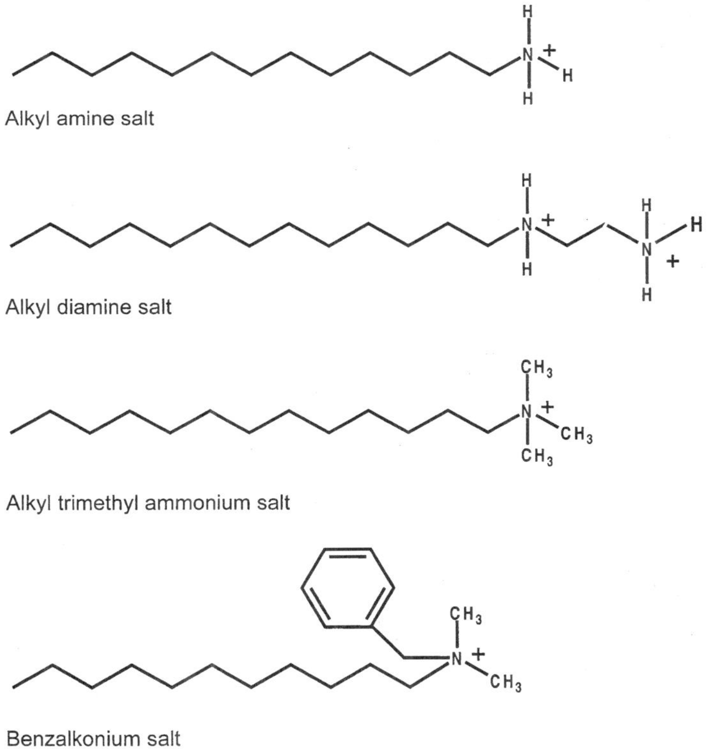

Alkyl amine salt

Alkyl diamine salt

Alkyl trimethyl ammonium salt

Benzalkonium salt

FIGURE 1.6 Chemical structure of some commonly used cationic surfactants.

but are still one of the most frequently used anionic surfactant types in drug delivery.

Cationic surfactants are frequently based on amine-containing polar head-groups (Figure 1.6). Due to their charged nature, the properties of cationic surfactants, e.g., surface activity or structure formation, are generally strongly dependent on the salt concentration, and on the valency of anions present. Cationic surfactants are frequently used as antibacterial agents, which may be advantageous also in certain drug delivery applications, such as delivery systems to the oral cavity. However, cationic surfactants are frequently also irritant and some times even toxic, and therefore their use in drug delivery is significantly more limited than that of nonionic, zwitterionic, and anionic surfactants.

Nonionic surfactants, i.e., surfactants with an uncharged polar headgroup, are probably the ones used most frequently in drug delivery applications, with the possible exception of phospholipids. In particular, nonionic surfactants used

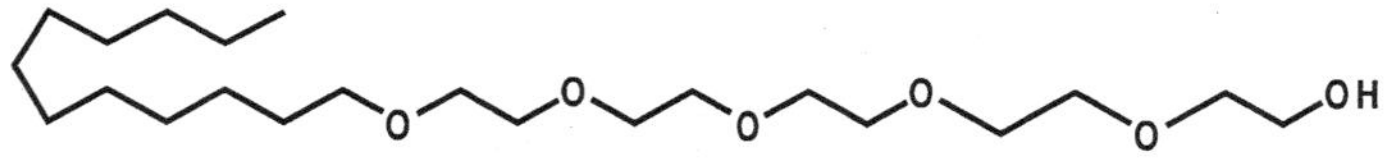

Alkyl ethoxylate

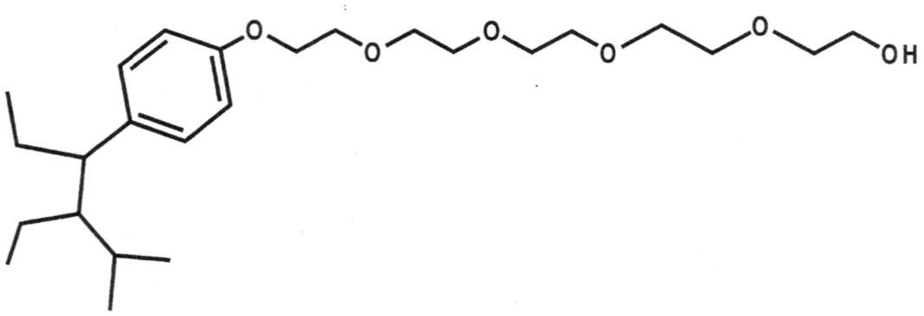

Nonylphenol ethoxylate

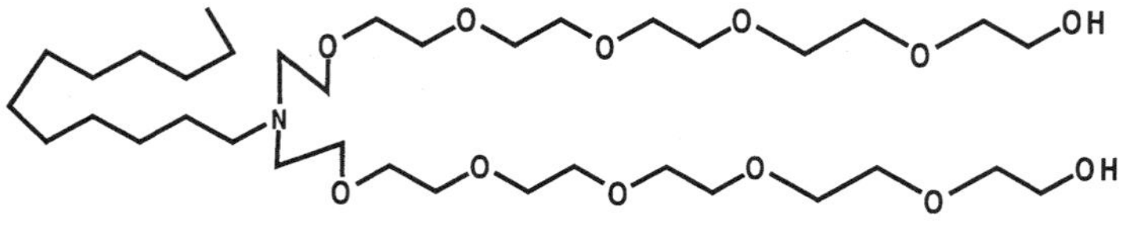

Amine ethoxylate

FIGURE 1.7 Chemical structure of some commonly used nonionic surfactants.

in this context are often based on oligo(ethylene oxide)-containing polar head groups (Figure 1.7). Due to the uncharged nature of the latter, these surfactants are less sensitive to salt, but instead quite sensitive to temperature, which may be used as a triggering parameter in drug delivery with these surfactants. The critical micellization concentration for such surfactants is generally much lower than that of the corresponding charged surfactants, and partly due to this, such surfactants are generally less irritant and better tolerated than the anionic and cationic surfactants.

Zwitterionic surfactants are less common than anionic, cationic, and non-ionic ones. Frequently, the polar headgroup consists of a quarternary amine group and a sulfonic or carboxyl group (Figure 1.8). Due to the zwitterionic nature of the polar headgroup, the surfactant charge changes with pH, so that it is cationic at low pH and anionic at high pH. Due to the often low irritating properties of such surfactants, they are commonly used in personal care products.

Contrary to zwitterionic single-chain surfactants, zwitterionic phospholipids such as phosphatidylcholine and phosphatidylethanolamine are extensively used in drug delivery (Figure 1.9). Reasons for this include their formation of interesting self-assemblied structures, liposomes in particular, as well as a frequently low toxicity and good biocompatibility.

During the last decade in particular, there has been a strong push to develop new surfactants of low toxicity and high biodegradability, particularly from renewable resources. In particular, carbohydrate polar headgroups have been found to be interesting in this respect (Figure 1.10).

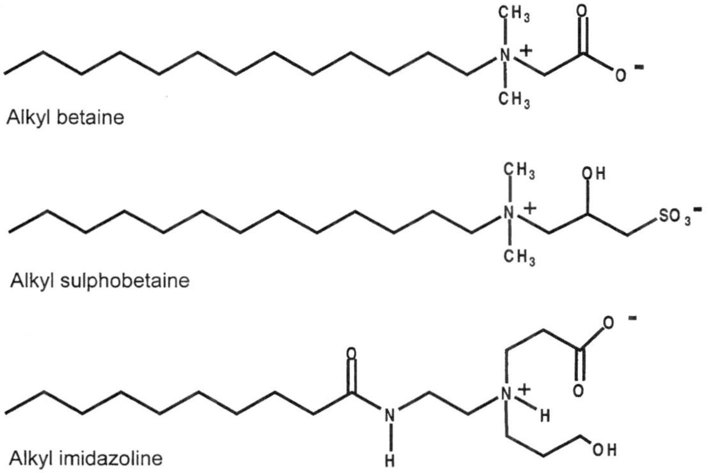

FIGURE 1.8 Chemical structure of some typical zwitterionic surfactants.

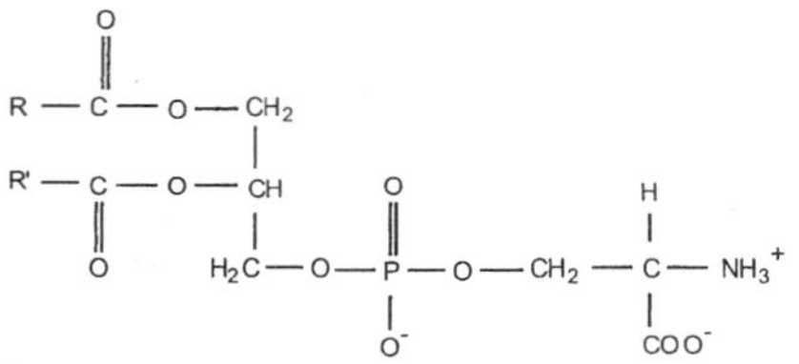

Phopsphatidyl serine

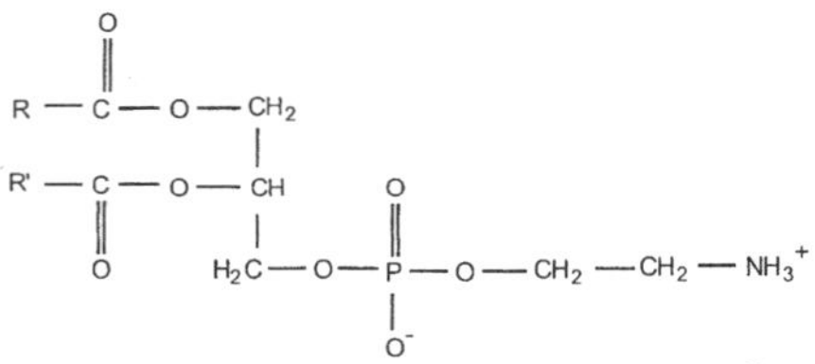

Phopsphatidyl ethanolamine

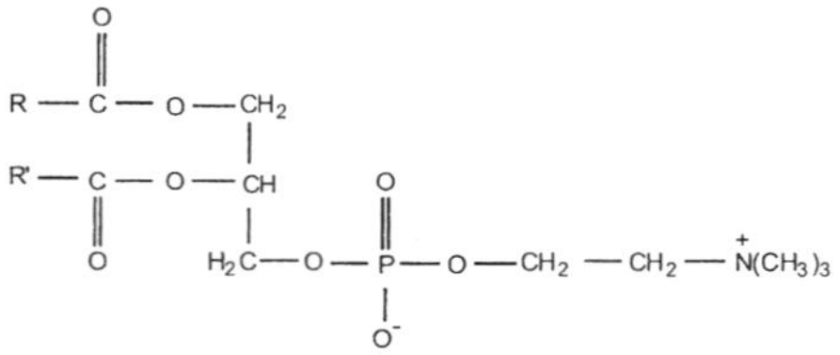

Phopsphatidyl choline

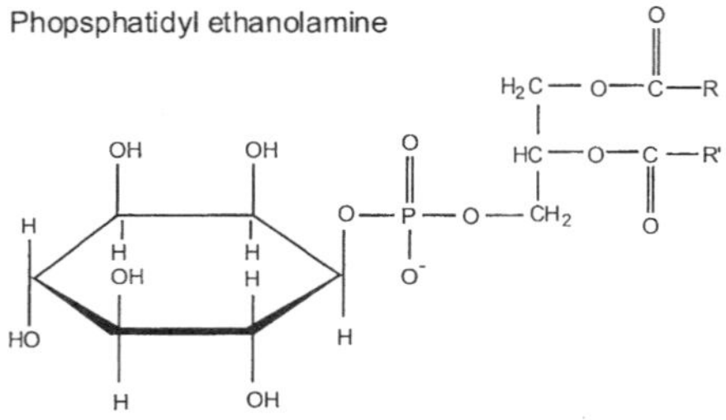

Phopsphatidyl inositol

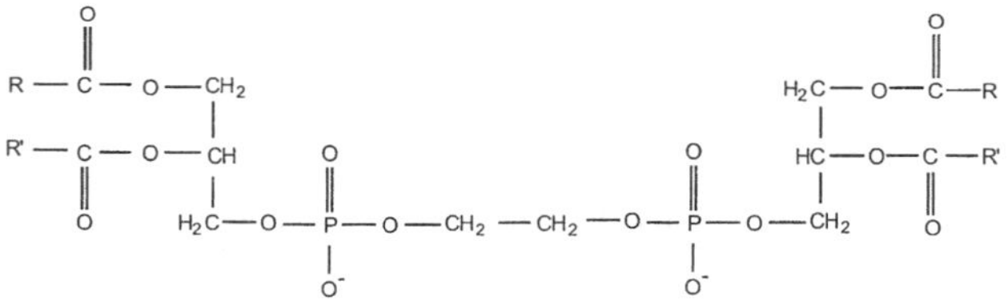

Diphopsphatidyl glycerol

FIGURE 1.9   Chemical structure of some commonly used phospholipids.

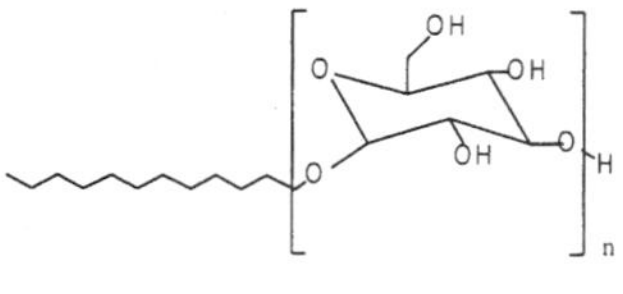

Alkyl polyglucoside (APG)

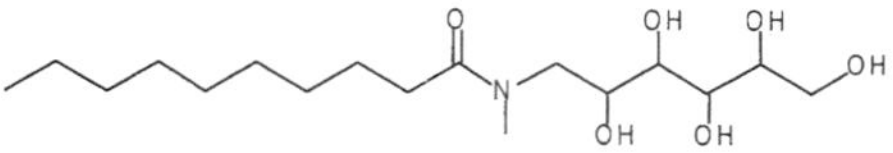

Alkyl glucamide

FIGURE 1.10   Chemical structure of a couple of carbohydrate-based surfactants.

Surfactants are useful as excipients in drug delivery formulations for a number of reasons. For example, through solubilization in the core of micelles or other types of surfactant self-assemblied structures the effective solubility of a hydrophobic drug may be increased, its hydrolytic degradation decreased, its toxicity decreased, and its bioavailibility improved. Also, the properties of the surfactant systems can allow advantageous effects relating to the drug release rate, extent and selectivity of drug uptake, etc. These and other aspects of the use of surfactants in drug delivery will be discussed in some detail in the following chapters.

1.2 INTRODUCTION TO POLYMERS

In analogy to surfactants, polymers find broad uses in drug delivery applications. Reasons for this include their surface activity, which makes them efficient stabilizers of colloidal drug delivery systems, their gel forming capacity, which allows

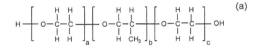

(a)

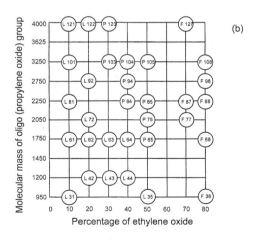

(b)

FIGURE 1.11 (a) Chemical structure of poly(ethylene oxide)-poly(propylene oxide)-poly(ethylene oxide) triblock copolymers. (b) Nomenclature of poly(ethylene oxide)-poly(propylene oxide)-poly(ethylene oxide) triblock copolymers of different composition and molecular weight. (Redrawn from Bahadur et al., Tenside Surf. Det. 1991, 28, 173.)

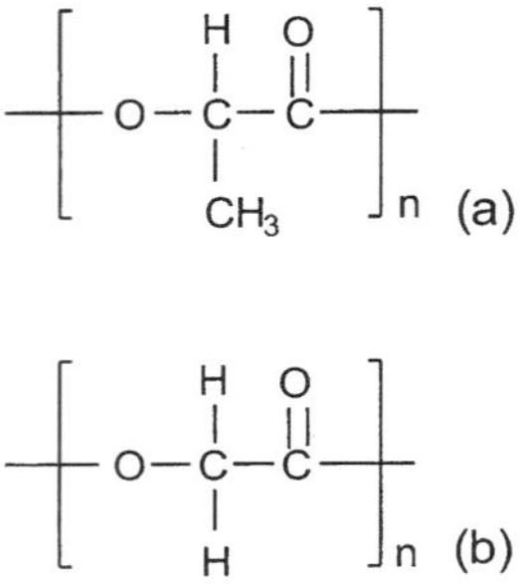

Figure 1.12 Chemical structure of (a) poly(lactic acid) and (b) poly(glycolic acid).

many opportunities in drug delivery, and their formation of self-assembly structures analogous to those formed by low molecular weight surfactants.

Several different types of polymers have been found to be of interest in drug delivery. First and foremost, block copolymers, consisting of blocks of two or several polymers, have been found to be useful, largely for the same reasons as low molecular weight surfactants. Particularly extensively used polymers within the drug delivery context are poly(ethylene oxide)-poly(propylene oxide) block copolymers, which are commercially available in a range of molecular weights and compositions (Figure 1.11).

An aspect which has been highlighted in relation to the use of polymers in drug delivery is their biodegradation. Due to the possibility to control the degradation rate of polymers over wide ranges through, e.g., the polymer structure and composition, biodegradation has been found to provide an interesting way to obtain a controlled drug release over a prolonged time, and to protect sensitive compounds from harsh environments, e.g., in the stomach. In particular, emphasis in this context has been placed on polymers consisting of, or containing, poly(lactic acid) or poly(glycolic acid) (Figure 1.12).

Another class of polymer which have found widespread use in drug delivery is the polysaccharides (Figure 1.13). In particular, this is due to the formation of gels in aqueous solutions containing also low amounts of polymer.

1.3 SURFACE ACTIVITY OF DRUGS

Drug molecules are frequently amphiphilic, and therefore also generally surface active. This surface activity depends on the molecular structure, and the balance between electrostatic, hydrophobic, and van der Waals forces, as well as on the drug solubility. Since the former balance depends on the degree of charging and electrostatic screening, the surface activity, and frequently also the solubility of

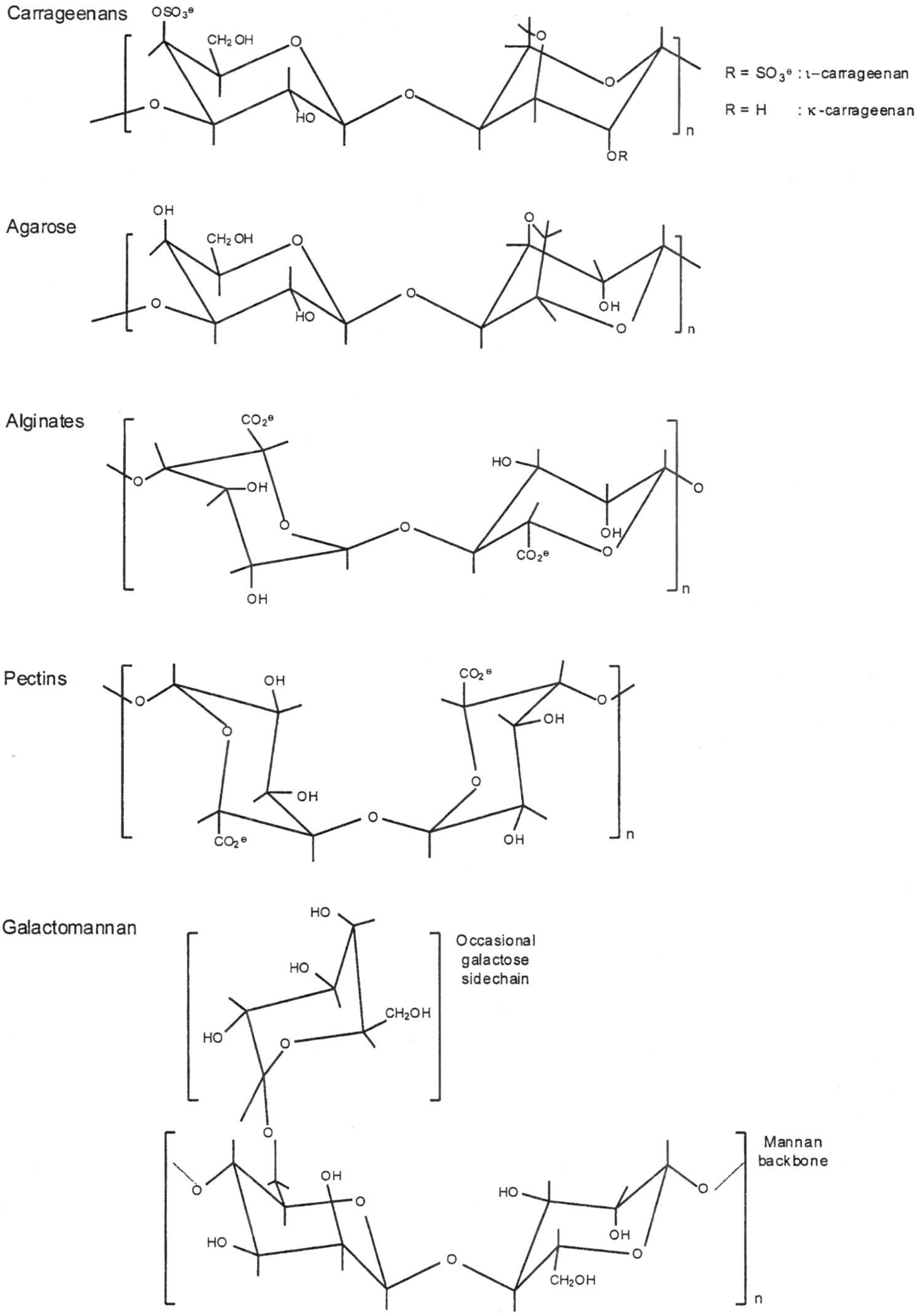

FIGURE 1.13 Chemical structure of some polysaccharides used in drug delivery.

Starch

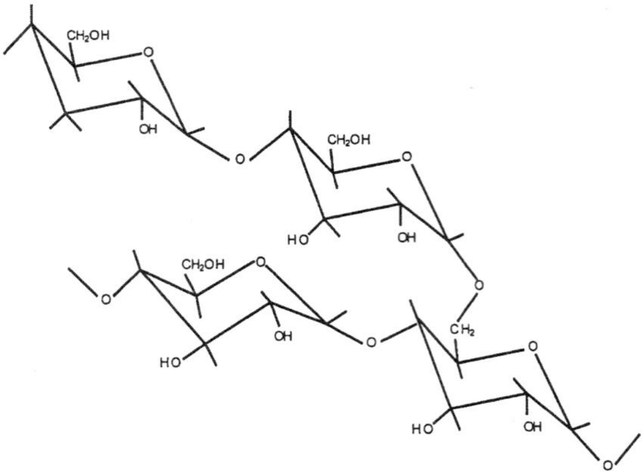

Xanthan

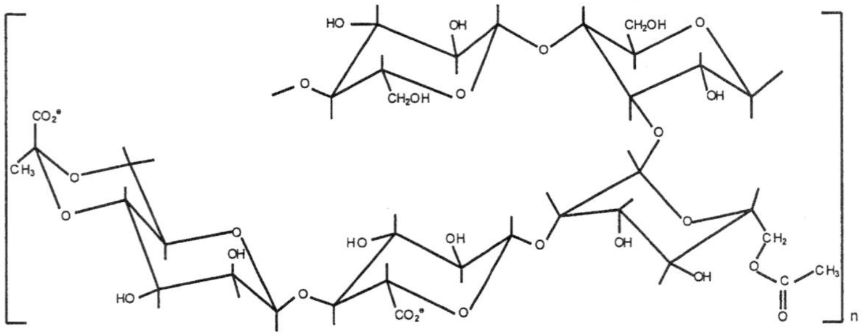

EHEC

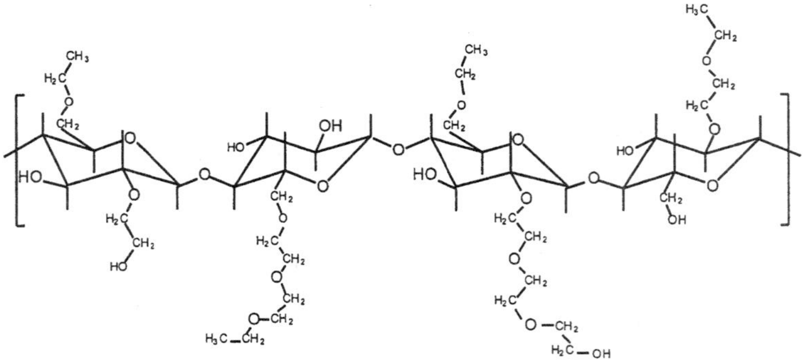

FIGURE 1.13   Continued.

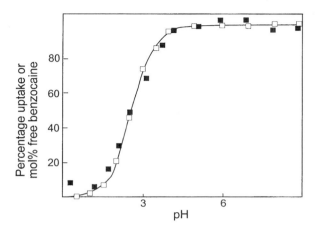

FIGURE 1.14 Adsorption of benzocaine at nylon 6 powder vs. pH at an ionic strength of 0.5 M and a temperature of 30°C (filled symbols), as well as the drug dissociation curve (open symbols). (Redrawn from Richardson et al., J. Pharm. Pharmac. 1974, 26, 166.)

a drug, often depends on pH. As an example of this, Figure 1.14 shows the adsorption of benzocaine at nylon particles and the corresponding drug dissociation curve. From the overlap of the pH-dependent adsorption and dissociation curves, it is evident that the surface activity in this case is largely dictated by the pH-dependent drug solubility. Thus, with decreasing solubility, accumulation at the surface, resulting in a reduction of the number of drug-water contacts, becomes relatively more favorable.

Considering the surface activity of drugs, one could perhaps expect that the action of a drug could be at least partly attributed to its surface activity. At least in some cases, e.g., neuroleptic phenolthiazines and local anesthetics, a correlation has indeed been found between the biological effect of drugs and their surface activity (Figure 1.15). In general, however, the surface activity of drugs may contribute to their biological action, but the relationship between surface activity and biological effect is less straightforward.

Also, larger drug molecules, such as oligopetides or proteins, are frequently surface active. The adsorption of such compounds is dictated by a delicate balance of a number of factors, including the molecular weight, the solvency (solubility), drug self-assembly, and the interactions between the drug and the surface. As an illustration of this, Figure 1.16 shows the adsorption of insulin as a function concentration of Zn^{2+}, which is known to induce insulin self-assembly. With an increasing concentration of Zn^{2+}, the surface activity increases as a result of protein aggregation. In fact, under some conditions only oligomeric insulin adsorbs,

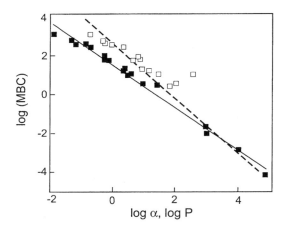

FIGURE **1.15** Correlation between the biological potency of local anesthetics, given as the minimum blocking concentration (MBC), and activated carbon adsorption affinity (α; filled squares), or octanol-water partition coefficient (open squares). (Redrawn from Abe et al., J. Pharm. Sci. 1988, 77, 166.)

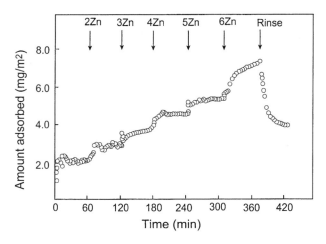

FIGURE **1.16** Amount of insulin adsorbed versus time at stepwise additions of Zn^{2+} (number of Zn^{2+}/hexamer) to an initially zinc-free human insulin solution. (Redrawn from Arnebrant et al., J. Colloid Interface Sci. 1988, 122, 557.)

whereas the unimers do not. This makes genetically engineered insulin forms containing amino acid substitutions which prevent the oligomerization interesting for preventing the adsorption in storage vials, which otherwise could result in problems relating to material loss and hence in a change in the amount drug administered.

Due to the surface activity of drugs, as well as the influence of interfacial interactions on the structure and stability of colloidal and self-assembled systems, the presence of the drug frequently affects the types of structure formed by surfactants and polymer systems, as well as their stability. This is important, since it means that the properties of the drug must be considered in the design of the drug carrier system, irrespectively of the carrier being an emulsion, a microemulsion, a micellar solution, or a liquid crystalline phase. This will be discussed and illustrated in some detail in the following chapters.

1.4 INTRODUCTION TO DRUG DELIVERY

Successful drug delivery requires consideration of numeous aspects. Depending on the route of administration, the indication at hand, the properties of the drug, and many other aspects, various strategies have to be developed. Without doubt the most generically important aspects of any therapy is its efficacy and safety. First and foremost, the drug concentration should be sufficiently high at the site of action in order to have a theapeutic effect, but at the same time it should not be too high, since this may result in detrimental side effects. For a safe and efficient therapy, the drug concentration should preferably lie essentially constant within this "therapeutic window" over the time of action (Fig. 1.17).

The goal of a constant drug concentration within the therapeutic window at the site of action over a suitable therapeutic time puts requirements not only on the drug but also on the drug formulation. The drug delivery system should preferably be designed such that a preferential accumulation of the drug is reached at the site of action, whereas the drug concentration elsewhere in the body should be as low as possible. The reason for this need of "targeting" is that a high concentration of the drug in tissues or cells other than those being targeted may cause problems related to side effects. A typical example of the latter is cancer therapy, where accumulation of chemotherapeutic agents in areas other than the tumor frequently causes severe side effects, some of which may be dose limiting, thereby limiting also the efficacy of the treatment. Furthermore, the drug should be stable against degradation during storage and administration, and the formulation designed such that drug degradation is minimized. Once the drug has performed its action, however, it should either be straightforwardly excreted or metabolized to harmless compounds.

There are also many other aspects to a drug delivery system, e.g., in relation to the route of administration. Naturally, the preferred situation is that the drug

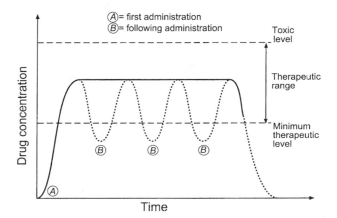

FIGURE 1.17   Schematic illustration of the drug level for an ideal sustained release formulation (solid line) as well as of a more typical situation demanding repeated administration (dotted line). Each administration is indicated.

is straightforwardly administrable by the patient himself/herself, without unpleasant sensations. However, depending on a number of different aspects also other routes may be chosen. The complete therapeutic strategy therefore involves choice not only of the drug but also of the drug delivery system and the administration route.

Different routes of administration (Table 1.1) put different requirements on the drug delivery system, and consequently different drug delivery systems tend to have their primary application within a given route of administration, and

TABLE 1.1   Some Different Routes of Drug Administration

Administration	Carrier in contact with
Oral	Gastrointestinal tract
Dermal	Skin
Topical	Skin
Buccal	Oral cavity
Parenteral	Blood
Occular	Eye
Nasal	Nose
Vaginal	Vagina
Rectal	Rectum/colon
Pulmonary	Lung

within a certain type of indication. For example, in oral drug delivery, the drug and the drug carrier have to pass through the stomach, with its quite low pH, which tends to affect both the drug stability and the drug solubility, as well as the properties of the drug carrier system. Also, the uptake in the intestine puts some rather demanding requirements on the drug and the drug formulation, not the least for hydrophobic drugs and/or large molecules (e.g., protein and peptide drugs). In topical administration the penetration over the stratum corneum poses a severe limitation in the therapy efficacy, which puts special demands on the drug delivery system. In intravenous drug delivery, the uptake of the drug and the drug carrier in the reticuloendothelial system frequently reduces the drug bioavailability and results in dose-limiting side effects.

In the following chapters, the main types of drug delivery systems based on surfactants and polymers will be discussed one at a time. For each type of delivery system, the basic concepts will first be covered, whereafter methods of analyzing such systems will be briefly outlined. Following this, various aspects of the use of the systems in drug delivery will be discussed in some detail.

BIBLIOGRAPHY

Alexandridis, P., B. Lindman (eds.), Amphiphilic Block Copolymers. Self-Assembly and Applications, Elsevier, Amsterdam, 2000.

Chien, Y. W. (ed.), Novel Drug Delivery Systems, Drugs and the Pharmaceutical Sciences, vol. 50, Marcel Dekker, New York, 1992.

Florence, A. T., D. Attwood, Physicochemical Principles of Pharmacy, Macmillan Press, London, 1989.

Jönsson, B., B. Lindman, K. Holmberg, B. Kronberg, Surfactants and Polymers in Aqueous Solution, Wiley, New York, 1998.

Kreuter, J. (ed.), Colloidal Drug Delivery Systems, Drugs and the Pharmaceutical Sciences, vol. 66, Marcel Dekker, New York, 1994.

Lee, V. H. L. (ed.), Peptide and Protein Drug Delivery, Advances in Parenteral Sciences, vol. 4, Marcel Dekker, New York, 1991.

Robinson, J. R., V. H. L. Lee (eds.), Controlled Drug Delivery: Fundamentals and Applications, Drugs and the Pharmaceutical Sciences, vol. 29, Marcel Dekker, New York, 1987.

Schmolka, I. R., in P. J. Tarcha (ed.), Polymers for Controlled Drug Delivery, CRC Press, Boca Raton, 1991.

2

Micelles

2.1 STRUCTURE AND DYNAMICS OF MICELLAR SYSTEMS

A notable feature of surfactants is their ability to self-associate to form micelles (Figure 2.1). Since micelles consist of surfactant molecules packing in a space-filling manner numerous parameters of the surfactant solution change at the critical micellization concentration (cmc). For example, since the micelles consist of many individual surfactant molecules, any parameter related to the size or diffusion in surfactant solutions can be used to detect the micellization, e.g., through scattering methods and nuclear magnetic resonance (NMR). Also, the micellar core contains little water (see below); hence solubilization of hydrophobic dyes is initiated at the cmc, and fluorescence investigations with probes sensitive for the polarity of the environment can be used to detect micellization. Also, a range of other techniques, such as conductivity (ionic surfactants), osmotic pressure, and surface tension, may be used to determine the cmc.

The main driving force for micelle formation in aqueous solution is the effective interaction between the hydrophobic parts of the surfactant molecules, whereas interactions opposing micellization may include electrostatic repulsive interactions between charged head groups of ionic surfactants, repulsive osmotic interactions between chainlike polar head groups such as oligo(ethylene oxide) chains, or steric interactions between bulky head groups.

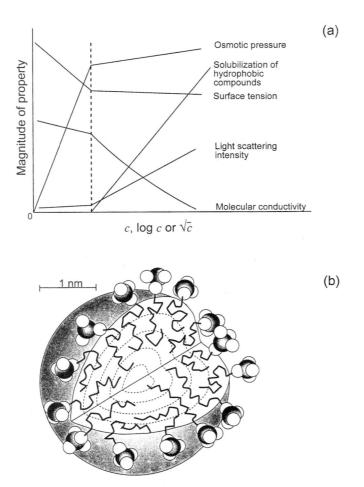

(a)

Osmotic pressure

Solubilization of
hydrophobic
compounds

Surface tension

Light scattering
intensity

Molecular conductivity

c, log c or $\sqrt{c}$

(b)

├─ 1 nm ─┤

FIGURE 2.1 (a) Schematic illustration of how a range of experimentally accessible parameters change with the surfactant concentration and how this can be used to detect the cmc. (b) Schematic illustration of a spherical micelle. (Redrawn from Israelachvili, Intermolecular and Surface Forces, Academic Press, 1992(b).)

Given the delicate balance between opposing forces, it is not surprising that surfactant self-assembly is affected by a range of factors, such as the size of the hydrophobic moiety, the nature of the polar head group, the nature of the counterion (charged surfactants), the salt concentration, pH, temperature, and presence of cosolutes. Probably the most universal of all these is the size of the hydrophobic domain(s) in the surfactant molecule. With increasing size of the hydrophobic domain, the hydrophobic interaction increases, thereby promoting micellization. As an illustration of this, Figure 2.2 shows the chain length dependence of the cmc for some different surfactants. As can be seen, the cmc decreases strongly with an increasing number of carbon atoms in the alkyl chain, irrespective of the nature of the polar head group. As a general rule, the cmc decreases a factor of 2 for ionic surfactants and with a factor of 3 for nonionic surfactants on addition of one methylene group to a surfactant alkyl chain. The extent of the decrease also depends on the nature of the hydrophobic domain, in terms of both structure (e.g., single chain vs. double chain surfactants) and composition (e.g., fluorinated surfactants), but qualitatively, the same effect is observed for all surfactants.

The dependence of the micellization on the nature of the polar head group is less straightforward than that of the alkyl chain length. Nevertheless, the cmc of nonionic surfactants is generally much lower than that of ionic ones, particularly at low salt concentrations, which is due to the repulsive electrostatic interaction between the charged head groups opposing micellization (Figure 2.2). For nonionic surfactant of the oligo(ethylene oxide) type, an increasing number of ethylene oxide groups at a constant alkyl chain length results in an increasing cmc as a consequence of an increasing osmotic repulsion between the oligo(ethylene oxide) chains when these grow larger (Figure 2.3). The length of the oligo(ethylene oxide) chains affects also the packing of the surfactant molecules in the micelle. More precisely, with an increasing length of the oligo(ethylene oxide) chain, the head group repulsion increases, which tends to increase the curva-

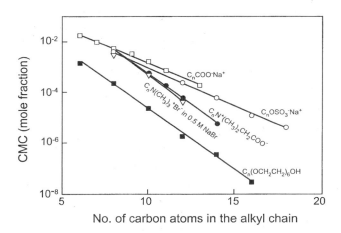

FIGURE 2.2 The dependence of the cmc with the length of the hydrophobic domain for a number of alkyl chain surfactants with different polar head group. (Redrawn from Lindman et al., Topics Current Chem. 1980, 87, 1.)

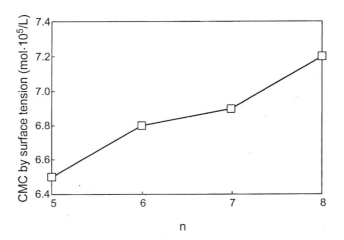

FIGURE 2.3 Effect of the length of the oligo(ethylene oxide) chain n on the cmc for a series of $C_{12}E_n$ surfactants. (Redrawn from Deguchi et al., J. Colloid Interface Sci. 1972, 38, 596.)

ture of the aggregates, and hence results in smaller and more spherical micelles. The latter effect can be observed, e.g., from the micellar size or aggregation number.

Cosolutes in general tend to affect the micellization in surfactant systems. Examples of such cosolutes include oils (or other hydrophobic compounds), salt, alcohols, and hydrotropes. Of these, salt plays a particularly important role, particularly for ionic surfactants. Thus, on addition of salt, the electrostatic repulsion between the charged head group is screened (Chapter 9). As a consequence, the repulsive interaction opposing micellization becomes relatively less important, and the attractive driving force for micellization therefore dominates to a larger extent. As a result of this, the cmc decreases on addition of salt (Figure 2.4).

For nonionic surfactants, on the other hand, addition of low or moderate concentrations of salt has little influence on the micellization due to the absence of charges in these systems. At very high salt concentrations ($\approx 0.1-1$ M), so-called lyotropic salt effects are typically observed. Depending on the nature of both the cation and the anion of the salt, the presence of the salt may either promote or preclude micellization.

For ionic surfactants, the presence of salt also affects the micellar size and aggregation number. In particular, screening of the repulsive electrostatic interaction through addition of salt facilitates a closer packing of the surfactant head groups, and therefore results in a micellar growth (Figure 2.5).

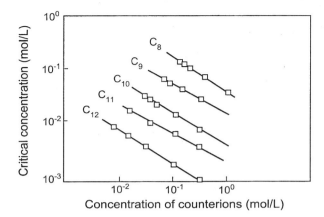

FIGURE 2.4 Effect of sodium chloride on the cmc of sodium alkyl sulfate surfactants. (Redrawn from Huisman, Proc. Koninkl. Ned. Acad. Wetenschap. B, 1964, 67, 367).

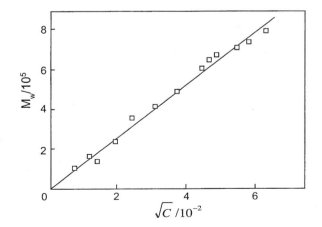

FIGURE 2.5 Effect of added salt on the micellar aggregation number for CTAB. (Redrawn from Mukerjee, J. Phys. Chem. 1972, 76, 565.)

Again, for nonionic surfactants, little or no such dependence is observed. Instead, many nonionic surfactants, notably those containing oligo(ethylene oxide) groups, display a sensitivity regarding temperature. With increasing temperature, surfactants and polymers containing oligo(ethylene oxide) or its derivatives display a decreased water solubility. At sufficiently high temperature, usually referred to as the lower consolute temperature (LCT) or the cloud point (CP), such molecules phase separate to form one dilute and one more concentrated phase (Chapter 8). Note that this behavior is opposite to what is observed for most other types of surfactants and polymers, which display increasing solubility/miscibility with increasing temperature.

The decreased solvency for the oligo(ethylene oxide) moieties with increasing temperature results in a decreased repulsion between the polar head groups in ethylene oxide-based surfactants, and hence micellization is favored at higher temperature. Consequently, the cmc displayed by these surfactants decreases with increasing temperature (Figure 2.6). For ionic surfactants, on the other hand, the temperature dependence is the opposite for entropic reasons. In parallel, the oligo(ethylene oxide) moieties contract with increasing temperature as a result of the decreasing solvency, and therefore can pack more densely at the interface. Together, this means that micellar growth is facilitated at the higher temperature (Figure 2.7).

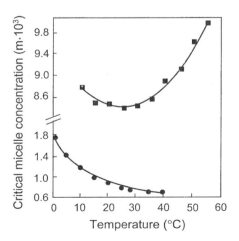

FIGURE 2.6 Effect of temperature on the cmc of $C_{10}E_5$ (circles). For comparison, the effect of temperature on the cmc for an ionic surfactant (SDS) is also shown (squares). (Redrawn from Elworthy et al., Solubilisation by Surface-Active Agents, Chapman & Hall, 1968.)

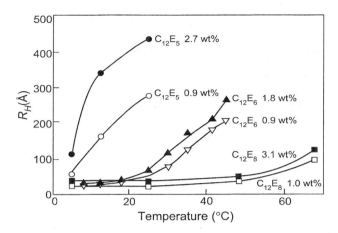

FIGURE 2.7 Effect of temperature on the micellar size R_H for $C_{12}E_n$ surfactants. (Redrawn from Nilsson et al., J. Phys. Chem. 1983, 87, 1377 and Brown et al., Chem. Scr. 1985, 25, 67.)

For ionic surfactants, but also for nonionic surfactants other than those based on oligo(ethylene oxide), the general rule is that the temperature dependence of the micellization and the structure of the micelles formed is rather minor.

Organic cosolutes in general play an important role in technical systems containing surfactants. This is the case not the least in drug delivery, where surfactants are used in order to facilitate the efficient and safe administration of a drug. The effect of a cosolute on the micellization in surfactant systems to a large extent depends on the nature of the cosolute. As illustrated above, salts have large effects on the micellization in ionic surfactant systems, but rather weak effects in nonionic surfactant systems. For uncharged cosolutes, the effect on the micellization in surfactant systems depends both on the nature of the cosolute and that of the surfactant, and both an increase and decrease of the cmc on addition of the cosolute is possible.

Of particular interest for the use of micellar systems in drug delivery are hydrophobic solutes, which are essentially insoluble in water but readily soluble in oil and therefore also in the hydrophobic core of micelles. As indicated above, the amount of a hydrophobic solute solubilized by a surfactant solution below the cmc is very limited. Above the cmc, on the other hand, the hydrophobic substance is solubilized in the micelles (Figure 2.8). Indeed, the capacity of surfactant systems to solubilize hydrophobic substances constitutes one of the single most important properties of such systems, as this forms the basis for the use of surfactants in numerous industrial contexts, including surfactant-assisted drug delivery.

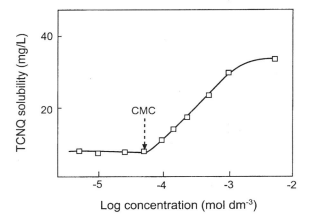

FIGURE 2.8 Solubility of 7,7,8,8-tetracyanoquinodimethane (TCNQ) in aqueous solution of $C_{12}E_8$ at 25°C. (Redrawn from Deguchi et al., J. Colloid Interface Sci. 1974, 49, 10.)

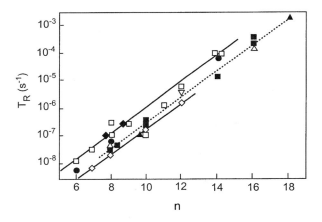

FIGURE 2.9 Effects of the alkyl chain length n of alkyl-based surfactants on the average residence time T_R for a surfactant molecule in a given micelle. Open squares: sodium alkylsulfates; filled diamonds: sodium alkylsulfonates; filled squares: sodium alkylcarboxylates; open diamonds: potassium alkylcarboxylates; open square: cesium decylcarboxylate; filled circles: alkylammonium chlorides; filled triangles: alkyltrimethylamine bromides; open triangles: alkylpyridinium chlorides; filled squares: alkylpyridinium bromides; reversed open triangle: dodecylpyridinium iodine. (Redrawn from Lang et al., in Zana, ed., Surfactants Solutions: New Methods of Investigation, Marcel Dekker, Inc. 1987.)

From simple space-filling considerations it is evident that the solubilization of a hydrophobic solute in the core of the micelles causes the latter to grow. At the same time, hydrophobic solutes may promote micellization and cause a decrease in the cmc. This is not entirely unexpected, since reducing the cmc in order to accomodate the oil in a one-phase system may offer an opportunity for free energy minimization for the system as a whole.

Finally, it is important to note that surfactant micelles are not static structures, but rather that the schematic illustration shown in Figure 2.1 represents an instant "snapshot" of such a structure. Thus, micelles are highly dynamic structures, where the molecules remain essentially in a liquid state. Also, the individual surfactant molecules are freely exchanged between micelles and between micelles and the aqueous solution. The residence time for the surfactant molecules in one given micelle is generally very short, but increasing about one order of magnitude for each ethylene group added to the surfactant hydrophobic tail (Figure 2.9).

2.2 BLOCK COPOLYMER MICELLES

Closely related to low molecular weight surfactants in many ways concerning self-assembly are block copolymers. This is particularly true for simpler block copolymer systems, such as diblock and triblock copolymers, which form not only micelles in dilute aqueous solution but also a range of liquid crystalline phases and microemulsions with oil and water. Such "polymeric surfactants" have found widespread use, not the least in drug delivery, as will be discussed in some detail below.

Although there has been extensive work on a range of block copolymer systems, much of this work has concerned solvent-based systems. During the last decade, however, a number of water-soluble block copolymer systems have been investigated concerning their physicochemical behavior, e.g., regarding self-association. In particular, much of the work has involved PEO-based copolymers [PEO being poly(ethylene oxide)], and these are also the ones of largest interest in the present context. A number of hydrophobic blocks have been investigated for PEO-based block copolymers, including poly(propylene oxide), poly(styrene), alkyl groups, poly(butylene oxide), poly(lactide), and poly(caprolactone). In particular, interest has focused on PEO/PPO block copolymers (PPO being polypropylene oxide), mainly due to their commercial accessibility in a range of compositions and molecular weights.

Composition and molecular weight are two of the prime parameters of interest for block copolymer systems. In analogy to low molecular weight nonionic surfactants, micellization is promoted by an increasing length of the hydrophobic block(s) and decreasing length of the hydrophilic one(s) (Figure 2.10). From the slope of the decrease in the cmc and in the micellar aggregation number with an increasing number of hydrophobic groups, the hydrophobicity of the hydrophobic

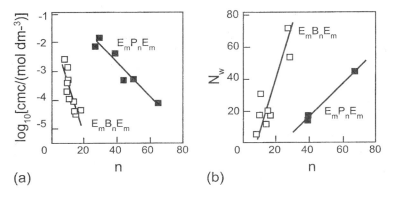

FIGURE 2.10 Effect of the length of the hydrophobic block n on the cmc (a) and micellar aggregation number N_w (b) of $E_mB_nE_m$ and $E_mP_nE_m$ triblock copolymers. (Redrawn from Booth et al., in Alexandridis et al., eds., Amphiphilic Block Copolymers: Self-Assembly and Applications, Elsevier, 2000.)

groups may be estimated. Such an analysis yields "hydrophobicity ratios" for propylene oxide (P), lactide (L), caprolactone (C), butylene oxide (B), and styrene (S) of $1:4:5:6:12$.

Also, the molecular architecture affects micellization in block copolymer systems. As can be seen in Figure 2.11, diblock (E_mB_n) copolymers self-associated more readily than triblock ($B_{n/2}E_mB_{n/2}$ and $E_{m/2}B_nE_{m/2}$) copolymers of the same total molecular weight and composition. The origin of this is that less efficient packing is achieved with the triblock copolymers, in the case of the BAB copolymer due to the hydrophilic block being a loop rather than a tail, and in the ABA case due to the presence of two rather than one hydrophilic tail.

The micellization of PEO-containing block copolymers is promoted by increasing temperature. As with the low molecular weight surfactants, this is due to a decreased solvency of the PEO domain(s). However, for PEO/PPO copolymers, the decreased aqueous solubility of the PPO domain(s) with increasing temperature also contributes to this behavior. Quantitatively, the temperature dependence of the cmc is quite strong for many PEO/PPO block copolymers. The concentration-induced aggregation at a fixed temperature, on the other hand, is frequently quite gradual, and the determination of the cmc in the traditional manner therefore difficult. The cmc values so determined frequently span widely, e.g., between different experimental methods used, but also display batch-to-batch variations. Therefore, the onset of self-assembly in such systems is often identified by a critical micellization temperature at a fixed polymer concentration (cmt), rather than by a cmc at fixed temperature (Figure 2.12).

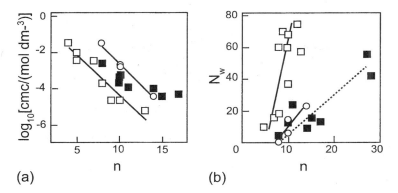

FIGURE 2.11 Effect of the number of butylene oxide groups n on the cmc (a) and micellar aggregation number N_w (b) for $E_m B_n$ (open squares), $B_{n/2} E_m B_{n/2}$ (circles), and $E_{m/2} B_n E_{m/2}$ (filled squares) copolymers. (Redrawn from Booth et al., in Alexandridis et al., eds., Amphiphilic Block Copolymers: Self-Assembly and Applications, Elsevier, 2000.)

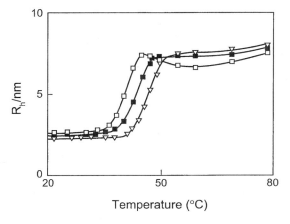

FIGURE 2.12 Temperature-dependent hydrodynamic radius R_h of Pluronic F68 at a bulk concentration of 51.7 (open squares), 25.0 (filled squares), and 12.5 (open triangles) mg · ml^{-1}. (Redrawn from Zhou et al., J. Colloid Interface Sci. 1988, 126, 171.)

There is also micellar growth with increasing temperature. However, in the general case, the increase in the micellar aggregation number is significantly stronger than that in the micellar radius, which indicates that the block copolymers pack more efficiently with increasing temperature. As with the EO-containing low molecular weight surfactants, this is an effect of the decreasing solvency of the polymer with increasing temperature. This also means that the hydration of the polymer molecules decreases with increasing temperature (Figure 2.13).

The effects of cosolutes on the self-assembly of PEO/PPO block copolymers are quite similar to those on low molecular weight PEO-containing surfactants. Thus, effects of salts on the micellization in these block copolymer systems are minor at low to medium salt concentration, whereas at high salt concentration ($\approx 0.1–1M$), lyotropic salt effects are observed. Furthermore, hydrophobic solutes may induce micellization. An illustration of this is given in Figure 2.14. As can be seen, the presence of lidocaine/prilocaine has little effect on the cmc for this copolymer system at pH $\ll$ pKa (7.86 and 7.89 for lidocaine and prilocaine, respectively), i.e., where these compounds are fully ionized and readily soluble in water, and therefore behaving as ordinary salt. On increasing pH, on the other hand, lidocaine and prilocaine become less soluble in water as a result of deprotonation, and at pH $\geq$ pKa behave essentially as sparingly soluble oils, thus promoting micellization and lowering cmt.

The localization of the solubilized molecule depends on the properties of the solubilizate, notably its hydrophobicity. The more hydrophobic the solubili-

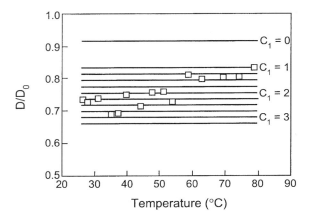

FIGURE 2.13 Effects of temperature on the number of water molecules bound per monomer C_1 in Pluronic F127 micelles, determined from the water self-diffusion (D/D_0). (Redrawn from Malmsten et al., Macromolecules 1992, 25, 5446.)

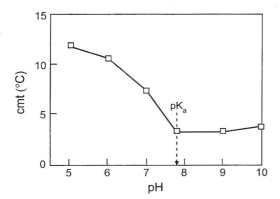

FIGURE 2.14 cmt as a function of pH from a formulation containing 5 wt% of active ingredient (50/50 mol/mol of lidocaine and prilocaine), 15.5 wt% Lutrol F127, and 5.5 wt% Lutrol F68. (Redrawn from Scherlund et al., Int. J. Pharm. 2000, 211, 37.)

zate, the more it tends to be localized in the core of the micelles. More amphiphilic molecules, on the other hand, tend to be located preferentially in the micellar interfacial layer.

An interesting difference between alkyl-based surfactants, on one hand, and PEO/PPO block copolymer, on the other, is that the hydrophobic moiety is significantly more polar in the latter case. This means that there is intermixing between the PEO and PPO blocks, but also that there is a significant amount of water present also in the core of the micelles formed by PEO/PPO block copolymers (Figure 2.15). With increasing temperature, however, there is a decreased hydration of the polymer.

Due to the partial polarity of the PPO block and the presence of water also in the micellar core, the solubilization capacity of PEO/PPO block copolymers differs somewhat from that of alkyl-based low molecular weight surfactants, where the water penetration to the micellar core is negligible. More specifically, while the solubilization of aromatic hydrocarbons may be significant in micelles formed by PEO/PPO block copolymers, that of aliphatic hydrocarbons is more limited. The amount solubilized also depends on the molecular volume of the solubilizate, and the larger the solubilized molecule, the lower the solubilization (Figure 2.16). Also, the structure of the copolymer affects the solubilization, and the solubilization capacity increases with an increasing molecular weight and an increasing PPO content of the block copolymer (Figure 2.17).

As with micelle formation as such, the solubilizing capacity of block copolymers also depends on the molecular architecture, with a lower degree of solubilization in tetrabranched PEO/PPO copolymers (Tetronics) than in PEO-PPO-PEO

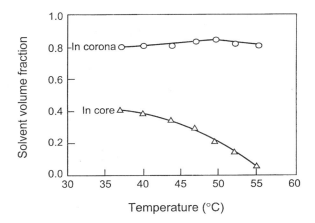

FIGURE 2.15 Volume fraction of water in the micellar core (triangles) and corona (circles) for a 2.5 wt% Pluronic L64 in D_2O. (Redrawn from Yang et al., Macromolecules 2000, 16, 8555.)

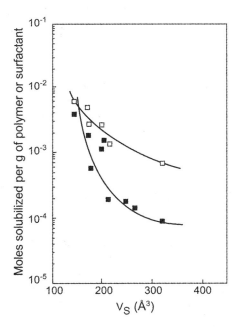

FIGURE 2.16 Effect of the molecular volume V_s on the extent of solubilization of hydrocarbons in SDS (open symbols) and Pluronic F127 (filled symbols) micelles. (Redrawn from Nagarajan et al., Langmuir 1986, 2, 210.)

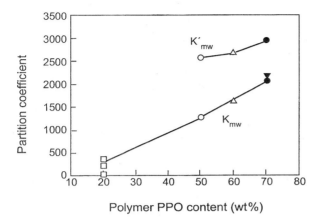

FIGURE 2.17 Relation between the micelle-water partition coefficient K_{mw} for naphthalene in PEO/PPO block copolymer micelles and the PPO content of the block copolymer. Shown also is K'_{mw}, the partition coefficient normalized with the polymer PPO content. (Redrawn from Hurter et al., Langmuir 1992, 8, 1291.)

copolymers (Pluronics). There are several reasons for the observed dependence of the polymer molecular weight, composition, and architecture on its solubilizing capacity, all relating to the micelle formation and structure. For solubilization to be efficient, the micelles formed should preferably be of a sufficiently high aggregation number and contain a sufficiently large and hydrophobic micellar core. Since micellization is promoted by an increasing PPO content and precluded by branching of the copolymer, the solubilization is improved with an increased PPO content, and is poorer for tetrabranched than for linear block copolymers.

As long as spherical micelles are formed, higher molecular weight block copolymers form larger micelles than low molecular weight ones, and are therefore expected to be more efficient solubilizers. However, spherical micelles are not always formed, and both the aggregation number and the shape of the micelles may change on solubilization, which affect the latter. As a general rule, however, larger micelles are more efficient solubilizers than small ones. For PEO/PPO block copolymers, where the block segregation is incomplete, and where also the micellar core contains some water, increasing the molecular weight also has another effect, in that the segregation between the blocks increases with the polymer molecular weight. This, in turn, results in a decreased polarity of the micellar core, thereby facilitating solubilization.

A striking difference between low molecular weight surfactants and many (unfractionated) block copolymers is that while the former are usually well defined and reasonably homogeneous and monodisperse, the latter frequently contain a range of molecular weights and compositions. Since fractions containing different molecular weights and compositions display different self-assembly, the overall micellization process for such systems is gradual. Furthermore, the composition of the micelles changes during this process, e.g., with an increasing polymer concentration. Thus, in the early stages of micellization, the micelles are dominated by the fractions which have the highest tendency to self-assemble (e.g., those with the highest content of the hydrophobic block, or diblock impurities in the case of triblock copolymers), whereas at higher total polymer concentration, the micellar composition approaches that of the overall average of the system. From an experimental point of view, this gradual transition makes the micellization more difficult to investigate for technical block copolymer (and surfactant) systems, and the cmc looses its strict meaning. Most likely, this has contributed to the rather widely differing cmc values reported for commercial block copolymers (e.g., the Pluronics) over the years.

Another difference between low molecular weight surfactants and block copolymers concerns the dynamics in micellar systems. As discussed above, the average residence time for surfactant molecules in micelles increases strongly with the number of methylene group in the hydrophobic tail(s). Due to the very large hydrophobic group(s) frequently present in block copolymers, block copolymer micelles are characterized by much slower kinetics than those formed by low molecular weight surfactants. For example, high molecular weight Pluronic copolymers display an exceedingly slow micellar dynamics. Thus, micelles can, at least in certain cases, be separated from the unmicellized molecules in size-exclusion chromatography experiments typically spanning over more than an hour. This is an astonishing result since it shows that the micelles do not disintegrate over the time of the experiment despite the free polymer concentration surrounding the micelles being below cmc. In fact, the possibility of separating micelles from unmicellized polymers for at least some block copolymer systems offers a way to follow the micellization process, and to determine the cmt (Figure 2.18).

From a practical drug delivery perspective, this slow disintegration kinetics offers some possibilities. For example, while micelles formed by low molecular weight surfactants disintegrate rapidly after parenteral administration of a surfactant solution unless the surfactant concentration is very high, drug-loaded block copolymer micelles may be administered in a similar way without disintegrating over an appreciable time period. Without any doubt, the slow disintegration kinetics of the micelles formed by at least some block copolymers has contributed significantly to their successful use in drug delivery (see below).

Although the vast majority of the work performed on block copolymer micelles in both basic studies and drug delivery work has been performed with PEO/PPO block copolymers, there is a current development to find new block copolymers for such uses. Over the last few years in particular, this has involved

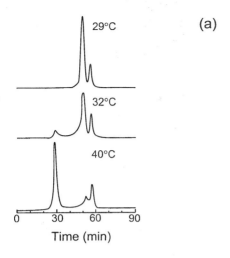

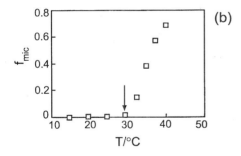

FIGURE 2.18 (a) Size exclusion chromatography trace for an aqueous Pluronic F127 solution at different temperatures. The peak appearing at an elusion time of 30 min corresponds to micelles, whereas the peaks at 50–60 min correspond to the nonmicellized polymers (with impurities). (b) Temperature dependence of the relative intensity of the peak corresponding to micelles f_{mic}. The arrow indicates the cmt. (Redrawn from Malmsten et al., Macromolecules 1992, 25, 5440.)

the development of biodegradable hydrophobic blocks, such as poly(lactide), poly(caprolactone), poly(β-benzyl-L-aspartate), poly(γ-benzyl-L-glutamate), poly(aspartatic acid), and poly(L-lysine). Such systems offer possibilities in drug delivery in that the degradation allows control of the drug release rate and other drug formulation performances, and the elimination of the polymer from the body is facilitated.

2.3 CHARACTERIZATION OF MICELLAR SYSTEMS

There are a number of aspects of surfactant and block copolymer micelles which are interesting to characterize in order to learn more about a particular system. The main one of these is without doubt the onset of micellization, i.e., the cmc or cmt. Once this has been determined, one may proceed to determine the size of the micelles formed, and the micellar aggregation number. In some cases, it may also be interesting to investigate other parameters, such as the shape of the micelles, the state of hydration, microviscocity in the micellar core, and the micellar dynamics.

As indicated above, there are numerous methods to determine the cmc or the cmt, including surface tension measurements, scattering experiments, NMR, fluorescence spectroscopy, calorimetry, osmotometry, conductivity, and solubilization experiments (Figure 2.1). Of these, three are discussed here, i.e., surface tension because this is the most frequently used method for cmc determinations, and scattering and NMR techniques because these are very versatile, and may provide information also about other aspects of micellar systems, such as the micellar size, the micellar aggregation number (scattering methods), the state of hydration (NMR), the counterion binding (NMR), and the location of solubilized molecules in micelles (NMR).

2.3.1 Surface Tension Measurements

Seemingly very simple surface tension measurements probably constitute the most frequently employed method for determining the cmc of surfactant and block copolymer systems. The origin behind this is that surfactants/block copolymers are surface active, and tend to adsorb at numerous surfaces, and so also at the air-water interface. On increasing the surfactant/block copolymer concentration (below cmc) the adsorption increases, which results in a surface tension reduction. Once the cmc is reached, all additionally added surfactant/copolymer molecules go to the micelles, whereas the free surfactant/copolymer concentration is essentially constant, as is the adsorption and the surface tension. Ideally, therefore, a plot of the surface tension vs. the surfactant/copolymer concentration displays a clear breakpoint, from which the cmc is readily identified (Figure 2.19).

In the case of polydisperse and/or heterogeneous surfactants/block copolymers the strict meaning of the cmc is lost, and also from a practical perspective determination of an effective cmc becomes more difficult. This is illustrated in Figure 2.19, where it is shown that the polydisperse/heterogeneous compound displays a more gradual decrease in the surface tension vs. concentration.

Surface tension measurements are also very sensitive to the presence of hydrophobic inpurities, and only an impurity level of the order of 0.1% of the surfactant may well cause a drastic deviation from the "ideal" curve displayed in Figure 2.19. The reason for this is that typical surface tension methods are

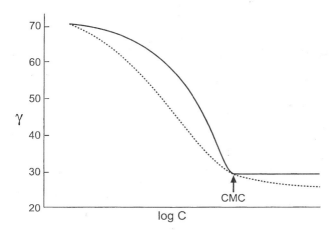

FIGURE 2.19 Schematic illustration of the surface tension γ of a surfactant/block copolymer versus the concentration *c* for a monodisperse and homogeneous sample (solid line) and a polydisperse and/or heterogeneous sample (dashed line).

based on the use of a macroscopic air-water surface (e.g., in a trough), and hence the bulk volume to surface area is large, and even minute amounts of impurities are sufficient to cause a dramatic accumulation at the interface, and hence large effects on the surface tension. From a more positive perspective, surface tension measurements constitute a critical test of the surfactant purity. If the surface tension curve looks nice, then the risk of any hydrophobic impurities is generally limited.

2.3.2 Light Scattering

Scattering of radiation from a surfactant solution offers possibilities to characterize the solution in a number of ways. In principle, both light, X-rays, and neutrons can be used for investigations of surfactant and block copolymer micelles, but due to its simplicity, light scattering is the technique most extensively used for such investigations. In so-called static light scattering, the scattering intensity is collected at different scattering angles for a series of samples of different concentrations. Frequently, the results are summarized in a so-called Zimm-plot, and information about the molecular weight M_w, radius of gyration R_g size, and second virial coefficient B (a measure of intermolecular interactions) is extracted from the reciprocal of the scattering intensity extrapolated to zero concentration, the angular dependence of the scattering intensity, and the concentration dependence of the scattering intensity, respectively (Figure 2.20).

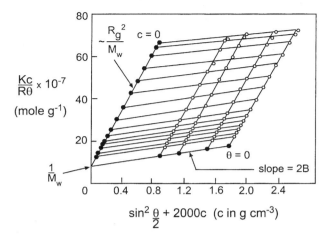

FIGURE 2.20 Typical Zimm-plot for static light scattering data, in which the scattering intensity is plotted as a function of concentration c and scattering angle θ.

In dynamic light scattering (often called also photon correlation spectroscopy), the time dependence of the light intensity fluctuations is analyzed in order to yield information about the diffusion coefficient, which in turn can be used to extract a micellar hydrodynamic radius (Chapter 9). Frequently, static and dynamic light scattering experiments are combined for a given system, which allows information to be extracted on both the micellar size, shape, and aggregation number.

2.3.3 NMR

Since both the microenvironment of a nucleus of a surfactant molecule and the overall mass transport properties change on micellization, NMR offers many opportunities when it comes to investigating both micellization and the properties of micellar systems. Probably the most extensively used of these is NMR self-diffusion measurements. Such measurements have several advantages:

1. A true self-diffusion coefficient is obtained.
2. No chemical labeling is required, and possible artefacts relating to fluorescence or radioactive labels can therefore be avoided.
3. The self-diffusion of essentially any number of components in a mixture can be followed simultaneously.
4. In contrast to, e.g., light scattering, there are no restrictions relating to optical clarity of the sample and use of dilute samples.
5. In contrast to experiments where the diffusion coefficient is determined

through following the concentration gradient of the diffusing species, NMR self-diffusion measurements are fast.

In the case of micellizing surfactants, self-diffusion measurements contain information on both free molecules and molecules in the micellar state. For low molecular weight surfactants, the micellar residence time is generally very short on the NMR time scale (≈ 100 ms), which means that there is extensive molecular exchange during an NMR experiment, and therefore the observed diffusion coefficient D_{obs} determined by NMR constitutes an average over the two states, i.e.,

$$D_{obs} = p_{mic}D_{mic} + p_{free}D_{free} \qquad (1)$$

where D_i and p_i are the diffusion coefficient and the fraction in state i. Since the diffusion coefficients of the free surfactant molecules can be determined from measurements below the cmc, since the diffusion coefficient of the micelles may be obtained through measurement of the diffusion coefficient of a hydrophobic molecule solubilized in the micellar core, and since the total concentration is known, the concentration of micelles and free surfactant micelles can be extracted. Furthermore, by simultaneously measuring the surfactant and counterion self-diffusion in the case of ionic surfactants, information about the degree of counterion binding, i.e., the fraction of counterions bound to the micelles, can be estimated. A typical result from such an analysis is shown in Figure 2.21.

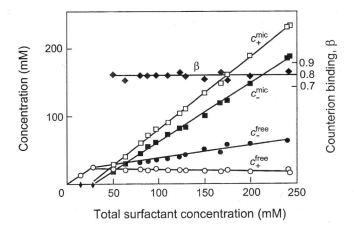

FIGURE 2.21 Concentrations of micellar (squares) and free (circles) surfactant molecules (open symbols), and counterions (filled symbols), as well as the degree of counterion binding (filled diamonds), as a function of the total surfactant concentration. The surfactant used was decylammonium dichloroacetate. (Redrawn from Stilbs et al., J. Phys. Chem. 1981, 85, 2587.)

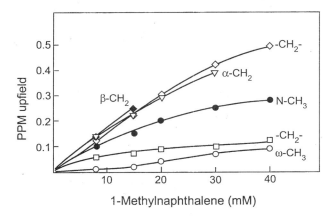

FIGURE 2.22 Effect of 1-methylnaphthalene on the chemical shift of CTAB protons. (Redrawn from Ulmius et al., J. Colloid Interface Sci. 1978, 65, 88.)

From the latter type of measurement one can conclude that:

1. Above the cmc, the concentration of micelles increases largely linearly with the total surfactant concentration, whereas the free monomer concentration is either constant (nonionic surfactants) or decreases somewhat (ionic surfactants).
2. Below the cmc, all surfactant molecules are in a nonmicellized form.
3. The degree of counterion binding for ionic surfactants is generally quite high ($\approx 70–90\%$).

Apart from self-diffusion measurements, there are also several other NMR techniques which may be used in order to characterize micellar systems. For example, measuring the chemical shift of surfactant molecules may provide information about both the extent of water penetration into the micellar core, and the precise location of solubilized molecules in micelles. As an example of the latter, Figure 2.22 shows the effect of an aromatic solubilisate, 1-methylnaphthalene, on the chemical shift of cetyltrimethylammunium bromide (CTAB) protons. As can be seen, the protons in the polar head group (α-, β-) of the surfactant experience a larger chemical shift than protons closer to the micellar core (ω-), which shows that the solubilizate is located close to the polar head groups, i.e., close to the micellar surface.

2.4 MICELLAR SYSTEMS IN DRUG DELIVERY

Solubilization of hydrophobic drugs in surfactant or block copolymer micelles offers a range of possibilities:

1. Through solubilization, larger quantities of sparingly soluble active substances may be incorporated in an aqueous solution.
2. Since the water concentration in the micellar core is low or very low, hydrolytic degradation may be reduced, hence resulting in an increased chemical stability of the drug.
3. Through the partitioning toward the micelles, the release rate of the drug may be controlled.
4. Micelles offer opportunities to affect the uptake of the drug in the body, and through solubilization of drugs they may result in decreased side effects and an increased efficiency of the drug.
5. Also in the absence of drug solubilization, surfactants may have beneficial effects, e.g., as adjuvants in vaccination.
6. Through incorporation of the drug in micelles, taste masking may be obtained.

Examples of such uses of surfactant and block copolymer micelles will be discussed below.

2.4.1 Solubilization of Drugs in Micellar Systems

Probably the most common reason for using surfactant and block copolymer micelles in relation to drug delivery is simply that the solubility of the drug in aqueous solution is insufficient. In this context addition of a surfactant above the cmc may strongly increase the solubility of the hydrophobic drug. As illustrated in Figure 2.8, the solubility of a hydrophobic solute (drug) increases strongly with the surfactant concentration as a result of the solubilization of the drug molecules in the micelles. It is noteworthy that the increased solubility with an increasing total surfactant concentration is generally largely linear. As shown in Figure 2.21, the concentration of micelles above the cmc increases essentially linearly with increasing total surfactant concentration. Thus, the solubility of the hydrophobic drug is directly related to the number of micelles (at least in the absence of solute-induced micellar growth or shape transitions).

The extent of solubilization depends on a number of parameters, such as the surfactant or copolymer structure, the micellar size and aggregation number, and the nature of the solubilizate. As an example of the former, Figure 2.23 shows the solubilization capacity for two different steroids of a series of $C_{16}E_n$ surfactants as a function of the length of the oligo(ethylene oxide) chain at constant length of the alkyl group. As the length of the oligo(ethylene oxide) chain increases, the repulsion between these polar head groups becomes more long range, and causes the micelles to become smaller. As a consequence of this, surfactants with longer oligo(ethylene oxide) chains are poorer concerning solubilization than those with shorter ones.

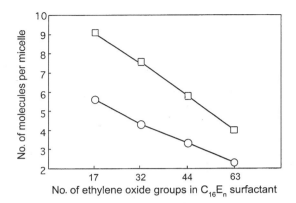

FIGURE 2.23 Effect of the length of the oligo(ethylene oxide) chain on the solubilization capacity of $C_{16}E_n$ surfactants for hydrocortisone (squares), and progesterone (circles). (Redrawn from Barry et al., J. Pharm. Pharmacol. 1976, 59, 220.)

The solubilization in micellar systems also depends on the nature of the solubilizate. Although some simple rules can be identified as discussed above, e.g., concerning the effects of solubilizate size and polarity for well-defined homologue series, it is not entirely simple to derive solid sets of rules concerning more complex solubilizates, such as drugs. To at least some extent, however, the rules from the simpler systems seem to hold also here. For example, for all the C_mE_n surfactants in Figure 2.23, the solubilization capacity for hydrophobic progesterone is lower than that for the more hydrophilic hydrocortisone.

Many drugs are moderately stable componds in aqueous solution, and undergo hydrolysis. Examples of hydrolytically sensitive compounds include esters and anhydrides. In particular, drugs containing ester groups tend to undergo hydrolysis such that the hydrolysis rate increases (1) at high or low pH, (2) at high temperature, and (3) at high water content. Such hydrolytic degradation may cause problems relating to storage stability of the formulation. Furthermore, since pH in the stomach is quite low, any hydrolytically labile drug which is administered orally risks displaying poor bioavailability. Also, the hydrolytic degradation products may not be well tolerated or even toxic, and their occurrence either in the formulation or in the biological system therefore is to be avoided. In all these cases, it is essential to reduce the hydrolytic breakdown of the drug. In the case of hydrophobic drugs this often involves the use of surfactant systems, such as micellar solutions, liquid crystalline phases, and microemulsions. In all such systems, the exposure of the hydrophobic and hydrolytically labile drug toward water is reduced, and hence the degradation rate decreases. As an example of this, Figure 2.24 shows the degradation rate of indomethacin, a nonsteroidal anti-

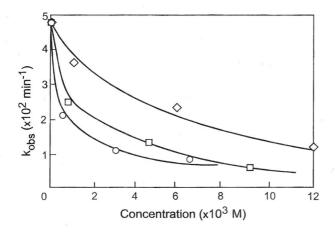

FIGURE 2.24   Degradation rate constant k_{obs} of indomethacin as a function of polymer concentration for Pluronic F68 (diamonds), F88 (squares), and F108 (circles) in aqueous solution. (Redrawn from Lin et al., Pharm. Acta Helv. 1985, 60, 345.)

inflammatory agent, in Pluronic block copolymer solutions. As can be seen, the degradation rate of this substance is reduced with an increasing copolymer (micelle) concentration for all polymers, which is a result of the solubilization of indomethacin in the block copolymer micelles, thereby shielding it from the aqueous environment.

In accordance with the discussion above, increasing the molecular weight of the block copolymer at a constant composition (F68→F88→F108) results in an increased block segregation, an increased micellization and solubilization capacity, reduced exposure of indomethacin to the aqueous environment, and hence also in a reduced degradation rate.

Since solubilization is a partitioning between the aqueous phase and the micellar microcontainers, both the equilibrium concentration in the aqueous surrounding and the release rate of the solubilized drug is reduced on solubilization. Therefore, solubilization may offer an opportunity to control the release rate of the drug, and specifically to obtain a sustained release over a prolonged time. Such controlled release may offer interesting opportunities, e.g., when (1) the drug is rapidly metabolized, (2) a low number of medication instances is desired, or (3) the drug is taken up slowly but degraded rapidly.

The release rate of a drug in a micellar solution depends on its state of solubilization, and hence on the properties of both the drug and the surfactant/block copolymer. The former of these is clearly seen, e.g., when investigating the release rate of a given drug as a function of ionization, e.g., achieved by varying pH. As an illustration of this, Figure 2.25 shows the pH-dependent release

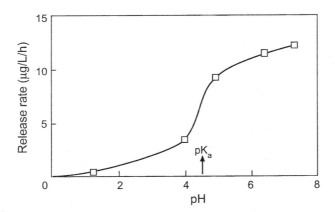

FIGURE 2.25 Release rate of indomethacin from PEO-PBLA micelles in aqueous solution at different pH. (Redrawn from La et al., J. Pharm. Sci. 1996, 85, 85.)

rate of indomethacin solubilized in PEO-poly(β-benzyl L-aspartate) (PBLA) block copolymer micelles, used as carriers in order to reduce irritation of the gastrointestinal mucosa and central nervous system toxicity. As can be seen, when this molecule obtains a charge as a result of increasing pH and following deprotonation, the release rate of this substance from the micelles increases drastically, with a transition point close to the pKa of the substance. Thus, at low pH indomethacin is uncharged, hydrophobic, and solubilized in the micelles, thus displaying a low release rate. At pH ≫ pKa, on the other hand, indomethacin is charged, and therefore not solubilized in the micelles to the same extent, and hence the release rate is fast.

Naturally, a sustained drug release rate from micellar systems only works as long as the micelles are sufficiently stable. In particular, on dilution of a micellar solution containing a solubilized drug following administration, the surfactant concentration after dilution must remain above the cmc in order to prevent the micelles from disintegrating. In this context, the long dilution-induced disintegration time displayed by at least some block copolymer micellar systems offers some possibilities.

2.4.2 Micelles in Intravenous Drug Delivery

As will be discussed in more detail in Chapter 4, intravenous administration of drugs may lead to their rapid clearence from bloodstream circulation, and accumulation in tissues associated with the rethiculoendothelial system (RES). As a result of this, the bioavailability of the drug in tissues not related to the RES may be limited, and dose-limiting toxic side effects may occur in RES-related tissues. In this context, the use of colloidal drug carriers, such as micelles, liposomes, and emulsion droplets may offer a way to reduce the RES uptake. In particular, PEO-containing block copolymers are quite attractive in this context; due to this, the generally small size of micelles, and the slow disintegration time of PEO-containing block copolymer micelles, such systems are quite interesting as drug carriers in intravenous drug delivery.

An area where a prolonged circulation time following intravenous administration is of interest is cancer therapy. In this area, the drug is desired to accumulate as much as possible in cancer-related tissues or cells in order to generate a sufficient effect, and to reduce toxic side effects. Through use of PEO-containing block copolymer micelles, a prolonged bloodstream circulation and a decreased RES uptake of solubilized cancer drugs can be achieved, which allows the dose to be further increased in order to reach a further improved therapeutic effect. An illustrative example of this is PEO-poly(aspartate) block copolymer conjugates with the anticancer drug adriamycin (ADR). This copolymer conjugate forms small micelles (15–60 nm), where ADR is located in the micellar core. Furthermore, the micellar disintegration time on dilution to $c <$ cmc is quite long (days). Therefore, the release rate of ADR from the block copolymer conjugate micelles is not limited by micellar disintegration after intravenous administration, but instead occurs as a result of the biodegradation of the aspartate segments. The conjugate micelles display a very long circulation time in the bloodstream and a slow uptake in liver, spleen, and marrow. Notably, the circulation time of the PEO-P(Asp(ADR)) conjugate is much longer than that of free ADR, as seen from the higher blood ADR concentration a given time after administration of the micellar system. For free ADR, on the other hand, a rapid clearance from bloodstream circulation is observed (Figure 2.26).

As is the case with many anticancer drugs, ADR may also cause side effects. This limits the upper concentration which can be used without causing detrimental effects. For intravenous administration of ADR in tumor-bearing mice, it has been found that at ADR concentrations higher than about 10 mg/kg, the mean survival time is drastically reduced, which is due to the occurence of serious side effects. For ADR solubilized in the block copolymer conjugates, on the other hand, the side effects occur at 1–2 orders of magnitude higher ADR concentration (Figure 2.27). Thus, the use of these micelles allows a substantially higher ADR concentration to be used in therapy without causing toxic side effects. Due to this and to the longer circulation time in the bloodstream, the cytotoxicity of the block copolymer conjugate micelles is superior to that of ADR in aqueous solution (Figure 2.28).

An interesting opportunity is to use the long circulation time displayed by PEO-containing block copolymer micelles and other colloidal drug carriers in

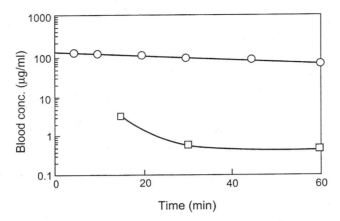

FIGURE 2.26 Blood concentration of ADR (squares) and PEO-P (Asp(ADR)) (circles) after intravenous injection in tumor bearing mice. (Redrawn from Yokoyama, Crit. Rev. Ther. Drug Carrier Syst. 1992, 9, 213.)

order to achieve a selective targeting to specific tissues or cell types. Areas where this is of interest include cancer therapy and drug delivery to the central nervous system, in the former case due to the occurence of side effects related to nonspecific drug uptake, and in the latter case due to the frequently poor bioavailability of drugs aimed for the central nervous system caused by the limited nonspecific

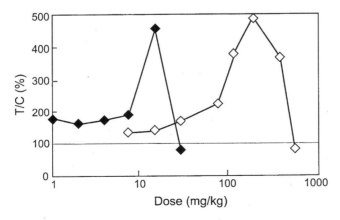

FIGURE 2.27 Mean survival (treated to control (T/C) ratio) of ADR (filled symbols) and PEO-P(Asp(ADR)) (open symbols) for tumor-bearing mice. (Redrawn from Yokoyama, Crit. Rev. Ther. Drug Carrier Syst. 1992, 9, 213.)

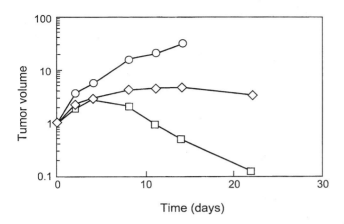

FIGURE 2.28 In vivo antitumor activity. Circles, diamonds, and squares refer to control, ADR (10 mg/kg), and PEO-P(Asp(ADR)) (200 mg/kg), respectively. (Redrawn from Yokoyama, Crit. Rev. Ther. Drug Carrier Syst. 1992, 9, 213.)

passage through the blood-brain barrier. As an illustration on the latter, Figure 2.29 shows results obtained on targeting PEO-PPO-PEO block copolymers to the brain when the copolymer was conjugated with antibodies to the antigen of brain glial cells (α_2-glycoprotein). Incorporation of haloperidol, a neuroleptic drug, into such micelles results in a drastically increased therapeutic effect. In particular, both the number of mouse migrations in a cell and grooming, the latter characterizing the rate of animal adaptation to unknown conditions, are lower for the antibody-containing carriers compared to the antibody-free ones. From this one can conclude that the neuroleptic effect of haloperidol is considerably increased in the former case, and that targeting in this case has improved the drug efficiency.

2.4.3 Reversed Micelles

In the same way that normal micellar systems can be used for solubilizing hydrophobic substances in an aqueous solution, reversed micellar systems may be used for solubilizing water-soluble drugs in an oil-continuous system. The reasons for doing this may be one of several:

1. The amount extensively water-soluble drugs which can be incorporated in an oil-continuous system may be increased. This, in turn, allows water-soluble drugs to be combined with the use of gelatin capsules.
2. Compared to a pure oil system, the function of sensitive structures requiring the presence of water (e.g., protein and peptide drugs) may be improved.

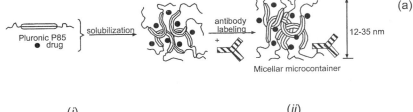

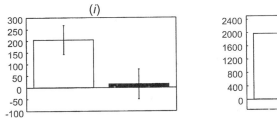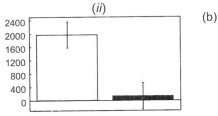

FIGURE 2.29 (a) Schematic illustration of the block copolymer carriers used for targeting to brain glial cells. (b) Therapeutic effect of haloperidol in mice as measured by horizontal mobility (i) and number of grooming incidents (ii) for haloperidol solubilized in Pluronic P85 micelles (open bars) and Pluronic P85-micelles modified with anti-α_2-glycoprotein (filled bars). (Redrawn from Kabanov et al., J. Controlled Release 1992, 22, 141.)

3. Compared to a pure aqueous system, the function of hydrolytically unstable hydrophilic substances may be improved.
4. The release rate of water-soluble drugs may be controlled.
5. Masking of bitter taste for extensively water-soluble drugs may be achieved.

Some of these aspects are discussed in the context of microemulsions (Chapter 5).

2.4.4 Comparison Between Micelles and Other Solubilizing Agents

Although micelles are frequently used for solubilizing sparingly soluble drugs, they are certainly not the only type of system which can be used for this purpose. Instead, systems not based on surfactants, e.g., cyclodextrins and covalent PEO modification of the drug, as well as other types of surfactant-containing systems, including liquid crystalline phases, microemulsions and emulsions, may be successfully employed for this purpose. The choice of system used for solubilization depends on numerous factors, including, e.g., (1) the amount of drug which needs to be solubilized, (2) the amount surfactant which can be tolerated, (3) requirements on long-term stability, (4) requirements on rheological properties, release rate, optical clarity, and other factors related to the administration of the drug.

TABLE 2.1 Main Advantages and Disadvantages with Different Systems for Solubilization of Hydrophobic Drugs

		Advantages		Disadvantages
Micelles	(i)	Low surfactant concentrations required	(i)	Sensitive to dilution
	(ii)	Good long-term stability		
Emulsions	(i)	Large solubilization capacity	(i)	Limited stability
			(ii)	Sometimes yield poor bioavailibility
			(iii)	Not straightforward to prepare
Microemulsions	(i)	Good long-term stability	(i)	Requires high surfactant concentrations
	(ii)	Good solubilization capacity		
Liquid crystalline phases	(i)	Good long-term stability	(i)	Difficult to prepare
	(ii)	Generally viscous	(ii)	Generally viscous
	(iii)	Good solubilization capacity		
Cyclodextrins	(i)	Good long-term stability	(i)	Limited solubilization capacity
			(ii)	Restrictions on drug size and shape
PEO-modification	(i)	Good long-term stability	(i)	Limited solubilization capacity
	(ii)	No risk for surfactant-induced activity loss for peptide drugs	(ii)	Limited reduction in hydrolysis

The main advantages and disadvantages of the different systems are summarized in Table 2.1. The solubilization capacity of surfactant and block copolymer micelles also finds other uses in pharmaceutical applications. For example, PEO-PPO-PEO block copolymers and low molecular weight surfactants are able to dissolve gallstones following oral administration. Furthermore, the resistance of Mycobacterium avium complex (MAC) to antibiotics is enhanced by its outer glycolipid layer. Therefore, PEO-PPO-PEO block copolymers have been used to solubilize these glycolipids, thereby resulting in a disruption of the glycolipid layer. Particularly, PEO-PPO-PEO block copolymers containing a high fraction of PPO have been found to be quite potent in increasing the efficiency of antibiotic therapy of MAC infections. Solubilization or disruption of the stratum corneum lipid structures is also frequently used in transdermal drug delivery in order to improve the topical bioavailability.

BIBLIOGRAPHY

Alexandridis, P., T. A. Hatton, Poly(ethylene oxide)-poly(propylene oxide)-poly(ethylene oxide) block copolymer surfactants in aqueous solutions and at interfaces: thermodynamics, structure, dynamics, and modeling, Colloids Surf. A, 96, 1–46 (1995).

Alexandridis, P., B. Lindman eds., Amphiphilic Block Copolymers. Self-Assembly and Applications, Elsevier, Amsterdam, 2000.

Brown W., ed., Dynamic Light Scattering: The Method and Some Applications, Calendron Press, Oxford, 1993.

Evans, D. F., H. Wennerström, The Colloidal Domain, Wiley, New York, 1999.

Florence, A. T., D. Attwood, Physicochemical Principles of Pharmacy, Macmillan Press, London, 1989.

Huglin, M. B., ed., Light Scattering from Polymer Solutions, Academic Press, London, 1972.

Israelachvili, J., Intermolecular and Surface Forces, Academic Press, London, 1992.

Jönsson, B., B. Lindman, K. Holmberg, B. Kronberg, Surfactants and Polymers in Aqueous Solution, Wiley, New York, 1998.

Kwon, G. S., Diblock copolymer nanoparticles for drug delivery, Crit. Rev. Ther. Drug Carrier Syst. 15:481–512 (1998).

Kwon, G. S., K. Kataoka, Block copolymer micelles as long-circulating drug vehicles, Adv. Drug Delivery Rev. 16:295–309 (1995).

Lindman, B., H. Wennerström, Micelles: amphiphile aggregation in aqueous solution, Topics Curr. Chem. 87:1–83 (1980).

Lucassen-Reynders, E. H., ed., Anionic Surfactants: Physical Chemistry of Surfactant Action, Surfactant Science Series, vol. 11, Marcel Dekker, New York, 1981.

Schick M. J., ed., Nonionic Surfactants. Physical Chemistry, Surfactant Science Series, vol. 23, Marcel Dekker, New York, 1987.

Shaw, D. O., ed., Micelles, Microemulsions and Monolayers, Marcel Dekker, New York, 1998.

Söderman, O., P. Stilbs, NMR studies of complex surfactant systems, Progr. NMR Spectroscop. 26:445–482 (1994).

Stilbs, P., Fourier transform pulsed-gradient spin-echo studies of molecular diffusion, Progr. NMR Spectroscopy 19:1–45 (1987).

Torchilin, V. P., Targeting of drugs and drug carriers within the cardiovascular system, Adv. Drug Delivery Rev. 17:75–101 (1995).

Yokoyama, M., Block copolymers as drug carriers, Crit. Rev. Ther. Drug Carrier Syst. 9:213–248 (1992).

Zana R., ed., Surfactant Solutions: New Methods of Investigation, Surfactant Science Series, vol. 22, Marcel Dekker, New York, 1987.

3

Liquid Crystalline Phases

3.1 ASSOCIATION STRUCTURES AND PACKING

Apart from micelles, surfactants and block copolymers may associate to form a range of different structures, including rods, lamellae, and bicontinuous interconnected structures. As with micelles, such systems are characterized by local disorder (''liquidlike'' behavior) and frequently also fast molecular dynamics. Simultaneously, however, long-range order exists, which may result in interesting rheological, mass-transport, and optical properties. A schematic illustration of different liquid crystalline structures is given in Figure 3.1.

Unfortunately, there is no universal notation system for liquid crystalline phases, and each phase goes under a number of different names in the scientific literature. The most common notations for the phases most relevant to the present context are given in Table 3.1.

The type of association structures formed in surfactant systems depends on a number of parameters, including (1) surfactant structure, (2) composition of the system, (3) presence of salt, oil, and cosolutes, and (4) temperature.

In order to understand the formation of these structures, it is helpful to consider the packing properties of the surfactant (block copolymer) molecules in the different structures (Figure 3.2). Thus, for flat lamellae, the surfactant molecules adopt essentially a cylindrical form, whereas in structures curved toward the oil (e.g., hexagonal and micellar structures) the surfactant molecule occupies a

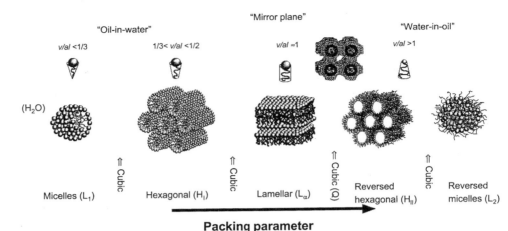

Packing parameter

FIGURE 3.1 Schematic illustration of association structures formed in surfactant and block copolymer systems, and the packing of surfactant molecules in different association structures. (Redrawn from Jönsson et al., Surfactants and Polymers in Aqueous Solution, Wiley, 1998.)

"cone," with the polar headgroup larger than the hydrophobic tail. For structures curved toward water (e.g., reversed hexagonal and reversed micellar structures), the opposite holds; i.e., the hydrophobic tail is larger than the polar head group (Figure 3.1).

In order to understand the type of surfactant packing preferred by the system, it is helpful to consider the critical packing parameter (cpp), defined as

TABLE 3.1 Different Notations for Liquid Crystalline Phases

Phase structure	Notations
Lamellar	lam, L_α, D, G, neat
Hexagonal	hex, H_1, E, M_1, middle
Reversed hexagonal	rev hex, H_2, F, M_2
Cubic (normal micellar)	cub, I_1, S_{1c}
Cubic (reversed micellar)	cub, I_2
Cubic (normal bicontinuous)	cub, I_1, V_1
Cubic (reversed bicontinuous)	cub, I_2, V_2
Micellar	mic, L_1, S
Reversed micellar	rev mic, L_2, S
Sponge phase	L_3, L_4

Source: From Jönsson et al., Surfactants and Polymers in Aqueous Solution, Wiley, 1998.

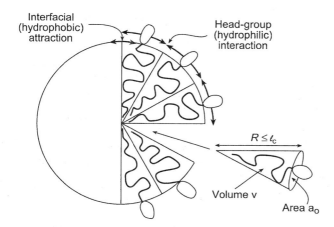

FIGURE 3.2 Schematic illustration of the parameters defining the cpp. (Redrawn from Israelachvili, Intermolecular and Surface Forces, Academic Press, 1992.)

$$\text{cpp} = \frac{v}{a \cdot l}$$

where v is the volume of the hydrophobic tail(s), a the polar head group area, and l (or l_c) the length of the hydrophobic chain(s) of the surfactant (Figure 3.2).

As can be seen in Figure 3.1, there is a direct correlation between the value of the cpp and the type of aggregate formed. For example, for a lamellar phase, the surfactant molecules occupy a cylindrical space and $v = a \cdot l$, that is, cpp = 1. The more the surfactant aggregate curves toward the oil (e.g., the progression lamellar → hexagonal → micellar), the smaller the value of cpp, i.e., the larger the headgroup area in relation to the surfactant volume. For reversed structures, the cpp increases in the order lamellar → reversed hexagonal → reversed micellar.

It follows that the packing of the surfactant molecules, and hence also the type of surfactant aggregate formed, depends on the values of a, v, and l, and that changing any of these parameters influences the structure of surfactant aggregates formed. As will be discussed below, these parameters may be practically altered in a number of ways (Table 3.2).

3.2 PHASE DIAGRAMS

Before we discuss the structures formed in surfactant and block copolymer systems in larger detail, it is useful to briefly consider the construction of phase diagrams, by which the phase behavior of surfactants is generally described. In the simplest case of relevance in the present context, a surfactant is mixed with

TABLE **3.2** Examples On How the Surfactant Packing May Be Practically Affected

		Increase		Decrease
a	(i)	Larger polar groups (nonionics)	(i)	Smaller polar groups (nonionics)
	(ii)	Low temperature (EO-surfactants)	(ii)	High temperature (EO-surfactants)
	(iii)	Charged polar group	(iii)	Presence of salt (ionics)
	(iv)	No salt present (ionics)		
I	(i)	Long hydrocarbon chains	(i)	Short hydrocarbon chains
v	(i)	Double-chain surfactants	(i)	Linear single-chain surfactants
	(ii)	Branched hydrophobic chains		

a solvent (notably water) only. Therefore, the system contains two components and is described by a binary phase diagram, indicating the different phases formed as a function of composition and temperature. In such a phase diagram, the ordinate shows the temperature, while the abscissa shows the fractional composition of the system, with one end representing pure surfactant in the absence of solvent and the other pure solvent in the absence of surfactant. Between the one-phase regions are two-phase regions, where the compositions of the two phases are given by the points where the tie-lines intersect the one-phase regions in the same way as for phase diagrams for simpler liquids (Figure 3.3).

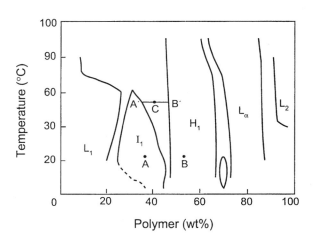

FIGURE **3.3** Typical example of a binary phase diagram. Points A and B are located in one-phase areas, whereas point C corresponds to a two-phase sample, where each phase has composition A' and B'.

In the general case, however, not only surfactant and water, but also "oil" is present in a typical surfactant system (compare, e.g., solubilized hydrophobic drugs in drug delivery). In such systems, the phase diagram used is generally referred to as *ternary*. A schematic illustration of a ternary phase diagram is given in Figure 3.4. At constant temperature, each surfactant/oil/water system displays a unique ternary phase diagram. Moreover, each point in the ternary phase diagram corresponds to a unique composition, which may be obtained by extrapolation to the "legs" of the triangle according to Figure 3.4. Since the system is now a three-component one, not only one- and two-phase areas are possible, but also three-phase triangles may occur. As before, the composition of the different phases in a two- or three-phase sample is given by the points where the tie-lines intersect the corresponding one-phase areas.

Note that ternary phase diagrams are strictly valid only when the system contains three components (surfactant, oil, and water). Therefore, it is not strictly valid if:

1. Several surfactants or a surfactant mixture is used.
2. The surfactant used is polydisperse and/or heterogeneous.
3. Further components are added in the form of salt or other cosolutes.

In such cases, a multidimensional phase diagram is needed to fully describe the system, which would be very time consuming to construct. In such cases, one usually fixes one or several of the composition parameters, and vary systemati-

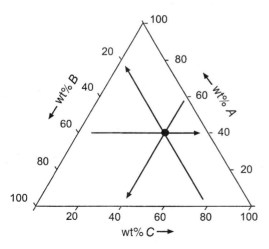

FIGURE 3.4 Schematic illustration of a ternary phase diagram. The composition of the sample indicated with the filled circle corresponds to 40 wt% A, 20 wt% B, and 40 wt% C.

cally, e.g., the cosolute concentration or the composition of the surfactant mixture.

3.3 ASSOCIATION IN NONIONIC SURFACTANT SYSTEMS

The structure of surfactant molecules has a major influence on their packing properties, and hence also on the types of self-association structures formed. For example, the self-association depends on whether or not the head group of the surfactant is charged. If it is charged, structure formation depends on the nature of the charge (e.g., whether it is titratable or not, or whether it is monovalent or divalent), whereas if it is uncharged, structure formation depends on parameters such as the bulkiness and length of the polar group. Also, the nature of the hydrophobic group affects the packing and the structures formed. In particular, the length, bulkiness, and branching of the hydrophobic group, as well as the number of such groups, is important for the self-association.

For nonionic surfactants, the main compositional parameters are the size and shape of the polar and nonpolar parts of the surfactant. It is illustrative here to consider $C_m E_n$ surfactants, since these have been extensively investigated and are available in essentially monodisperse homologue fractions, so that the effects of composition on the self-assembly may be clearly seen (Figure 3.5).

By comparing binary phase diagrams for $C_{12}E_n$, where $n = 5$, 6, and 8, it can be seen that increasing the size of the polar head group for a fixed hydrophobic group results in:

1. A decrease in the lamellar phase on going from $C_{12}E_5$ to $C_{12}E_6$, and an almost complete elimination of this phase in the case of $C_{12}E_8$
2. A progressive increase in the extension of the hexagonal phase
3. An increased stability of the micellar phase compared to the hexagonal phase
4. Occurrence of a discrete cubic phase for $C_{12}E_8$ but not for the other surfactants

Hence it is clear that increasing the length of the oligo(ethylene oxide) chain when keeping the hydrophobic group constant results in a transition toward structures more curved toward the oil, e.g., lamellar $\rightarrow$ hexagonal $\rightarrow$ micellar. This can be understood from the oligo(ethylene oxide) chains repelling each other. In order to minimize this repulsion, the oil-water interface curves toward the oil, which results in a larger area available for each oligo(ethylene oxide) chain, and hence in a lower repulsion. The larger the oligo(ethylene oxide) chains, the larger the curvature needs to be to reduce this repulsion.

Although water penetration to the interior of micelles and other self-assembled structures is very limited for alkyl-based surfactants, there is oil-water contact, e.g., in the case of the outermost alkyl group of an alkyl chain. Since this

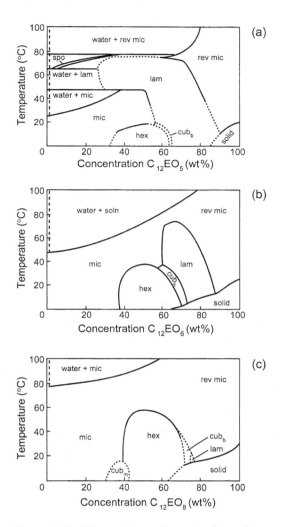

FIGURE 3.5 Binary phase diagrams (two-phase regions not shown) for mixtures of water and $C_{12}E_n$, where $n = 5$, 6, and 8. (Redrawn from Mitchell et al., J. Chem. Soc. Faraday Trans. I 1983, 79, 975.)

contact is unfavorable, and since the higher the curvature toward oil the more significant this contact, the increased interfacial curving of surfactant aggregates comes with an energy penalty. Therefore, increasing the cohesion between the hydrophobic groups, e.g., by increasing the length of the alkyl chain in the case of $C_m E_n$ surfactants, tends to oppose the effects of an increasing length of the

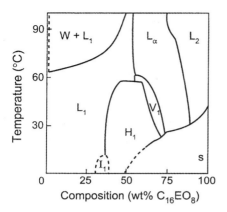

FIGURE 3.6 Binary phase diagram for $C_{16}E_8$. (Redrawn from Mitchell et al., J. Chem. Soc. Faraday Trans. I 1983, 79, 975.)

oligo(ethylene oxide) chain. This is illustrated in Figures 3.5 and 3.6, where it can be seen that increasing the alkyl chain length from 12 to 16 at a constant length of the oligo(ethylene oxide) chain results in the opposite effects compared with increasing the length of the latter and keeping the alkyl chain fixed. Thus, with an increasing alkyl chain length the micellar phase is disfavored in relation to the hexagonal phase, whereas the latter is disfavored compared with the lamellar phase.

As discussed in Chapter 2, increasing the temperature in aqueous solutions of C_mE_n or other oligo(ethylene oxide) surfactants or copolymers eventually results in phase separation ("clouding"). This is clearly shown also in the phase diagrams in Figure 3.5 and 3.6. In parallel, structures more curved toward oil are disfavored compared with less curved ones with increasing temperature. For example, increasing the temperature for either $C_{12}E_5$ or $C_{12}E_6$ results in a transformation from hexagonal to lamellar phase, and for the former surfactant also from the micellar to the lamellar phase. This is due to a contraction of the oligo(ethylene oxide) chains on increasing the temperature, which favors a closer packing of these chains, and therefore also aggregates less curved toward the oil. Naturally, these transitions are completely analogous to the micellar growth observed at increasing the temperature for surfactants containing oligo(ethylene oxide) (Chapter 2).

In order to describe the relative importance of the hydrophilic and the hydrophobic groups in a surfactant, the so-called hydrophilic-lipophilic balance (HLB) is sometimes used. Although the HLB concept is used for both ionic and nonionic surfactants, it is most useful for nonionic ones where long-range

TABLE 3.3 Group Contribution to HLB Numbers and Definition of HLB of Surfactants

Hydrophilic group numbers		Hydrophobic group numbers	
-SO$_4$Na	35.7	-CF$_3$	−0.870
-CO$_2$K	21.1	-CF$_2$-	−0.870
-CO$_2$Na	19.1	-CH$_3$	−0.475
-N (tertiary amine)	9.4	-CH$_2$-	−0.475
Ester (sorbitan ring)	6.3	-CH-	−0.475
Ester (free)	2.4		
-CO$_2$H	2.1		
-OH (free)	1.9		
-O-	1.3		
-OH (sorbitan ring)	0.5		

HLB = 7 + Σ (hydrophilic group numbers) + Σ (hydrophobic group numbers).
Source: From Jönsson et al., Surfactants and Polymers in Aqueous Solution, Wiley, 1998.

electrostatic interactions are not present, and the self-assembly properties are largely dependent on the surfactant composition. The HLB for any given surfactant may be calculated from its chemical structure (Table 3.3).

Based on empirical experience, some rules of thumb can be stated regarding the relation between the surfactant function, on one hand, and their HLB number, on the other. As can be seen in Table 3.4, solubilization capacity for hydrophobic molecules is best for surfactants with intermediate to high HLB numbers. Such surfactants also display the most efficient emulsification of oil in water (o/w), whereas for emulsification of water in oil (w/o) a more hydrophobic surfactant,

TABLE 3.4 Relation Between Surfactant Function and HLB Number

HLB number	Function
3–6	Emulsification (w/o)
7–9	Wetting
8–18	Emulsification (o/w)
13–15	Detergency
15–18	Solubilization

e.g., containing short oligo(ethylene oxide) groups and/or long hydrocarbon tail(s), should be used.

The HLB concept has been found to give a fair indication of the performance also of mixed surfactant systems. In such cases, the effective HLB for the mixture is simply obtained from the weighted average (in terms of mol%) of the HLB of the components in the mixture. Clearly, however, this yields only a rough first indication on the properties of the surfactant system, since the same system can display strongly temperature-related and other effects.

3.4 ASSOCIATION IN IONIC SURFACTANT SYSTEMS

As discussed in relation to micelle formation in Chapter 2, ionic surfactants differ significantly from nonionic ones in several respects. First, the presence of the charged head group causes a significant head group repulsion which precludes self-assembly (indicated, e.g., by a higher cmc) and favors maximizing the distance between the head group charges through formation of structures curved toward the oil. Second, since the electrostatic interaction is screened by addition of salt, the latter drastically affects the structures formed in ionic surfactant systems, whereas those formed by nonionic ones are less affected by salt.

This difference between ionic and nonionic surfactants is also evident in the formation of liquid crystalline phases, as can be seen straightforwardly from the phase diagrams. Shown in Figure 3.7 is the binary phase diagram for sodium dodecyl sulfate (SDS), an extensively used surfactant, also in drug delivery.

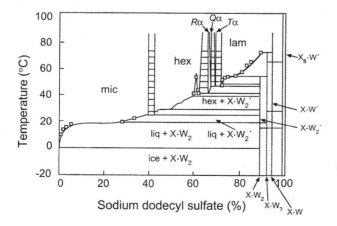

FIGURE 3.7 Binary phase diagram for the SDS/water system. (Redrawn from Laughlin, The Aqueous Phase Behavior of Surfactants, Academic Press, 1994.)

Focusing on the liquid crystalline phases and ignoring the rich crystallization behavior, it can be seen from Figure 3.7 that SDS only forms phases with zero curvature (i.e., a lamellar phase) and phases where the aggregates are curved toward the oil (micellar and hexagonal phases). This is a consequence of the electrostatic repulsion between the negatively charged head groups, which tends to curve the interface toward the oil phase in order to maximize the average distance between the charges, thereby minimizing this repulsion (effectively increasing the head group area and reducing the cpp). At higher surfactant concentrations, there is a transition from micelles to less curved self-assembled structures (rods, lamellae), which is due to both the increased chemical potential and an electrostatic screening of the headgroup interaction through the surfactant itself.

On addition of salt, the repulsive electrostatic interaction between the charged headgroups is screened, which means that aggregates curved toward the oil (e.g., micelles) become less favored compared with those with lower curvature (e.g., lamellae), and hence, addition of salt to an ionic surfactant system leads to a progression micelles $\rightarrow$ hexagonal phase $\rightarrow$ lamellar phase, analogous to the micellar growth displayed in micellar solution (Chapter 2). Since the screening increases with increasing salt concentration and with the valency of the counterions, the effect on the phase behavior in ionic surfactant systems goes in the same direction (i.e., cpp increases with increasing salt concentration and counterion valency).

In the other extreme, addition of oil or any substance readily soluble in the interior of surfactant aggregates, but poorly soluble in the aqueous solution, results in an effective increase in the hydrophobic volume, and therefore also in an increase in the cpp. This means that on addition of "oil," this is solubilized in the surfactant aggregates, thus resulting in micellar structural changes as well as phase transitions, e.g., in the sequence micellar $\rightarrow$ hexagonal $\rightarrow$ lamellar $\rightarrow$ reversed hexagonal $\rightarrow$ reversed micellar.

Some molecules, e.g., moderately hydrophobic ones containing one or several polar groups, e.g., cosurfactants, tend to distribute to the oil-water interface when added to a surfactant/water system. Therefore, their effects on the surfactant structures depend on both the effect on the head group interaction and the hydrophobic volume. Just to illustrate one possible outcome of this, Figure 3.8 shows results on the effect of an intermediate-length n-alcohol (decanol) on the phase behavior of an ionic surfactant. As can be seen, addition of decanol favors aggregates with a lower curvature toward the oil phase, which is due to a screening of the electrostatic repulsion between the head groups. In the language of the cpp, addition of decanol causes v to increase while A increases less or even decreases (the latter through screening of the head group electrostatic repulsion). Again, this is analogous to the micellar growth of ionic surfactant micelles on addition of medium-chain or long-chain n-alcohols.

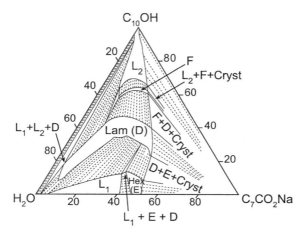

FIGURE 3.8 Phase behavior of the sodium octanoate/decanol/water system. In particular, note the progression micellar (or hexagonal)—lamellar—reversed micellar phase on addition of decanol at a fixed sodium octanoate/water ratio. (Redrawn from Laughlin, The Aqueous Phase Behavior of Surfactants, Academic Press, 1994.)

3.5 CUBIC PHASES

Apart from the hexagonal, reversed hexagonal, and lamellar phases, cubic phases are frequently occurring in surfactant systems, and are also quite interesting for drug delivery. Such cubic phases can consist of either micelles or reversed micelles close packed in a cubic symmetry, or of a bicontinuous structure. Depending of the structure, the mean curvature of these structures can vary considerably, and hence cubic phases are found over the entire surfactant concentration range (Figure 3.9).

Cubic liquid crystalline phases are interesting for drug delivery for a number of reasons:

1. The bicontinuous cubic phases can solubilize large amounts of both hydrophilic and hydrophobic drugs.
2. Through controlling the microstructure, the drug release rate can be controlled over a wide range.
3. Through control of the microstructure, protein drugs (e.g., enzymes) can be immobilized, thereby allowing them to function at the same time as they are not exposed to proteolytic enzymes, antibodies, etc.
4. The cubic phases are generally characterized by a high stiffness. This offers opportunities for fixation of the formulation at a desired site after administration and in situ formation.

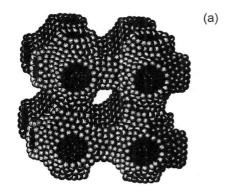

(a)

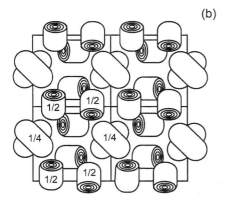

(b)

FIGURE 3.9 Two different possible cubic liquid crystalline structures, i.e., a bicontinuous one (a) and one consisting of close-packed slightly elongated micelles (b). [Redrawn from Evans et al., The Colloidal Domain, VCH, 1994 (a) and Fontell et al., Mol. Cryst. Liquid Cryst., 1985, 1, 9(b).]

3.6 LIQUID CRYSTALLINE PHASES FORMED BY PEO-PPO-PEO BLOCK COPOLYMERS

Just as low molecular weight surfactants containing oligo(ethylene oxide), PEO/PPO block copolymers display a rich self-association behavior, and form not only micelles and reversed micelles but also a range of liquid crystalline phases (Figure 3.10).

The effect of ''oil'' in PEO/PPO block copolymer systems can be straightforwardly deduced from a ternary phase diagram. As can be seen in Figure 3.10,

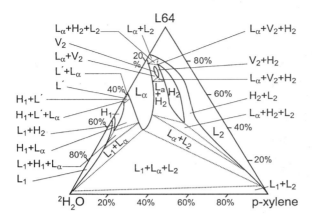

FIGURE 3.10 Ternary phase diagram for the system Pluronic L64 (EO$_{13}$PO$_{30}$EO$_{13}$)/H$_2$O/p-xylene at 25°C. The phase boundaries of the one-phase regions are drawn with solid lines, while the boundaries of the two-phase regions and the three-phase triangles are indicated with dotted lines. (Redrawn from Alexandridis et al., Macromolecules 1995, 28, 7700.)

the normal progression with increasing oil content observed with oligo(ethylene oxide)-containing surfactants appears also in PEO/PPO block copolymer systems, e.g., micellar → hexagonal → reversed micellar (surfactant/water = 45/55) or lamellar → reversed hexagonal → reversed micellar (surfactant/water = 75/25). Just as for low molecular weight surfactants, this curvature regression is due to solubilization of the oil in the block copolymer aggregates, thereby increasing the hydrophobic volume and increasing the cpp.

As with low molecular weight nonionic surfactants, the copolymer composition constitutes one of the most interesting parameters for self-assembly in PEO/PPO block copolymer systems. However, contrary to, e.g., the C$_m$E$_n$ surfactants, the relation between the copolymer composition and the phase behavior is less straightforward as a result of polymer polydispersity and heterogeneity, and less than perfect molecular weight agreement between polymers with different composition. However, some conclusions can nevertheless be drawn. As can be seen from Figure 3.11, Pluronic F38, which contains a high PEO fraction, and thus long oligo(ethylene oxide) chains and a short oligo(propylene oxide) chain, does not form reversed structures such as reversed micellar or reversed hexagonal phases, but only a lamellar phase and phases curved toward the oil (micellar, discrete cubic, and hexagonal phases). Pluronic L121, containing a low fraction of oligo(ethylene oxide) and a high fraction of oligo(propylene oxide), on the other hand, forms only a lamellar phase and the reversed hexagonal, reversed

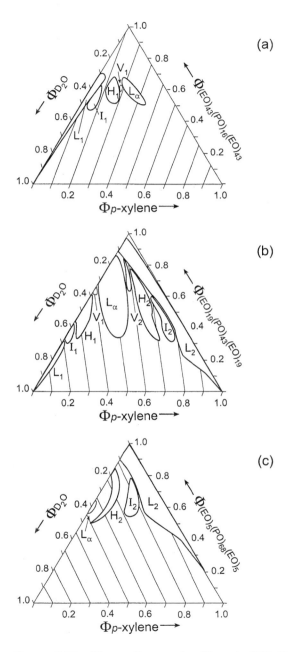

FIGURE 3.11 Phase diagram for Pluronic F38 ($EO_{43}PO_{16}EO_{43}$), Pluronic P84 ($EO_{19}PO_{43}EO_{19}$), and Pluronic L121 ($EO_5PO_{68}EO_5$) together with p-xylene and water. (Redrawn from Svensson et al., Langmuir 2000, 16, 6839.)

cubic, and reversed micellar phases, but no phases curved towards the oil phase. Pluronic P84, finally, lying between these two extremes forms both reversed and normal type of aggregates. Overall, therefore, the effects of the composition are analogous to those found in low molecular weight nonionic surfactant systems of the $C_m E_n$ type.

The effects of the polymer molecular weight on the phase behavior of block copolymers at a constant composition is another parameter of interest. As can be seen in Figure 3.12, the lower the molecular weight of the polymer, the more the disordered phases (i.e., the micellar and the reversed micellar) dominate, whereas at high molecular weight the ordered phases become relatively more stable. The origin of this effect is that for a system characterized by an incomplete segregation between the blocks, such as PEO/PPO copolymers, the segregation increases with increasing molecular weight. This, in turn, favors the formation of ordered liquid crystalline phases.

The segregation between the blocks and between PPO and water may be

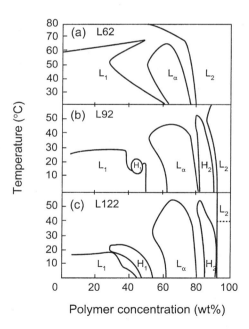

FIGURE 3.12   Binary phase diagram for Pluronic L62, Pluronic L92, and Pluronic L122 together with water. These polymers all contain 20% oligo(propylene oxide), but have different molecular weights (Fig. 1.11). (Redrawn from Svensson et al., Macromolecules 1999, 32, 637.)

increased also by increasing the temperature. In analogy to the molecular weight dependence and the effect of block segregation on the formation of liquid crystalline phases, an increased temperature for concentrated or moderately concentrated PEO/PPO copolymer/water systems induces a transition from micelles to rods and to lamellae. Of particular importance in relation to drug delivery, such a temperature-induced transition from a micellar solution to a discrete cubic phase occurs in the binary $EO_{99}PO_{65}EO_{99}$ (Pluronic F127)/water system. The liquid crystalline phase is not perfectly ordered for kinetic reasons, and therefore this system is often referred to as a "gel" (Figure 3.13). However, since it is more closely related to liquid crystalline phases than to, e.g., polysaccharide gels or gels formed by polymer/surfactant mixtures, they are discussed in the present chapter rather than in Chapter 8.

The temperature-induced transition in the Pluronic F127 system from micellar solution to a (disordered) cubic liquid crystalline phase is extremely abrupt, and results in a dramatic thickening on increasing the temperature, e.g., from room to body temperature (Figure 3.14). The precise value of the transition temperature can be fine-tuned, e.g., by varying the polymer concentration, or through addition of a second (co)polymer, salt, surfactant, or other cosolute. On cooling the highly elastic system under the transition temperature, the system becomes reversibly low-viscous once more. Given this, the capacity for this system to solubilize hydrophobic drugs, the commercial availability of this copolymer, and its relatively low toxicity, it is not surprising that this system has been found to

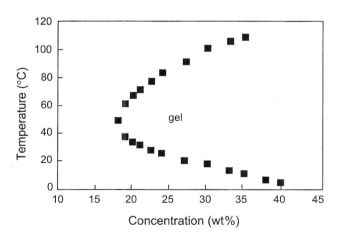

FIGURE 3.13 Phase behavior for the Pluronic F127/water system. (Redrawn from Malmsten et al., Macromolecules 1992, 25, 5440.)

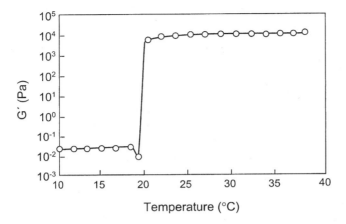

FIGURE 3.14 Elastic modulus G' for a 25 wt% aqueous Pluronic F127 solution versus temperature. (Redrawn from Scherlund et al., Int. J. Pharm. 1998, 173, 103.)

offer a range of opportunities in drug delivery, as will be exemplified and discussed below.

3.7 CHARACTERIZATION OF LIQUID CRYSTALLINE PHASES

Before characterizing liquid crystalline phases formed by surfactants and block copolymers, it is important that these are prepared in a proper way. Particularly for stiffer liquid crystalline phases the equilibration may be exceedingly slow (sometimes weeks or even months). One way to shorten the equilibration time is to repeatedly centrifuge samples back and forth in order to improve the mixing. Even with this procedure some cubic phases may take a few weeks to equilibrate. This has at least two direct implications. First, in situ transformations into liquid crystalline states in a drug delivery application frequently do not result in perfect liquid crystalline phases, but rather in only partially ordered ones, or in multiphase systems where one of the phases constitutes the equilibrium state. Second, if true equilibrium properties are desired in order to investigate, e.g., phase diagrams or structural aspects in such systems, care should be taken to ensure that the system is chemically stable over this time.

   Once prepared, there are several ways to investigate liquid crystalline systems in order to identify the phases and to map the phase diagram, and for investigating the microstructure of the phases formed. Below, only a couple of these methods are discussed in brief, with the aim of giving as first feeling to the type of investigations underlying the phase diagrams discussed in the present chapter.

3.7.1   X-Ray Diffraction

The most frequently used method for investigating liquid crystalline phases formed by surfactant and block copolymer systems is without doubt X-ray diffraction. Since liquid crystals possess long-range structural order, interaction with electromagnetic radiation of a suitable wavelength may result in the generation of diffraction patterns. These are characterized by constructive interference when Bragg's law is fulfilled, i.e., when

$$n\lambda = 2d \sin \Theta \tag{3.1}$$

where λ is the wavelength, Θ is the diffraction angle, d is the distance between lattice planes, and n the diffraction order ($n = 1, 2, 3, \ldots$). As done conventionally in X-ray diffraction, the "Miller indices" $h, k,$ and l denote the number of parallel planes which intersect with each unit cell axis, and are used to identify the symmetry of the liquid crystalline phase (Table 3.5).

When the composition of the sample is known together with the nature of the liquid crystalline phase, X-ray diffraction data can be used to extract information about the characteristic dimensions in the liquid crystalline structure.

3.7.2   NMR

NMR offers a range of possibilities for investigating liquid crystalline phases. Apart from the methods discussed in Chapter 2, it is particularly one which should be mentioned in the context of investigations of liquid chrystalline phases formed by surfactants and block copolymers. Thus, deuterium (^{2}H) NMR spectroscopy offers a powerful technique for investigating phase equilibria, since the occurrence of different phases can be straightforwardly identified with this method. Also, macroscopic phase separation, which in viscous liquid crystalline samples may be a very slow process, is not required. The basis for this method is that isotropic phases yield a narrow singlet resonance signal of quadrupolar nuclei such as ^{2}H, whereas anisotropic phases result in so-called quadrupolar splitting, thereby yielding a doublet resonance signal. Furthermore, anisotropic phases may

TABLE 3.5   Relation Between the First Reflections for Different Liquid Crystalline Phases

Cubic	$1:1/\sqrt{2}:1/\sqrt{3}:1/\sqrt{4}:1/\sqrt{5}:1/\sqrt{6}:1/\sqrt{8}:\ldots$
Lamellar	$1:1/2:1/3:1/4:\ldots$
Hexagonal	$1:1/\sqrt{3}:1/\sqrt{4}:1/\sqrt{7}:\ldots$

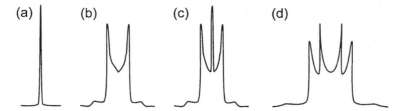

FIGURE 3.15   Typical ^{2}H-NMR spectra of (a) isotropic phases (e.g., micellar and cubic phases); (b) an anisotropic liquid crystalline phase, where the magnitude of the splitting increases with the degree of anisotropy, and therefore being larger for a lamellar phase than for a hexagonal one; (c) a two-phase sample consisting of the phases present in samples (a) and (b); and (d) a two-phase system containing two anisotropic phases (e.g., a lamellar phase and a hexagonal phase).

be separated through the magnitude of the splitting. Moreover, mixtures of several phases yield ^{2}H-NMR signals which are made up through superposition of signals the individual phases. From this, not only the nature of the phase in the case of a single-phase system, but also the composition of a multiphase systems may be determined (Figure 3.15).

3.7.3   Polarizing Microscopy

As a result of their molecular ordering, anisotropic liquid crystalline phases, such as the hexagonal, the lamellar, and the reversed hexagonal phases, are optically birefringent. This property can be used for studying such phases with polarizing microscopy. The lamellar phase usually yields mosaic patterns under the polarizing microscope, whereas the hexagonal phases normally show nongeometric textures. The occurence of crystals may also be identified by this method. On the other hand, isotropic phases (e.g., micellar and reversed micellar solutions and cubic phases) are nonbirefringent and generate a dark background when investigated under the polarizing microscope.

3.8   LIQUID CRYSTALLINE PHASES AS DRUG DELIVERY SYSTEMS

3.8.1   General Considerations

Liquid crystalline phases offer a number of useful properties for drug delivery. First, they allow drug solubilization, and with a proper choice of self-association structure, both water-soluble and oil-soluble drugs may be incorporated also in rather high concentrations. This, in turn, offers possibilities to increase the drug solubility, to decrease drug degradation, and to control and sustain the drug release rate. Second, liquid crystalline phases frequently display a rather high viscosity, which may also offer opportunities when the drug formulation needs to be localized, e.g., intramuscularly, on the skin or in the oral cavity.

Before considering specific applications of the use of liquid crystalline phases in drug delivery, however, it is helpful to consider the effect of the drug on the structures formed in liquid crystalline surfactant and block copolymer systems. In the general case, the drug may be present in the water phase, solubilized in the hydrophobic core of the aggregates, or present at the oil/water interface together with the surfactant. Depending on the preferred location of the drug, it affects the association structures differently. For example, if the drug is charged, highly water soluble, and not surface active, it behaves essentially as a salt, and hence screens electrostatic interactions in ionic surfactant systems. If the drug is hydrophobic and poorly water soluble, it may be solubilized in the interior of the surfactant aggregates, and hence act as an oil, thus promoting structures less curved toward the oil or more curved toward water.

An illustration of this is given in Figure 3.16, showing the effect of the local anesthetic drug lidocaine, present either in its base form or in the form of

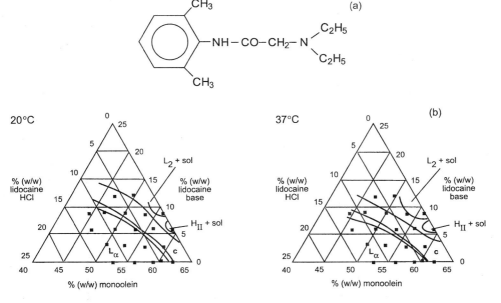

FIGURE 3.16 (a) Chemical structure of lidocaine. (b) Phase diagrams for the system lidocaine base/lidocaine-HCl/monoolein at 35% water. (Redrawn from Engström et al., Int. J. Pharm. 1992, 79, 113.)

the corresponding HCl salt, on the phases formed in the monoolein/water system. As can be seen from the chemical structure of lidocaine, this drug contains both a polar and a nonpolar domain, and is therefore surface active. Considering this, one would expect lidocaine to accumulate in the monoolein layers. Furthermore, since lidocaine base is more hydrophobic than the HCl salt form, the former has a larger tendency to distribute toward the oil in the monoolein/water system. As can be seen in Figure 3.16, lidocaine base causes a transition from a cubic phase (which is slightly curved toward water) to a reversed hexagonal and then toward a reversed micellar phase, whereas lidocaine-HCl causes a transition from the cubic phase to the lamellar phase. Thus, addition of lidocaine-HCl to the monoolein/water system results in the drug being located in the monoolein layers, where the charge of the drug molecules induces a repulsive interaction. This causes the system to maximize the distance between the charges, and hence induces a transition from the cubic phase, curved slightly toward the water, to a lamellar phase. On addition of lidocaine base, on the other hand, no charges are introduced in the monoolein layer, and hence the effect on the head group interaction is minor, at the same time as the hydrophobic volume increases. This causes a transition toward structures more curved toward water (i.e., cubic → reversed hexagonal → reversed micellar) (Figure 3.17).

Irrespective of the nature of the drug and the surfactant, the general rule is that the drug does indeed affect the phase behavior and the structures formed in surfactant systems. In the development of liquid crystalline formulations, the surfactant system should therefore be "tuned" to display the desired properties

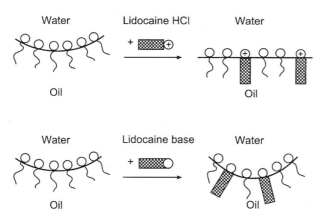

Figure 3.17 Schematic illustration of the effects of lidocaine base and lidocaine-HCl on the packing of monoolein. (Redrawn from Engström et al., Int. J. Pharm. 1992, 79, 113.)

in the presence of the drug, e.g., through varying the nature of the surfactant, the surfactant concentration, pH, or some other parameter.

Due to their frequently high viscosity and stiffness, liquid crystalline phases are often difficult to prepare and handle from a practical perspective. For example, mixing is difficult, and administration complicated (compare, e.g., intramuscular injections of thick formulations), of limited patient compliance (compare, e.g., oral administration of "gel-like" formulations) or inefficient. Therefore, the in situ transition from a low-viscous state to the required high-viscous liquid crystalline phase after administration is of major importance for the use of liquid crystalline phases for drug delivery. There are several parameters which may be used for triggering such a transition in situ after administration, including

1. Temperature (The body temperature is higher than the storage temperature.)
2. Dilution (The formulation is often in contact with excess water after administration.)
3. Salt (The physiological electrolyte concentration may be used to screen electrostatic interactions in the formulation.)
4. pH (The physiological pH at the administration site may be used to either reduce or increase electrostatic interactions in the formulation.)
5. Calcium ion concentration (Strong binding of Ca^{2+} to carboxyl groups may be used to change the electrostatic interaction in the formulation after administration.)

3.8.2 Temperature-Induced Phase Transitions

Of the transition mechanisms listed above, probably the one most extensively used in drug delivery is temperature. There are many systems which display such temperature-induced "thickening," based both on liquid crystalline phases and other systems (compare, e.g., polymer-surfactant systems; Chapter 8). An example in relation to temperature-induced formation of liquid crystalline phases is the monoolein/water system (Figure 3.18). As can be seen, the binary monoolein/water system displays a lamellar phase which may be converted to a bicontinuous cubic phase (Q) on increasing the temperature in a certain composition range. Since the cubic phase is much more viscous than the lamellar phase, there is a pronounced temperature-induced thickening of the system with increasing temperature. Although the situation becomes more complex in the presence of a drug, Figure 3.19 shows results obtained with an analogous system.

Another example of a system displaying a temperature-induced thickening is the previously discussed Pluronic F127/water system. This is also a good example on how "tuning" of the formulation may be obtained in order to meet the formulation requirements. As shown in Figure 3.14, this systems displays a dra-

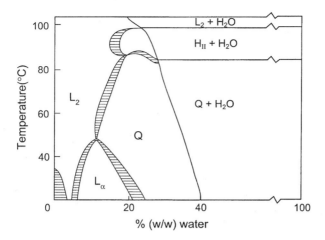

FIGURE 3.18 Binary phase diagram for the monoolein/water system. (Redrawn from Hyde et al., Z. Kristallogr. 1984, 168, 213.)

matic increase in elasticity with increasing temperature due to a transition from a micellar solution to a (partly disordered) cubic liquid crystalline phase. The transition temperature depends on the polymer concentration (Figure 3.13), but can also be controlled by adding a second PEO/PPO copolymer and varying the composition at a fixed total polymer concentration (Figure 3.20).

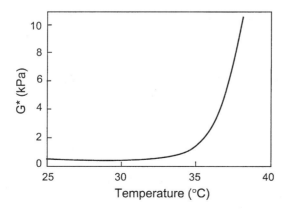

FIGURE 3.19 Complex modulus G^* versus temperature for a formulation containing 2.4 wt% lidocaine base, 2.6 wt% lidocaine-HCl, 60 wt% monoolein, and 35 wt% water. (Redrawn from Engström et al., Int. J. Pharm. 1992, 86, 137.)

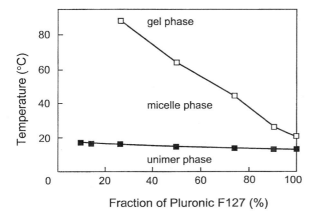

FIGURE 3.20 Transition temperature for a mixture of Pluronic F127 and Pluronic F68 as a function of composition at a fixed total copolymer concentration of 21 wt%. (Redrawn from Scherlund et al., Int. J. Pharm. 2000, 211, 37.)

Addition of a drug also affects the transition temperature. This is exemplified in Figure 3.21, showing the effect of adding a 1:1 mixture of the local anesthetic drugs lidocaine (pKa = 7.86) and prilocaine (pKa = 7.89) to a Pluronic F127/F68 mixture. At pH 5, where lidocaine/prilocaine are highly charged (pH ≪ pKa), these substances act essentially as electrolytes, and have little effect on the transition temperature. At pH > pKa, on the other hand, lidocaine/prilocaine are both uncharged and poorly water soluble, which induces a strong concentration-dependent decrease in the transition temperature.

For this particular system, the formulation composition may be controlled by the total polymer concentration, the copolymer mixture composition, the drug concentration and pH in order to meet the performance requirements of the formulation, e.g., regarding a combined effect of a suitable release rate, loading capacity, and transition temperature.

3.8.3 Dilution-Induced Phase Transitions

Another way to induce in situ formation of liquid crystalline phases in drug delivery applications is by simple dilution. Since excess water frequently surrounds the formulation after administration, there is often a dilution of the formulation. This may be used in order to achieve an in situ formation of a stiff liquid crystalline phase for drug delivery purposes. Similarly to temperature-induced transitions, dilution-induced ones are of general applicability, and could be used for a range of administration routes. Salt- or pH-dependent transitions, on the other hand, are more dependent on the site and route of administration.

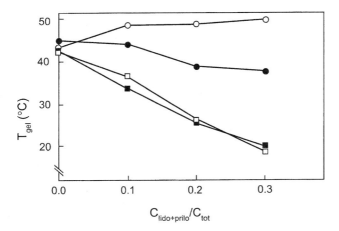

FIGURE 3.21 The effect of the concentration of lidocaine/prilocaine (1/1) on the transition temperature of a system containing 15.5 wt% Pluronic F127 and 4% Pluronic F68. The pH was 5 (open circles), 7 (filled circles), 8 (open squares), and 10 (filled squares). (Redrawn from Scherlund et al., Int. J. Pharm. 2000, 194, 103.)

Going back to the monoolein/water system (Figure 3.18), we see that this system offers an opportunity for such a dilution-induced transition. Thus, at low water content this system forms a reversed micellar phase. On dilution with water, on the other hand, this is transformed to a cubic phase via a lamellar phase. Given the high stiffness of the cubic phase, the system thus undergoes a dramatic thickening simply by dilution with water. Furthermore, the cubic phase is in equilibrium with excess water, which means that it does not dissolve by continued exposure to water, therefore making it interesting for controlled release or depot formulations.

Also Pluronic-based systems display such dilution-induced transitions to form stiff liquid crystalline phases after administration. For example, Figure 3.22 shows the partial phase behavior of a formulation containing Pluronic F68, a medium-chain (C_8) oil (Akoline MCM), water, and a 1:1 mixture of lidocaine and prilocaine. Note that the phase diagram is a pseudo-three-component phase diagram since the oil phase actually consists of three components, since salt is present in the system in order to controll pH, and since both the Akoline MCM and the Pluronic F68 are polydisperse and heterogenous chemicals, each containing a number of different fractions. The interpretation of the phase behavior is therefore not entirely straightforward. Nevertheless, from the phase diagram it seems that a dilution-induced thickening transition can be obtained by starting at the low-viscous intermediate phase (*), which according to the phase diagram

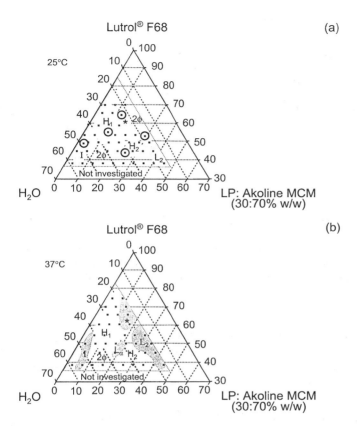

FIGURE 3.22 Phase diagram for the Pluronic F68/water/Akoline MCM/lidocaine (l)-prilocaine (p) system. (Redrawn from Scherlund et al., Eur. J. Pharm. Sci. 2001, 14, 53.)

should turn into a hexagonal phase, then a cubic phase, and finally a micellar solution.

Indeed, such a transition can be inferred also from a dramatic thickening of the system on addition of even small amounts of water, by an initial occurence of optical birefringence after water addition, and a final dissapearance of the birefringence and a complete dissolution of the sample at longer times in excess water (Figure 3.23).

As will be discussed more extensively in Chapter 5, also dilution-induced transitions not involving liquid crystalline phases have found applications in drug delivery. Probably the most prominent example of this is the Sandimmune formu-

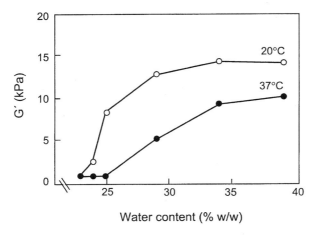

FIGURE 3.23 The elastic modulus G' as a function of water content for a formulation with an initial composition of Pluronic F68/water/LP/Akoline MCM of 64/23/3.9/9.1. (Redrawn from Scherlund et al., Eur. J. Pharm. Sci. 2001, 14, 53.)

lation used for cyclosporine. This is based on a reversed micellar solution, which can be filled in gelatin capsules, and which on exposure to excess water switches into a normal micellar solution (or an o/w microemulsion) with cyclosporine solubilized in the micelles.

3.8.4 Use of Liquid Crystalline Phases in Drug Delivery

The solubilization of drugs in liquid crystalline phases offers advantages analogous to those obtained through solubilization in micellar systems. As with micellar solutions, the release rate from a formulation containing a drug solubilized in a liquid crystalline phase depends strongly on the localization of the drug molecules in the self-assembled structure, i.e., on whether it is localized in the hydrophobic domain(s), the aqueous domain(s), or the surfactant layer. For liquid crystalline phases curved toward the oil (e.g., discrete cubic or hexagonal phases), an increased drug partitioning to the hydrophobic domain(s), achieved, e.g., through hydrophobic modifications of the drug, results in a decreased release rate (Figure 3.24). For oil-continuous systems, on the other hand, the reverse occurs.

A notable feature of many liquid crystalline phases is their ability to incorporate rather large amounts of of molecules spanning from very hydrophilic to very hydrophobic, and from very small to very large. As an illustration of this, Table 3.6 shows a number of substances which have been successfully incorporated in the cubic liquid crystalline phase formed in the monoolein/water system.

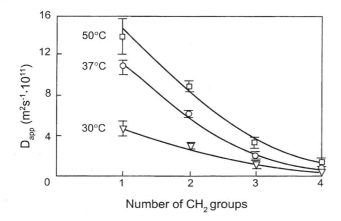

FIGURE 3.24 Apparent diffusion coefficient D_{app} of p-hydroxybenzoate esters from a 25% Pluronic F127 gel as a function of ester chain length at different temperatures. (Redrawn from Gilbert et al., Int. J. Pharm. 1986, 37, 223.)

Liquid crystalline phases are of interest also from the point of view of absence of "drug" release. This is the case, e.g., for certain potent enzymes, which, if not effectively immobilized, could result in detrimental side effects. Although the incorporation of such pharmaceutically potent proteins in liquid crystalline phases has not been studied in any detail yet, it is interesting to note that such liquid crystalline systems have the capacity of solubilizing proteins. Examples of proteins which have been successfully incorporated into (cubic) liquid crystalline phases include lysozyme, α-lactalbumin, bovine serum albu-

TABLE 3.6 Substances Successfully Incorporated into the Cubic Liquid Crystalline Phase Formed in the Monoolein/Water System

Compound	M_w	wt%
Sodium chloride	58	0.9
Lidocaine	270	5
Gramicidin	1141	6
Desmopressin	1069	4
Insulin	6000	4
Bovine serum albumin	67000	18

Source: From Engström, Lipid Technol. 1990, 2, 42.

min, pepsin, α-chymotrypsin, cytochrome *c*, glucose oxidase, lactate oxidase, urease, and creatinine deiminase. Liquid crystalline phases should therefore have potential in this context.

Apart from an effectively enhanced solubility of sparingly soluble drugs and the resulting sustained and controlled release of the drug after administration, a reason for seeking solubilizing drugs into liquid crystalline phases is to improve their chemical stability. The protective properties of these systems make them interesting, e.g., for oral administration of substances sensitive to acid-catalyzed hydrolysis, or in oral administration of protein and peptide drugs, which without such protection have only a very limited bioavailability, primarily due to their proteolytic degradation. For the latter type of systems care must be taken to ensure that the surfactants or block copolymers used in the liquid crystalline system do not cause any detrimental activity loss of the peptide/protein due to conformational changes caused by surfactant binding (Chapter 8).

3.9 LIQUID CRYSTALLINE PHASES IN DRUG DELIVERY APPLICATIONS

3.9.1 Administration to the Oral Cavity

Administration of drugs to the oral cavity poses a challenge for several reasons. For example, a localized effect is generally desired, e.g., when anesthetizing the region closest to a particular tooth or preventing periodontal disease in a particular tooth pocket. Often, the localization needs to take place in a confined space, e.g., between teeth or in a periodontal pocket. Furthermore, the formulation is often exposed to considerable mechanical stress through masticatory movements, which tend to preclude the precise localization of a drug formulation for a prolonged time. Also, the localization is precluded through the abundant mucus production in the oral cavity, which makes bioadhesion more difficult. These requirements suggest that low-viscous systems which can be easily injected, e.g., by a syringe, and subsequently undergo a thickening transition and thereby become effectively localized in a given region within the oral cavity, should be of interest for drug delivery to the oral cavity.

An example of an approach based on this principle is given in Figure 3.25 for an in situ–thickening formulation containing Pluronic F127/Pluronic F68 and lidocaine/prilocaine intended for local anesthetics in the oral cavity in relation to scaling procedures. Apart from the requirements mentioned above, such a formulation should also have a fast onset and long-term stability properties. As discussed above, this system undergoes a transition from a low-viscous micellar state to a stiff (partly disordered) liquid crystalline phase on increasing the temperature. Through varying the polymer composition, concentration and pH, a temperature responsive formulation of a 1 : 1 mixture of lidocaine and prilocaine

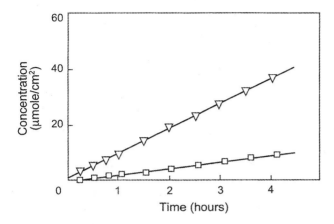

FIGURE 3.25 Release curves for a block copolymer formulation containing lidocaine/prilocaine, Pluronic F68, and Pluronic F127 (triangles) and a commercially available bench mark formulation EMLA® cream; (squares). (Redrawn from Scherlund et al., Int. J. Pharm. 2000, 194, 103.)

mixture with excellent drug release rate and long-term stability could be obtained. As shown in Figure 3.25, the release rate for block copolymer system is significantly higher than that of a benchmark emulsion formulation, which is parallelled by a faster onset for this formulation.

Also, liquid crystalline phase formulations have been used for administration to the oral cavity for treatment of periodontal disease. Although this indication is slightly different from that of local anesthetics, the requirements on the formulation properties are comparable, and consequently liquid crystalline formulations are of interest. In particular, formulations consisting of monoolein, sesame oil, and metronidazole benzoate have been investigated in this context. By administering such systems as suspensions, which transform into either a cubic or a reversed hexagonal phase on water uptake, the excess water present in the oral cavity can be used in order to trigger a transition from relatively low viscous, and hence easily administered initial formulation, into the stiffer cubic and reversed hexagonal phases in situ. In particular, the reversed hexagonal phase displays favorable sustained release properties (Figure 3.26).

3.9.2 Administration to the Skin

As will be discussed more in Chapters 4 and 5, the protective properties of the stratum corneum frequently result in a low drug bioavailability following topical administration. Therefore, drug delivery systems for application to the skin fre-

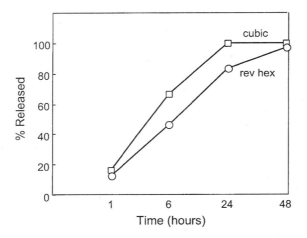

FIGURE 3.26 Release of metronidazole benzoate from the cubic (squares) and reversed hexagonal (circles) phase. (Redrawn from Norling et al., J. Clin. Periodontol. 1992, 687, 19.)

quently aim at improving the drug transport over the stratum corneum. Sometimes such formulations are based on so-called penetration enhancers, whereas in others, they are based on surfactant systems, e.g., in the form of liposomes and microemulsions. In yet other occasions, an increased penetration is not necessarily aimed for, but instead a localized effect on the skin or a skin protective effect is sought.

Irrespective of the purpose of a surfactant-based formulation in topical drug delivery, however, it is important to note that the formulation composition, and hence also its structure, changes after application to the skin due to differentiated evaporation of the formulation components. More precisely, the amount of the more volative components (e.g., water) is gradually reduced after administration. This has implications for both the drug penetration and skin irritation. For example, if the formulation after evaporation consists of a (reversed) microemulsion structure, solubilization of lipid biomembranes can be substantial, which may lead to good skin penetration of the drug but may also cause skin irritation. If, on the other hand, the remaining system is a lamellar liquid crystalline phase, skin irritation is less likely, but the drug uptake may be less efficient. In any case, a controlled dermal application of such formulations requires knowledge of the phase behavior of the system, and of the effects of evaporation on the structures formed.

An area where the protective effects of temperture-thickening systems has been found to be of some interest is wound dressings in the treatment of thermal burns. There are several properties such formulations should fulfill:

1. Application should be uncomplicated.
2. The dressing should adhere to the uninjured skin surrounding the wound and be strong enough to resist mechanical damage such as lifting and slipping, but also come off easily when removed.
3. Since small areas of nonadherence leads to fluid-filled pockets where bacteria may proliferate, the adherence should be uniform.
4. Large amounts of fluid are lost through evaporation and exudation in burn wounds, which results in body temperature fall as well as in metabolic disturbances. For this reason, but also since this assists epithelization, dressings should absorb fluid and maintain a high humidity at the wound.
5. Wound dressings should also provide a bacterial barrier, which could be achieved either by the dressing itself or by the inclusion of antibacterial agents, the release of which should preferably be sustained.

A number of different types of dressings have been investigated for this purpose, including preformed polymer films, spray-on films, gels, foams, and composites. Due to their reversed thermoreversible thickening, with consequent straightforward application and removal, their solubilization capacity, and their high water content, PEO/PPO block copolymer systems have also been investigated in this context. In particular, Pluronic F127 has been found to display some attractive features as carrier for bacteriocidal silver nitrate and silver lactate. For example, Figure 3.27 shows results obtained after full thickness thermal burns in rats, and as can be seen the mortality rate after treatment with the Pluronic

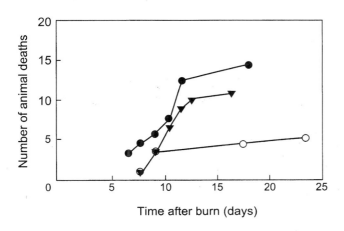

FIGURE 3.27 Mortality after full thickness skin thermal burns in rats for Pluronic F127 + silver nitrate (open circles), Pluronic F127 (filled triangles), and control (filled circles). (Redrawn from Nalbandian et al., J. Biomed. Mater. Res. 1972, 6, 583.)

F127 formulations containing the bacteriocidal components is much lower than that in the control group. The dressings have been found to be efficient against both *Pseudomonas aeruginosa* and *Proteus mirabilis*. The Pluronic F127-based dressings have therefore been proposed as artificial skin against electrolyte imbalances, heat loss, and bacterial invasion.

3.9.3 Parenteral Administration

Injectable in situ thickening formulations are interesting also for parenteral administration, e.g., in the form of intramuscular or subcutaneous depot formulations with the aim of achieving controlled drug release over a prolonged time. Also in this context, formulations based on liquid crystalline phases offer some possibilities. For example, antitumor treatment using IL-2 has shown positive results for several cancers in both experimental animal models and in humans. Unfortunately, the use of high-dose IL-2 therapy is precluded due to the toxicity associated with it. However, the antitumor effect of IL-2 has been found to be correlated to the time IL-2 remains in the serum rather than with the peak serum IL-2 concentration. Therefore, a sustained release formulation of IL-2 could be expected to allow a high therapeutic efficiency and at the same time result in reduced toxic side effects. Indeed, Pluronic F127/water formulations displaying in situ thickening after intramuscular administration have been found to result in a reduced peak serum IL-2 concentration and in a longer circulation of IL-2 than the corresponding aqueous IL-2 solution (Figure 3.28). Such formulations are therefore interesting for IL-2 intramuscular therapy.

3.9.4 Rectal Administration

Another application area for systems displaying in situ thickening, such as liquid crystalline phases formed by PEO/PPO block copolymers, is rectal administration. As an example of this, Figure 3.29 shows results on the rectal administration of indomethacin, the usefulness of which is severely reduced by gastrointestinal side effects. Although the bioavailability of the Pluronic F127–based formulation, as determined from the integration of the plasma concentration over time, is comparable to that of suppositories, the Pluronic F127–based formulation offers several advantages:

1. For the suppository there is a pronounced peak in the plasma concentration after less than 1 hour. Since high peak plasma concentrations are associated with indomethacin side effects, e.g., on the nervous system, and since the the Pluronic F127 formulation displays no such peak plasma concentration, side effects should be reduced for the latter.

2. Histopathological investigation have shown that damage to the mucosal membrane by the copolymer rarely occurs in the rectum.

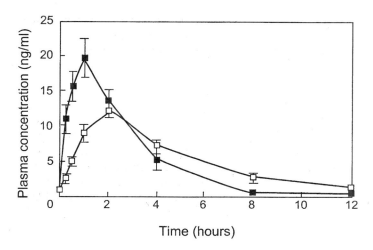

FIGURE 3.28 Plasma IL-2 concentration following intramuscular injection in rats of an aqueous IL-2 solution (filled symbols) and an IL-2/Pluronic F127/water formulation (open symbols). (Redrawn from Wang et al., Int. J. Pharm. 1995, 113, 73.)

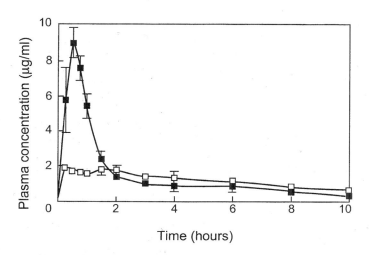

FIGURE 3.29 Plasma concentration of indomethacin after rectal administration to rabbits from a suppository (filled symbols) and a Pluronic F127/water formulation (open symbols). (Redrawn from Miyazaki et al., Chem. Pharm. Bull. 1986, 34, 1801.)

3. Individual differences following rectal administration of the gel formulation are smaller than those for the other formulation.
4. Solubilization of indomethacin results in a decreased hydrolysis rate of this substance.

3.9.5 Nasal Administration

Nasal administration offers several advantages in drug delivery, such as avoidance of first-pass effects, fast absorption, and a way within protein and peptide drug delivery to avoid poor bioavailability through proteolytic degradation in the gastrointestinal tract. Similar to the oral cavity, however, bioadhesion is desired, and in situ thickening a way to achieve an increased drug formulation efficiency. Given this, liquid crystalline phases forming in situ are interesting for nasal drug delivery.

BIBLIOGRAPHY

Alexandridis, P., B. Lindman (eds.), Amphiphilic Block Copolymers. Self-Assembly and Applications, Elsevier, Amsterdam, 2000.

Engström, S., L. Engström, Phase behavior of the lidocaine-monoolein-water system, Int. J. Pharm. 79:113–122 (1992).

Engström, S., L. Lindahl, R. Wallin, J. Engblom, A study of polar lipid drug carrier systems undergoing a thermoreversible lamellar-to-cubic phase transition, Int. J. Pharm. 86:137–145 (1992).

Evans, D. F., H. Wennerström, The Colloidal Domain, Wiley, New York, 1999.

Ganem-Quintanar, A., D. Quintanar-Guerrero, B. Buri, Monoolein: a review of the pharmaceutical applications, Drug Dev. Ind. Pharm. 26:809–820 (2000).

Glatter, O., O. Kratky, Small-Angle X-Ray Scattering, Academic Press, London, 1982.

Israelachvili, J., Intermolecular and Surface Forces, Academic Press, London, 1992.

Jönsson, B., B. Lindman, K. Holmberg, B. Kronberg, Surfactants and Polymers in Aqueous Solution, Wiley, New York, 1998.

Laughlin, R. G., The Aqueous Phase Behavior of Surfactants, Academic Press, 1994.

Lucassen-Reynders E. H., ed., Anionic Surfactants. Physical Chemistry of Surfactant Action, Surfactant Science Series, vol. 11, Marcel Dekker, New York, 1981.

Schick, M. J., ed., Nonionic Surfactants. Physical Chemistry, Surfactant Science Series, vol. 23, Marcel Dekker, New York, 1987.

Schmolka, I. R., in P. J. Tarcha (ed.), Polymers for Controlled Drug Delivery, CRC Press, Boca Raton, 1991.

Seddon, J. M., Structure of the inverted hexagonal (H_{II}) phase, and non-lamellar phase transitions of lipids, Biochim. Biophys. Acta 1031:1–69 (1990).

Zana, R., ed., Surfactant Solutions: New Methods of Investigation, Surfactant Science Series, vol. 22, Marcel Dekker, New York, 1987.

4

Liposomes

Liposomes or vesicles have ever since their discovery attracted scientists in the field of physical chemistry, biophysics, and biochemistry, not the least due to their structural similarity to phospholipid membranes in living cells (Figure 4.1). Also in the context of drug delivery, liposomes have attracted considerable attention due to their capacity to solubilize oil-soluble substances and to encapsulate water-soluble drugs. Although liposomes may be formed by a range of different surfactants and block copolymers, and although some interest in the context of drug delivery has been placed on liposomes formed by nonionic surfactants ("niosomes"), liposomes formed by phospholipids have attracted most interest and found most widespread use in drug delivery applications.

4.1 PREPARATION AND PROPERTIES OF LIPOSOME SYSTEMS

The structure of liposomes can differ widely depending on both composition and process conditions. In particular, the size of the liposomes generated can range from very small to considerable. They may also contain either one or several bilayer structures. This structural diversity has resulted also in a plethora of names for different types of liposomes. Some of the names found in the literature on the topic are provided in Table 4.1.

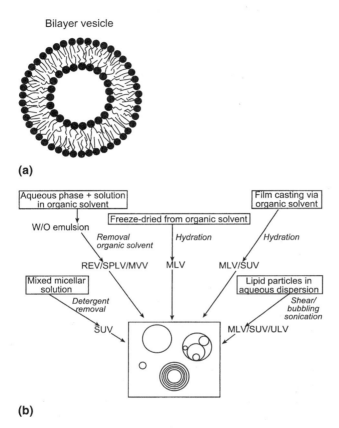

(a)

(b)

FIGURE 4.1   Schematic illustration of (a) the structure of a unilamellar liposome, and (b) some commonly used preparation methods for liposomes. [Redrawn from Israelachvili, Intermolecular and Surface Forces, Academic Press, 1992 (a), and Crommelin et al., in Kreuter, ed., Colloidal Drug Delivery Systems, Marcel Dekker, 1994 (b).]

There are a numbers of techniques which can be used for generation of liposomal systems (Figure 4.1). Different preparation techniques yield different liposome type and size, and depending on, e.g., the stability requirements or the administration route, a particular preparation method may therefore be required or preferred. Once prepared, there are several properties which are of interest and importance for liposomal systems. In particular, the stability of liposomes toward aggregation and fusion is of major importance, as is the leakage rate of solubilized or encapsulated drugs.

TABLE 4.1 Nomenclature of Liposomes

Based on liposome structure	
MLV	Multilamellar large vesicles (>0.5 μm)
OLV	Oligolamellar vesicles (0.1–1 μm)
UV	Unilamellar vesicles (all sizes)
SUV	Small unilamellar vesicles (20–100 nm)
MUV	Medium-sized unilamellar vesicles
LUV	Large unilamellar vesicles (>100 nm)
GUV	Giant unilamellar vesicles (>1 μm)
MVV	Multivesicular vesicles (usually >1 μm)
Based on preparation method	
REV	Vesicles prepared by reverse-phase evaporation
MLV-REV	Multilamellar vesicles prepared by reverse-phase evaporation
SPLV	Stable plurilamellar vesicles
FATMLV	Frozen and thawed MLV
VET	Vesicles prepared by extrusion
FPV	Vesicles prepared by French press
FUV	Vesicles prepared by fusion
DRS	Vesicles prepared by dehydration-rehydration
BSV	Bubblesomes

Source: From Crommelin et al., in Kreuter, ed., Colloidal Drug Delivery Systems, Marcel Dekker, 1994.

Depending on the nature of the polar head group, phoshoplipid liposomes may be either charged or uncharged. For charged liposomes, the colloidal stability is determined largely by the magnitude and range of electrostatic interactions, as discussed in some detail in relation to polymer particles in Chapter 9. Also for zwitterionic phospolipids with a zero net charge, such as phosphatidylcholine (PC) and phosphatidylethanolamine (PE), phospholipid liposomes repel each other, thereby providing colloidal stability to such systems. The origin of this repulsive interaction between liposome bilayers, and between phospholipid lamellae in lamellar liquid crystalline phases, is thermal fluctuations in the membranes and hydration interactions (Figure 4.2).

The simplest type of thermal fluctuations are the so-called protrusions, i.e., molecular motions of individual surfactant or phospholipid molecules normal to the plane of the membrane. If two such membranes approach each other to distances close enough so that the individual protrusions are precluded, this generates a repulsive interaction, which is analogous to the steric or osmotic effect in polymer systems. Apart from these individual molecular motions, there are also

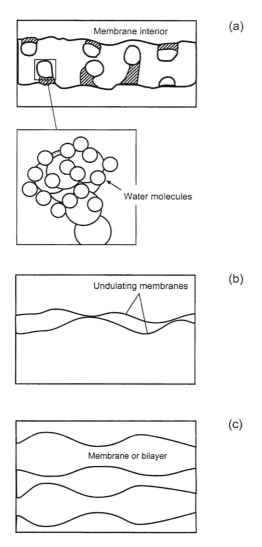

Figure 4.2 Schematic illustration of (a) molecular protrusions, (b) undulations, and (c) peristaltic fluctuations in surfactant or phospholipid bilayers. (Redrawn from Israelachvili, Intermolecular and Surface Forces, Academic Press, 1992.)

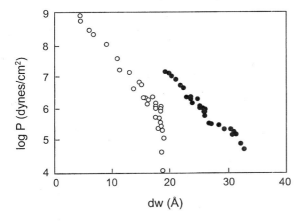

FIGURE 4.3 Effect of chain melting on the hydration repulsion. Results are shown for dipalmitoyldiphosphatidylcholine (DPPC) at 50°C (filled circles) and 25°C (open circles), which is above and below the melting transition for this system (41°C), respectively. (Redrawn from Rand et al., Biochim. Biophys. Acta 1989, 988, 351.)

collective fluctuations, relating to bending fluctuations and area variation variations of the surfactant or phospholipid bilayer. Again, a repulsive interaction is generated when these fluctuations are precluded due to the proximity of a second bilayer/liposome.

Protrusions, undulations, and peristaltic fluctuations are all facilitated by an increased ''membrane fluidity.'' Consequently, the repulsive interaction between zwitterionic lipid bilayers is stronger and more long range above the chain melting temperature (Figure 4.3).

With increasing temperature, there is also a decrease in the surface shear viscosity as a result of the increased ''fluidization'' of the lipid membrane. Interestingly, the major decrease occurs around the pretransition, whereas at the chain melting transition, the surface shear viscosity is already quite low (Figure 4.4).

With increasing temperature, there is also a monotonous increase in the vesicle surface area. Addition of cholesterol reduces the area change at the main transition and broadens the temperature range over which the transition occurs. The net effect is that, even at temperatures well below the chain melting temperature in the absence of cholesterol, the bilayer is still in a liquidlike state in the presence of high concentrations of cholesterol (Figure 4.5).

Addition of cholesterol also affects the membrane elasticity. Specifically, increasing the cholesterol content in a lipid membrane results in an increased elastic modulus of the membrane. Thus, despite cholesterol making lipid bilayers

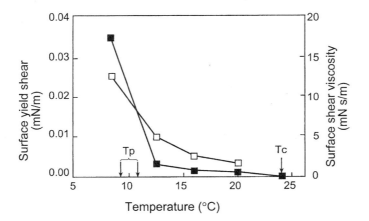

FIGURE 4.4 Effect of temperature on the surface shear viscosity (open symbols) and the surface yield shear (filled symbols) derived from micropipet aspiration of dimyristoyldiphosphatidylcholine (DMPC) vesicles below the main transition T_c and pretransition T_p temperature. (Redrawn from Evans et al., J. Phys. Chem. 1987, 91, 4219.)

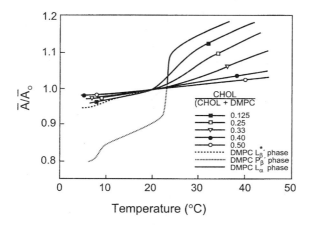

FIGURE 4.5 Relative area A/A_0 vs. temperature for DMPC/cholesterol mixtures. Liposome areas are normalized with the liposome area at 20°C. The structure of the L_α, L_β', and P_β' phases is shown in Figure 4.12c. (Redrawn from Needham et al., Biochemistry 1988, 27, 4668.)

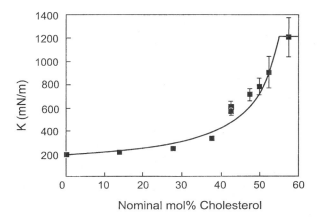

FIGURE 4.6 Elastic area expansion modulus K vs. cholesterol concentration for stearoyloleoylphosphatidylcholine (SOPC)/cholesterol mixtures. (Redrawn from Needham et al., Biophys. J. 1990, 58, 997.)

increasingly fluid by reducing the melting transition, the membrane elasticity increases simultaneously (Figure 4.6).

Within drug delivery, it is sometimes desirable to modify the surface properties of liposomes. For example, in analogy to other types of charged colloids, liposomes may be destabilized at high elecrolyte concentrations. As will be discussed further below, this might be advantageous in some applications. For pH-sensitive liposomes in gene therapy, for example, such a stabilization-destabilization transition is desired. In other contexts, however, such destabilization behavior is less advantageous.

Also, in applications where liposomes are administered intravenously, the adsorption of serum proteins is of major importance. As discussed below, adsorption of certain serum proteins (opsonins) at the liposome surface causes the liposome bloodstream circulation time to decrease, and results in problems with both poor drug bioavailability and the occurrence of dose-limiting side effects. In such cases liposomes may be surface modified by PEG-containing lipids in order to reduce the serum protein adsorption (Figure 4.7).

With an increasing PEO (or PEG) chain density, the protein adsorption at such liposomes decreases as a result of a repulsive osmotic interaction, and masking of attractive protein-liposome interactions. As will be discussed in some detail below, a decreased serum protein adsorption results in a prolonged bloodstream circulation, in a more even tissue distribution of drugs administered intravenously through colloidal drug carriers, and in a number of positive effects originating from this. An additional benefit with PEO-modified liposomes is that the interac-

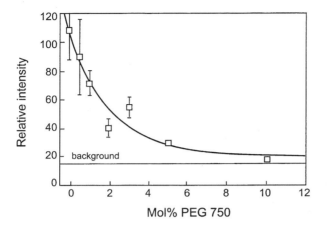

FIGURE 4.7   Dependence of the binding of avidin at liposomes (higher intensity means higher degree of binding) containing 5 mol% biotin incorporated in the vesicle membrane as a function of the concentration of PE-PEO$_{750}$. (Redrawn from Needham et al., in Janoff, ed., Liposomes: Rational Design, Marcel Dekker, 1998.)

tion between the liposomes is nonelectrostatic. This, in turn, makes the liposome stability against flocculation largely independent of both pH and electrolyte concentration.

In the context of serum protein adsorption it can also be noted that incorporation of cholesterol in liposome membranes results in a decrease in the serum protein adsorption. Although the mechanism behind the effects is not entirely clear at present, an increased hydration repulsion with increasing concentrations of cholesterol seems a plausible origin of this. Irrespective of the mechanism of the reduced serum protein adsorption, however, it results in a prolonged bloodstream circulation time (Figure 4.8).

4.2   SOLUBILIZATION AND RELEASE FROM LIPOSOMES

One of the most interesting properties of liposomes is their capacity to incorporate both water-soluble and oil-soluble substances. The incorporation of oil-soluble substances in liposomes is rather similar to that in micellar solutions, liquid crystalline phases, or microemulsion systems. Incorporation of water-soluble drugs and other substances in the inner liposome water compartment, on the other hand, is slightly more complex, and affects the liposome preparation process. After incorporation, nonentrapped drugs are removed, e.g., by ultrafiltration or chromatography. The capture efficiency of liposomal systems depends on a number of factors. For example, smaller liposomes contain a smaller inner volume, and

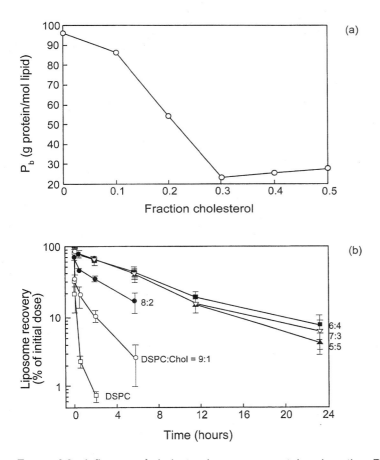

FIGURE 4.8 Influence of cholesterol on serum protein adsorption P_b (a) and the plasma clearance time (b) of distearolyphosphatidylcholine (DSPC) liposomes. In (b), results are shown for a DSPC in the absence of cholesterol (open squares), as well as for mixed liposomes consisting of a DSPC/cholesterol ratio of 9/1 (open circles), 8/2 (filled circles), 7/3 (open triangles), 6/4 (filled squares), and 5/5 (filled triangles). (Redrawn from Semple et al., Biochemistry 1996, 35, 2521.)

hence their capture efficiency is poorer than that of larger liposomes. Also, multi-lamellar liposomes are less efficient in their capture of water-soluble, non-membrane interacting, substances than unilamellar ones.

Liposomes may also be loaded after their formation, which is usually referred to as active liposome loading. The simplest driving force for such loading is through a drug concentration gradient generated by addition of the drug to a preformed liposome dispersion. The higher the drug concentration on the outside of the liposomes, the higher the concentration gradient, and the stronger the driving force for drug transfer from the outer to the inner side of the liposomes. Hence the loading kinetics and efficiency increases with concentration for water-soluble, non-membrane interacting, substances. Another approach is to use a pH gradient, by which a strong gradient may be achieved without the need for high drug concentrations. One such approach, the so-called ammonium sulfate technique, is shown in Figure 4.9. Thus, as NH_3 passes through the membrane from the inside to the outside, the pH drops on the inner side of the liposome mebrane. This, in turn, results in an ionization of the drug (which should be a weak base), and hence there is a gradient for drug transport over the membrane.

The release of drugs solubilized or incorporated in liposomes may be controlled in a number of ways. As discussed in Chapters 2 and 3, the release of encapsulated and solubilized drugs can be controlled by the drug structure and charge, where the latter can be controlled by pH and the salt concentration. However, the structure of the carrier system also strongly affects the drug release rate. For liposomes, a number of alternative approaches for controlling the drug release rate based on the properties of liposomes have been employed:

1. Release controlled by the composition of the lipid bilayers. For example, bilayers in the gel state or bilayers containing high levels of cholesterol are less permeable in general, and therefore result in a slower drug release.

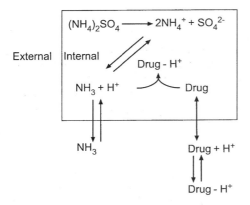

FIGURE 4.9 Schematic illustration of how an ammonium gradient can induce a pH gradient and promote loading of weak bases in liposomes. (From Crommelin et al., in Kreuter, ed., Colloidal Drug Delivery Systems, Marcel Dekker, 1994.)

2. Release controlled by pH. For example, decharging of the liposomes may result in flocculation, which in turn may result in an increased drug release rate.
3. Release induced by removal of bilayer components. For example, delipidated albumin can destabilize liposomes by competition for liposome components necessary for liposome stability.
4. Release induced by complement. For example, liposome-induced generation of the complement component(s) C5-9, the ''membrane-attack complex,'' may cause lysis of the liposomes similar to cell lysis.

Due to the two latter mechanisms, but also others related to the interaction between liposomes and serum proteins, the release of encapsulated material from liposomes is generally significantly higher in serum than in, e.g., buffer solution (Figure 4.10).

4.3 METHODS FOR INVESTIGATING LIPOSOME SYSTEMS

A number of methods discussed in Chapters 2, 3, and 9, such as different scattering techniques and NMR, are quite useful also for liposome systems. Apart from these, there are also a few techniques which may provide further information about the liposome system, and which may help understanding and control the use of liposomes in drug delivery.

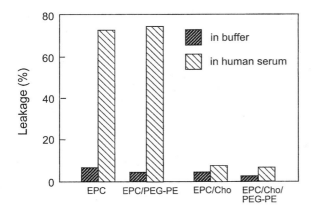

FIGURE 4.10 Comparison of the leakage of propidium from liposomes in buffer and in human serum for a number of different liposome compositions. EPC = egg phosphatidylcholine, PEG-PE = poly(ethylene glycol)-phosphatidylethanolamine, Cho = cholesterol. (Redrawn from Silvander et al. Chem. Phys. Lipids 1998, 97, 15.)

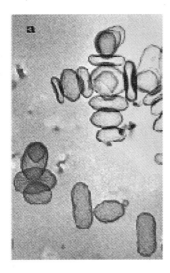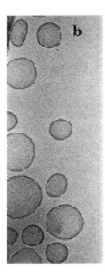

FIGURE 4.11   Cryo-TEM images of liposomes formed by DSPC/cholesterol without (a) and with (b) 5% PEO_{2000}-DSPE. (Redrawn from Edwards et al., Biophys. J. 1997, 73, 258.)

4.3.1   Cryo-TEM

Cryogenic transition electron microscopy (cryo-TEM) is an interesting method for investigating and visualizing not only liposomes but also micelles, micro-emulsions, emulsions, and liquid crystalline phases. Through use of samples prepared in thin films formed in a grid through vitrification, this method allows such systems to be investigated without any staining, gold coating, and the like. With cryo-TEM the liposome structure in terms of size and number of layers can be directly obtained. As an illustration of this, Figure 4.11 shows liposomes formed by DSPC and cholesterol. As can be seen, the liposomes are unilamellar. Furthermore, they are not entirely spherical, but rather elongated. On addition of PEO_{2000}-DSPE, on the other hand, the liposomes are seen to become more spherical, which most likely is due to the higher repulsion between the PEO chains in the flat regions than in the highly curved ones.

4.3.2   Differential Scanning Calorimetry

Calorimetry offers a direct way to observe self-assembly and phase transitions in surfactant systems. Of particular interest to studies of liposomes is probably differential scanning calorimetry (DSC), in which the heat generated in a system is followed with temperature. Through comparison between the sample and a

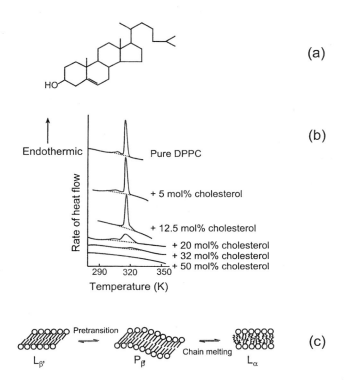

FIGURE 4.12 (a) Chemical structure of cholesterol. (b) DSC scans for DPPC liposomes as a function of the cholesterol content. (c) Schematic illustration of the
pretransition and the melting transition. (Redrawn from Ladbroke et al., Biochim.
Biophys. Acta 1968, 150, 333.)

reference system, melting and other transitions in liposome systems may be monitored. As an illustration of this, Figure 4.12 shows DSC scans for DPPC liposomes. For pure DPPC, two transitions are observed, the first of which (the pretransition) corresponding to a disordering of the lipid membranes in the absence
of chain melting, whereas the second one is very pronounced and corresponds
to chain melting. On addition of cholesterol, the pretransition decreases and the
main melting transition is reduced. The origin of this effect is that cholesterol
distributes toward the lipid membrane, and induces disordering there.

4.3.3 Drug Release

The release of a component encapsulated in liposomes offers rather sensitive and
highly relevant information relating to the permeability of the lipid bilayers,

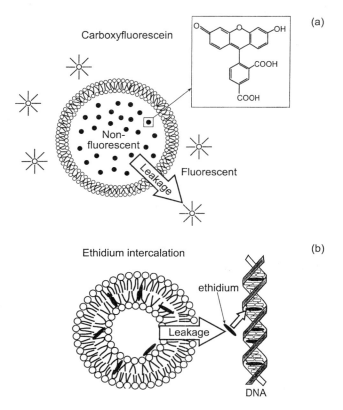

FIGURE 4.13   Schematic illustration of the use of (a) carboxyfluorescein and (b) ethidium for probing release from liposomes.

which in turn can be coupled to structural parameters in liposome systems. Two frequently used methods for studying leakage are based on carboxyfluorescein self-quenching and ethidium intercalation with DNA, respectively (Figure 4.13). Carboxyfluorescein is highly soluble in water and may readily be localized to the inner aqueous compartment of liposomes at the same time as external carboxyfluorescein is effectively removed. At high concentration, the fluorescence of carboxyfluorescein is reduced due to self-quenching, and hence solutions containing liposomes with (moderate to high amounts) encapsulated carboxyfluorescein display very low fluorescence. Carboxyfluorescein molecules which penetrate the lipid bilayer(s), on the other hand, experience a limited quenching due to their low concentration outside the liposomes, and therefore fluoresce. Therefore, the release of carboxyfluorescein from liposomes can be straightforwardly followed simply by monitoring the fluorescence intensity of liposomal systems containing carboxyfluorescein. At the end of such experiments, the liposomes are destroyed through addition of a micelle-forming surfactant, which results in a release of all carboxyfluorescein, thus allowing ''100% release'' to be identified and thereby also allowing translation from the fluorescence intensity curve to a percent released curve.

Ethidium, on the other hand, is a hydrophobic substance, which is incorporated in the lipid membrane(s) of liposomes, and which results in fluorescence upon intercalation with DNA (Figure 4.13b). If ethidium is incorporated in liposomes and DNA is added to the aqueous continuum surrounding the liposomes, the fluorescence intensity will increase over time as a result of ethidium release from the liposomes and following intercalation.

As an illustration of other types of leakage studies in liposome systems, Figure 4.14 shows the release rate as a function of temperature. As can be seen, the release of Na$^+$ is promoted as the temperature is increased to approach the

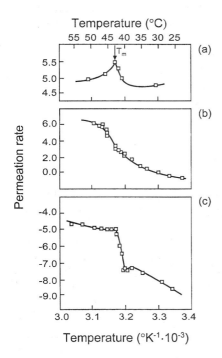

FIGURE 4.14 Temperature-dependent permeation of Na$^+$ (a), water (b), and H$^+$/OH$^-$ (c) over DPPC bilayers. T_m indicates the transition temperature for this phospholipid system. (Redrawn from Deamer et al., Chem. Phys. Lipids 1986, 40, 167.)

melting transition, which clearly illustrates the importance of the chain melting for the release of encapsulated material. Note, however, that the effect of temperature on membrane permeability is rather complex, as illustrated by the large difference in temperature-dependent release of Na^+, water, and H^+/OH:

4.3.4 Fluorescence Spectroscopy

Apart from different types of release methods, fluorescence spectroscopy can yield valuable information about liposome systems also in other ways, including aggregation numbers and estimates of lifetimes of individual lipid molecules in a liposome. Fluorescence spectroscopy can also yield information about the localization of a solubilized molecule., e.g., in a lipid membrane in a liposome. This can be achieved by measuring the fluorescence anisotropy, where a larger value of the anisotropy indicates a larger degree of orientation, e.g., as a result of a preferential localization close to the lipid-water interface.

For example, 1,6-diphenyl-1,3,5-hexatriene (DPH) and 4-heptadecyl-7-hydroxycoumarin (HC) are two hydrophobic fluorescent probes which are solubilized in the lipid membrane(s) of liposomes. As can be seen in Figure 4.15, HC displays a significantly higher fluorescence anisotropy than DPH, which shows that HC is localized to the lipid-water interface to a higher extent than DPH. This, in turn, is due to the higher polarity of part of HC compared to the more apolar DPH. Note, finally, that with increasing temperature, the anisotropy due to both componds decreases as a result of the lipid membrane(s) becoming more fluid.

4.4 LIPOSOMES IN DRUG DELIVERY

For several decades now, liposomes have been considered promising for drug delivery, e.g., due to their capacity to encapsulate water-soluble and solubilize oil-soluble drugs, thereby, e.g., controlling the drug release rate, the drug degradation, and the drug bioavailability. Liposomes, similarly to other colloidal drug carriers, may also have advantageous effects, e.g., for directed intravenous administration to certain tissues, e.g., liver, spleen, and marrow, as adjuvants in vaccines formulations, etc.. However, as a formulation base they also suffer from numerous weaknesses, e.g., related to complicated preparation, sterilization difficulties, poor storage stability, limited to poor solubilization capacity for more hydrophobic drugs, and difficulties to control the drug release rate. Nevertheless, during the last decade or so, the development of so-called Stealth liposomes, i.e., liposomes surface modified by PEO derivatives, as well as other developments, have resolved several of these issues.

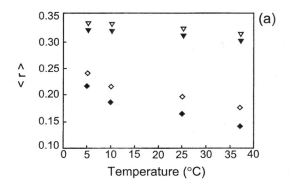

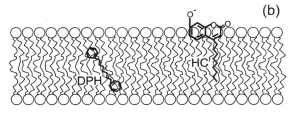

FIGURE 4.15 (a) Fluorescence anisotropy ⟨r⟩ of HC (triangles) and DPH (diamonds) in egg phosphatidylcholine/cholesterol liposomes vs. temperature. Open and filled symbols represent presence and absence of 5% PEG-PE, respectively. (b) Schematic illustration of the location of DPH and HC in the lipid membrane. (Redrawn from Silvander et al. Langmuir 2000, 16, 3696.)

4.4.1 Intravenous Administration

Intravenous administration of drugs is the route of choice, e.g., when the patient is unconscious, or when an acute treatment is necessary. Also, as discussed in Chapter 5, in the context of oral administration of protein and peptide drugs, a range of substances are poorly absorbed when given orally, e.g., as a consequence of their degradation in the gastrointestinal tract or poor uptake due to their physicochemical properties. In such cases, parenteral administration offers an efficient way of administration.

On intravenous administration of a drug, there is frequently a need for colloidal drug carriers, such as micelles, o/w emulsions, or liposomes. Reasons for this include, e.g.,

- Solubilization of sparingly soluble drugs and hence increasing its solubility in the bloodstream
- Reduced drug toxicity

- Reduced biological or chemical degradation of the drug
- Achievement of controlled or sustained release
- Decreased immunological reactions
- Prolongation of the drug circulation time and achievement of a more even tissue distribution
- Targeting to selective tissues or cell types

When a colloidal drug carrier is administered intravenously, it is cleared rapidly from bloodstream circulation by the reticuloendothelial (RES) system, and accumulated in RES-related tissues, such as liver, spleen, and marrow. The drug accumulation in RES-related tissues may be favorable in certain instances, e.g., when the site of action of the drug is in one or several of these tissues. In the general case, however, the RES uptake poses a problem for intravenous administration of colloidal drug carriers:

1. Due to the efficiency of RES, the uptake of the colloidal drug carriers is generally rapid, and therefore the bloodstream circulation time of the latter short. This risks resulting in a low bioavailability in tissues other than RES-related ones.
2. Through the RES uptake, most of the drug is accumulated in RES-related tissues. Therefore, the local concentration of the drug in these tissues may be quite high, resulting in a dose-limiting local toxicity.

Therefore, in the general case, a long circulation time and an even tissue distribution is advantageous from a therapeutic point of view.

The uptake of colloidal drug carriers by the reticuloendothelial system is governed by macrophages through a process called phagocytosis. In this, the colloidal carrier is attached to the macrophage surface, which is followed by a series of processes, resulting in the engulfment of the drug carrier (Figure 4.16). The initial attachment of the colloidal drug carrier at the surface of a macrophage and the subsequent triggering of phagocytosis is a complex process, which is not entirely understood at present. It has been found that the uptake of colloidal drug carriers by the RES depends on a range of factors, e.g., the size and surface properties of the carrier, e.g., hydrophobicity, charge, and chemical functionality. In particular, the uptake increases with an increasing particle size, hydrophobicity (although for very hydrophobic particles, a decrease uptake is observed), and charge (Figure 4.17), but is also dependent on, e.g., the specific chemical functionality of the carrier.

The uptake of colloidal drug carriers by macrophages is initiated by adsorption of certain serum proteins, so-called opsonins, at the carrier surface. These include, e.g.,

- Immunoglobulins, which may facilitate the uptake of colloidal drug carriers through interaction with the complement system or by a direct

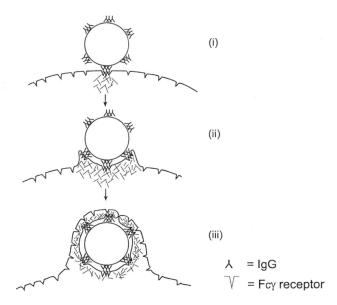

λ = IgG

$\mathbb{V}$ = Fcγ receptor

FIGURE 4.16 Scematic illustration of receptor-mediated phagocytosis of colloidal drug carriers by macrophages. (i) A colloidal drug carrier has attracted IgG adsorption and binds to the receptor at the macrophage surface. (ii) The carrier is engulfed. (iii) Membrane fusion leaves the macrophage surface intact. (Redrawn from Paul, Fundamental Immunology, Raven Press, 1993.)

interaction between the adsorbed IgG molecules and receptors present at macrophage surfaces

- Complement proteins such as C3 and C1q, which may activate the complement cascade
- "Adhesion" proteins such as fibrinogen and fibronectin
- The Hageman factor
- C-reactive protein (CRP)

Phagocytocis depends on the adsorption of opsonins at the drug carrier surface in a complex way, where the composition of the adsorbed layer, as well as surface-induced activation play a role. However, the extent of phagocytosis and RES uptake also depends on the total amount of serum proteins adsorbed at the drug carrier surface. More precisely, there is an inverse correlation between the serum protein adsorption, on one hand, and the bloodstream circulation time, on the other. Thus, the higher the total serum protein adsorption, the faster the clearance from bloodstream circulation (Figure 4.18).

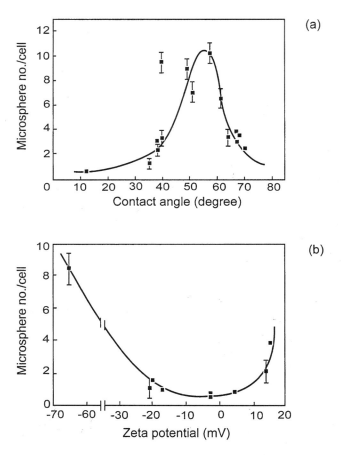

FIGURE 4.17 Effect of the particle surface energy (higher contact angle means more hydrophobic particles) (a) and surface charge (higher zeta potential means more highly charged particles) (b) on the phagocytosis by macrophages. (Redrawn from Tabata et al., Adv. Polym. Sci. 1990, 94, 106.)

From Figure 4.18, it follows that if the drug carrier can be made to adsorb little or no serum protein, its circulation time in the bloodstream is prolonged. For different colloidal drug carriers, this can be achieved in different ways. For example, phospholipids are usually used for preparation of liposomes for intravenous administration. Through choice of the structure of the polar headgroup of the phospholipid, a desired protein adsorption may be achieved. In particular, phospholipids which carry a zero net surface charge (e.g., PC or SM), or where

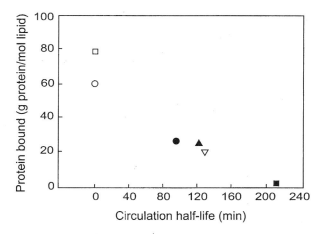

FIGURE 4.18 Correlation between total amount of protein adsorbed and circulation time before plasma clearance of LUVs containing trace amounts of [³H]cholesterylhexadecyl ether administered intravenously in mice. Results are shown for liposomes containing ganglioside GM1 (filled square), phosphatidylcholine (PC; filled triangle), phosphatidylinositol (PI; filled circle), sphingomyelin (SM; open triangle), phosphatidic acid (PA; open square), and diphosphatidylglycerol (DPG; open circle). (Redrawn from Chonn et al., J. Biol. Chem. 1992, 267, 18759.)

the charge is shielded by an outer group (e.g., GM1 or PI), the serum protein adsorption is low and the circulation time is long. For phospholipids carrying a bare charge (e.g., PA or DPG), on the other hand, the serum protein adsorption is substantial, and the bloodstream circulation time short. Therefore, through choice of the phospholipid or phospholipid mixture composition, the clearance rate may be tuned (Figures 4.18 and 4.19).

A particularly efficient way of reducing serum protein adsorption at colloidal drug carriers is to use different types of surface modifications based on PEO derivatives. Thus, provided that the PEO-based coating of the drug carrier is sufficiently thick and dense, the adsorption of essentially all serum proteins is reduced dramatically. This results in a drastically prolonged bloodstream circulation time, a decreased accumulation in RES-related tissues, and an increased accumulation of the drug also in tissues and cells not related to the RES (Figure 4.20).

In order to understand the positive effects of PEO-based coatings, it is instructive to briefly consider the effect of PEO-based coatings on serum protein adsorption. Thus, the adsorption of such proteins to any surface can be the result of several different driving forces, but in general, the electrostatic, hydrophobic,

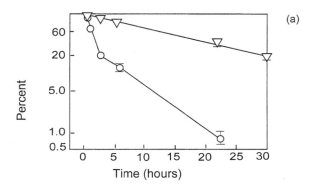

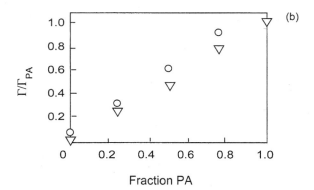

FIGURE 4.19   (a) Clearance of SUV liposomes consisting of distearoylphosphati-dylcholine (DSPC) (triangles) and of DSPC/distearoylphosphatidic acid (DSPA) (circles) from bloodstream circulation after injection in mice. (b) Adsorption of fi-brinogen (triangles) and apolipoprotein B (circles) at PC/PA mixed phospholipid surfaces versus the phospholipid mixture composition (Γ/Γ_{PA}). Note that the protein adsorption, and hence the bloodstream circulation time, may be tuned by varying the PC/PA ratio. (Redrawn from Senior, Crit. Rev. Ther. Drug Carrier Syst. 1987, 3, 123 (a) and Malmsten, in Malmsten, ed., Biopolymers at Interfaces, Marcel Dek-ker, 1998 (b).)

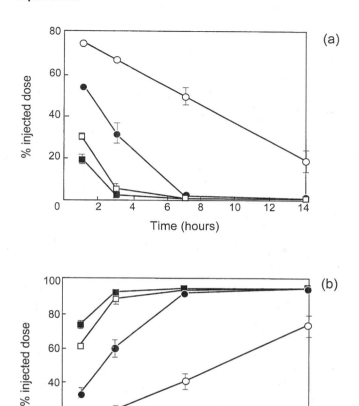

FIGURE 4.20 (a) Blood clearance and (b) uptake in liver and spleen observed for liposomes containing PE-PEO phospholipids. Results are shown for PEO_{750}-PE (open squares), PEO_{2000}-PE (filled circles), and PEO_{5000}-PE (open circles) following intravenous injection in mice. Filled squares show results obtained for the uncoated liposomes. (Redrawn from Mori et al., FEBS Lett. 1991, 284, 263.)

and van der Waals interactions (Chapter 9) dominate and drive the adsorption. Since PEO-based surface coatings are uncharged, hydrophilic, and also contain a lot of water (the latter reducing van der Waals attractive interactions between the surface and the protein), this reduces the adsorption driving force. Furthermore, the PEO chains give rise to a repulsive steric interaction which opposes protein adsorption to a PEO-modified surface. Together, these two contributions result in a very low serum protein adsorption. However, for the attractive interactions between the serum proteins and the underlying carrier to be fully screened, the PEO layer needs to be sufficiently thick, and hence a minimum PEO molecular weight of the order of 1000–2000 is generally required. Furthermore, if the PEO chain density is not sufficiently high, small serum proteins may "slip through" the PEO layer, and also the repulsive osmotic interaction may be insufficient to withstand a strongly attractive protein-carrier interaction (Figure 4.7).

Surface modification of colloidal drug carriers to introduce PEO chains may be achieved in several different ways. For liposomes, introduction of a PEO-modified phospholipid (e.g., PEO-PE) in the liposome offers particularly interesting opportunities (Figure 4.20). This technique has the advantage that the PEO chains are firmly anchored at the colloid surface, which eliminates the risk of colloid destabilization and opsonization enhancement through collision-induced desorption or desorption on dilution. Another possibility is to coat preformed liposomes with a PEO-containing block copolymer, the main advantage of which is its simplicity, although care must be taken when using this approach to reduce dilution-induced desorption of the protective surface coating. Yet another possibility is to attach PEO through a covalent link in one end of the PEO chains. Similarly to the PEO-PE modification, the latter has the advantage of resulting in an effectively irreversible PEO anchoring to the carrier surface. On the other hand, the approach is more complex than the use of PEO-PE, and therefore often less interesting from a practical point of view.

Analogous to PEO-containing block copolymer micelles (Chapter 2), PEO-containing liposomes offer significant opportunities in cancer therapy:

1. Through the increased bloodstream circulation time, the accumulation in tissues not related to the RES is increased. This is favorable if the tumor is not localized in RES-related tissues. If it is located in RES-related tissues, on the other hand, non-Stealth liposomes should be used.
2. In parallel to the improved bioavailability achieved by the prolonged bloodstream circulation, the occurrence of detrimental side effects in RES-related tissues is reduced, which in turn allows a higher dose to be used.

3. Solubilization or encapsulation of toxic cancer drugs contributes to the reduced toxicity.

By the use of PEO-containing liposomes, enhanced antitumor capacity and reduced toxicity of the encapsulated drug can be reached for a variety of tumors. As an example of this, Figure 4.21 shows how PEO-modified liposomes can be successfully used for administration of a cytotoxic drug (doxorubicin). As can be seen, the PEO-modified liposomes display a longer bloodstream circulation time than the corresponding nonmodified liposomes. Furthermore, the prolongation of the circulation time in blood correlates to a decrease of accumulation in RES-related tissues such as liver, and a correspondingly increased accumulation in the tumor.

Another illustration of the potential of liposomes in cancer therapy is given in Figure 4.22, showing results on the inhibition of lung metastases in mice bearing malignant fibrosarcoma by treatment with liposomes containing C-reactive protein (CRP). As can be seen, PEO-modified liposomes result in a significantly prolonged survival, whereas the CRP/no liposome and no CRP/liposome controls gave results identical to those obtained for the untreated control group. This illustrates that an efficient drug and an efficient drug carrier are both necessary for a successful therapy in this case.

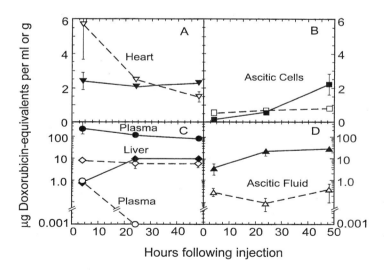

FIGURE 4.21 Doxorubicin in tumor-bearing mice, either as free drug (open symbols/dashed lines) or in DSPE-PEO liposomes (filled symbols/solid lines). (Redrawn from Papahadjopoulos et al., Proc. Natl. Acad. Sci. USA 1991, 88, 11460.)

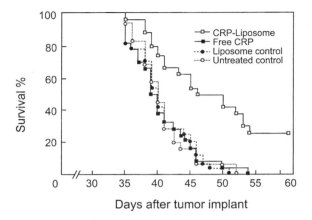

Days after tumor implant

Figure 4.22 Prolongation of survival of tumor-bearing mice by treatment with CRP in a liposome formulation. Results are shown for the untreated control (open circles), liposomes containing no CRP (filled circles), free CRP in the absence of liposomes (filled squares), and liposome-bound CRP (open squares). (Redrawn from Deodhar et al., Cancer Res. 1982, 42, 5084.)

4.4.2 Targeting

An issue related to the use of colloidal drug carriers in intravenous administration is that of directly targeting the drug, or rather the drug carrier, to a specific tissue or cell type in order to increase the drug bioavailability and to reduce adverse side effects. Particularly, PEO-modified liposomes (or block copolymer micelles; Chapter 2) are quite promising in this respect:

1. Due to the PEO chains, serum protein adsorption to the carrier surface is very low, and hence the risk that the recognition moiety is "buried" by unspecific protein adsorption is limited.
2. A long circulation time and relatively even tissue distribution is a prerequisite for any specific binding to a localized recognition moiety. If the tissue distribution is dominated by unspecific mechanisms, labeling of the drug carrier with a specific recognition moiety has little effect.

If a biospecific molecule, e.g., a suitable antibody (fragment), a peptide sequence or a lectin, is covalently attached to such a carrier, the long bloodstream circulation in principle should facilitate targeting to a localized antigen. As also discussed in relation to block copolymer micelles in Chapter 2, specific targeting of intravenously administered long-circulating carriers modified by a recognition moiety for a localized species is indeed possible. As another illustration of this,

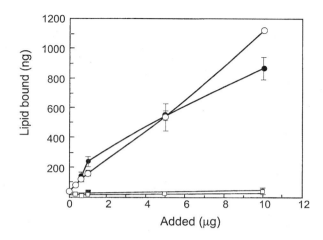

FIGURE 4.23 Binding to mouse pulmonary artery endothelial cells of two liposome preparations functionalized with relevant antibodies (filled and open circles, respectively), functionalized with an irrelevant antibody (open squares) or uncoated liposomes (filled squares). (Redrawn from Holmberg et al., J. Liposome Research 1990, 1, 393.)

Figure 4.23 shows results on the binding of liposomes to mouse pulmonary artery endothelial cells. As can be seen, the amount lipid bound to these cells is significant with two different relevant antibodies, whereas the binding of both the bare liposomes and liposomes modified with an irrelevant antibody is negligible. One should be aware, however, that although beneficial therapeutic effects have been observed for conjugated PEO-containing liposomes and micelles, the presence of the recognition moiety on the carrier surface may also be detrimental, e.g., causing the long circulation time in the absence of such entities to decrease drastically.

4.4.3   Topical Administration

Another area where liposomes have found use is in topical drug delivery. A major problem concerning topical drug delivery is that the drug may not reach the site of action at a sufficient concentration to be efficient, which mainly is due to the barrier properties of the stratum corneum (see also Chapter 5). To overcome this problem, topical formulations may contain so-called penetration enhancers, such as propylene glycol, dimethylsulfoxide, and Azone (Table 4.2).

Although the use of penetration enhancers may yield an improved drug transport, they may also result in an increased systemic drug level, which is not always desired, and may cause irritative or even toxic effects. As discussed in

TABLE **4.2**   Characteristics of the Ideal
Dermal Penetration Enhancer

Pharmacologically inert
Non-toxic
Immediate in action
Reversible in action
Chemically and physically compatible with
   the drug and with the skin
Cosmetically acceptable

Chapter 5, one way to reach an increased drug penetration without the use of penetration enhancers is to use microemulsions. Another approach for this is to use liposomes or other types of lipid suspensions. Based on liposomes, favorable results have been found for a number of drugs, including local anesthetics, retinoids, and corticosteroids. As an illustration of this, Figure 4.24 shows results on the effect of cortisol entrapped in liposomes. As can be seen, an improved cortisol penetration is found for the liposome formulation compared to the control formulation. Since the therapeutic effect of cortisol in a range of indications, e.g., acute dermatoses, is limited by the cortisol penetration (i.e., the local cortisol

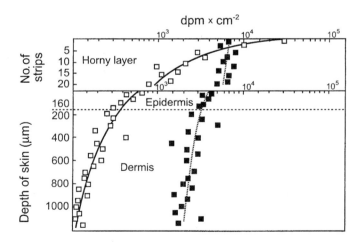

FIGURE **4.24**   Concentration (dpm/cm^2) profile of cortisol following topical administration with an ointment (open squares) and liposomes (filled squares) formulation. (Redrawn from Lasch et al., Biomed. Biochim. Acta 1986, 10, 1295.)

concentration), this makes liposome formulations advantageous for this use of cortisol.

For drugs incorporated in lipid drug carriers, the drug penetration is strongly dependent on that of the drug carrier. For such carriers in general, and liposomes in particular, passage through pores in the stratum corneum should be favored by easily deformable bilayers, since these better can accomodate local stresses occurring during passage (Figure 4.25). Given this, it could be expected that different types of liposomes have different capacity to penetrate the stratum corneum, and specifically, that highly deformable bilayers should be advantageous for skin penetration. In fact, a class of highly deformable liposomes, so-called transfersomes have been identified as being exceptionally deformable and displaying quite efficient transfer over the stratum corneum of drugs spanning widely in lipophilicity and molecular weight, also in relation to transcutaneous delivery of protein and peptide drugs (Figure 4.26).

The kinetics of action of topically administered drugs depends on both the penetration rate of the drug carrier, the drug release rate, the rate of drug redistribution and action after passage, and the drug clearance rate. Naturally, the onset of the driving force for penetration depends on the chemical potential gradient

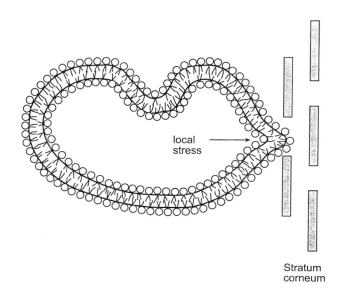

local stress

Stratum corneum

FIGURE 4.25 Schematic illustration of the early stage of liposome passage through a pore in the stratum corneum. (Redrawn from Cevc, in Lipowsky et al., eds., Handbook of Physics of Biological Systems, Vol. 1, Elsevier, 1995.)

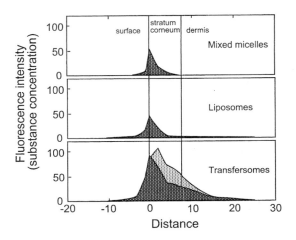

FIGURE 4.26   Relative penetration capability of fluorescent labeled mixed micelles, liposomes, and transfersomes into intact skin. (Redrawn from Cevc, Crit. Rev. Ther. Drug Carrier Syst. 1996, 13, 257.)

over the skin, and hence on the evaporation from the topically administered formulation. Generally, unless the formulation is very concentrated, significant evaporation must occur before the driving force for penetration is sufficiently large. This, in turn, induces a lag time before the drug action may be substantial (hours). Note in Figure 4.27 that there is a lag time of about 4 hours prior to the occurrence of the labeled substances in the blood. Also, the time processes are comparable for all substances, indicating that the transfer of the deformable liposomes (with its content) is the main way of skin penetration for these polypeptide/ protein systems. This is also indicated by the sizeable fraction of lipids (typically 6–8%) found also in bloodstream circulation.

    A range of substances have been investigated regarding topical administration using liposome and transfersome systems. These include, e.g.,

    Analgesics
    Antibiotics
    Antifungals
    Cyclosporine
    Nonsteroidal anti-inflammatory agents
    Steroids
    Tamoxifen
    Virustatics

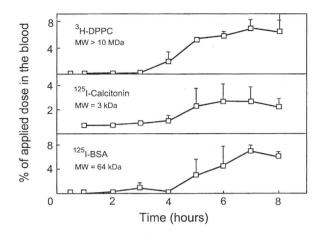

FIGURE 4.27 Kinetics of penetration through intact skin of transfersome preparations containing radioactively labeled phospholipids (^{3}H-DPPC), ^{125}I-Calcitonin, and ^{125}I-BSA. (Redrawn from Cevc, Crit. Rev. Ther. Drug Carrier Syst. 1996, 13, 257.)

but also biological macromolecules, such as

> Superoxide desmuthase
> Insulin
> Interferon
> Antibodies
> Other proteins
> Other biopolymers

For example, tamoxifen is an antiestrogen, which is used extensively for treatment of breast cancer. In order to reduce side effects such as thrombosis and depressions, it would be of interest to develop a regioselective formulation. In this context, topical administration of a formulation based on transfersomes loaded with tamoxifen has been found to be promising (Figure 4.28). As can be seen, the epicutaneously administered formulation gives quite comparable results with the subcutaneously injected one at high tamoxifen concentration, and better than the latter at low drug concentrations. In fact, less than 5% of the drug remains on the skin surface.

Also for polypeptide and protein drugs, topical formulations based on liposomes may offer some opportunities. As an illustration of this, Figure 4.29 shows results obtained with highly deformable liposomes containing insulin after appli-

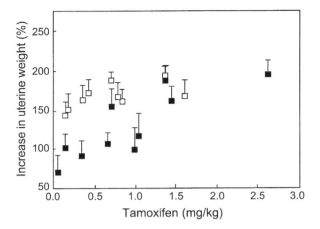

FIGURE 4.28 Biological effect, as measured by the growth of the uteri in young specimen, versus the concentration of tamoxifen administered either epicutaneously in a transfersome formulation (open squares) or subcutaneously dissolved in soybean oil (filled squares). (Redrawn from Cevc, Crit. Rev. Ther. Drug Carrier Syst. 1996, 13, 257.)

cation to intact skin. As can be seen, this results in hypoglycemia after 90–180 minutes, depending on the carrier composition. The decrease in the blood glucose concentration is about 35% of that of subcutaneously administered insulin, but the cumulative effect significantly larger. Less deformable mixed micelles and liposomes, on the other hand, gave rather poor results.

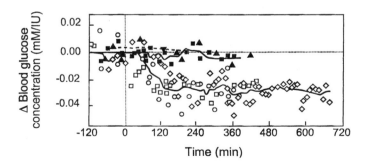

FIGURE 4.29 Effect on blood glucose level after application to intact skin of insulin incorporated in a formulation consisting of highly deformable liposomes (open symbols), mixed micelles (filled squares), and liposomes (filled triangles). (Redrawn from Cevc, Crit. Rev. Ther. Drug Carrier Syst. 1996, 13, 257.)

4.4.4 Gene Therapy

Today, diseases caused by genetic lesions are treated by drugs which suppress or eliminate the symptoms of the disease, whereas no treatment of the lesion in itself is provided. There is some hope, however, that recent advances in molecular biology in general, and relating to the human genome in particular, will provide possibilities to replace defect gene sequences. Such methodologies are generally referred to as gene therapy. Examples of diseases where gene therapy may offer possibilities include, e.g., cystic fibrosis, Alzheimers disease, Parkinson's disease, AIDS, and cancer. For gene therapy to work, however, the replacement or insertion gene sequence must be delivered into the cell nucleus, which poses a considerable drug delivery problem. Thus, for a DNA sequence to reach its site of action, it must pass a number of compartments. Subsequently it is transcribed to mRNA, and expressed in protein synthesis. This entire process is usually referred to as transfection. A schematic illustration of this is given in Figure 4.30.

First, the DNA, often in a complexed form (see below) adheres to the cell surface. After this, internalization into the cell occurs, generally by endocytosis, which is followed by release into the cytoplasm. From here, the DNA (or DNA-containing carrier) can either diffuse to the nucleus membrane or be transported by active intracellular trafficking. Then it must cross the cell nucleus membrane, before transcription to mRNA, and final expression to proteins in the cytoplasm. Clearly, the whole process is a very complex one, and the different conditions in the different compartments generally render the transfection rate very low.

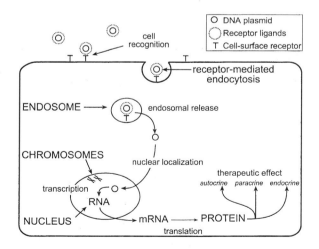

FIGURE 4.30 Schematic illustration of gene transfection. (Redrawn from Rolland, Crit. Rev. Ther. Drug Carrier Syst. 1998, 15, 143.)

For several reasons, drug carriers offer opportunities in gene therapy. First, DNA is a highly charged polyelectrolyte, and at extracellular and intracellular electrolyte concentrations highly stretched. For high molecular weight DNA, therefore, the mere size of the DNA contributes to reducing the transfection rate. Second, DNA is highly negatively charged, which generates a repulsive electrostatic interaction between DNA and the negatively charged cell surface, again resulting in a low transfection rate.

Thus, there is a need for carrier systems which promote the transfer of DNA into the cell nucleus in order to improve the transfection rate. In the first approach investigated, virus vectors were used and found to be quite efficient. Viral vectors, however, are not optimal from a safety perspective, and therefore considerable efforts have been directed to find simpler and safer carrier systems. In particular, the latter have been based on complex formation between DNA and oppositely charged lipids (often in the form of liposomes), surfactants, and polyelectrolytes.

Although both positively and negatively charged lipids, as well as titrating ones, have been investigated in the context of gene therapy, particular systems based on cationic lipids have been found to be of interest (Figure 4.31).

The complex formation between DNA and cationic lipid/liposome systems depends on a range of parameters, such as lipid charge, pH, salt concentration, and DNA/lipid concentration ratio. In particular, the latter is important, since it offers a powerful way to alter the size and charge of the complexes formed. For example, by increasing the relative concentration of cationic lipids/liposomes the negative charge of the complexes formed decreases monotonously, and at sufficiently high lipid/DNA ratio, the complexes formed are positively charged (Figure 4.32).

Furthermore, the size of the complexes formed depends strongly, although in a less direct way, on the DNA/lipid ratio. Thus, at charge neutralization, the stability of complex particles is limited due to the absence of significantly repulsive electrostatic interactions, and hence there is particle flocculation, resulting either in macroscopic phase separation or occurrence of very large particles. For complexes carrying either a net positive or a net negative charge, on the other hand, an electrostatic repulsive interaction between the particles stabilizes these against flocculation, and hence quite small particles may form (at least in the absence of bridging flocculation) (Figure 4.33).

Further information about the complexation between DNA and cationic liposomes may be obtained by fluorescence measurements. For example, ethidium bromide, which intercalates between DNA base pairs, can be used as a fluorescence probe. As such, it is sensitive to quenching, and therefore also the the proximity between ethidium bromide molecules and to DNA conformational changes. As can be seen in Figure 4.34, the fluorescence intensity for a system containing DNA and ethidium bromide decreases upon addition of cationic lipo-

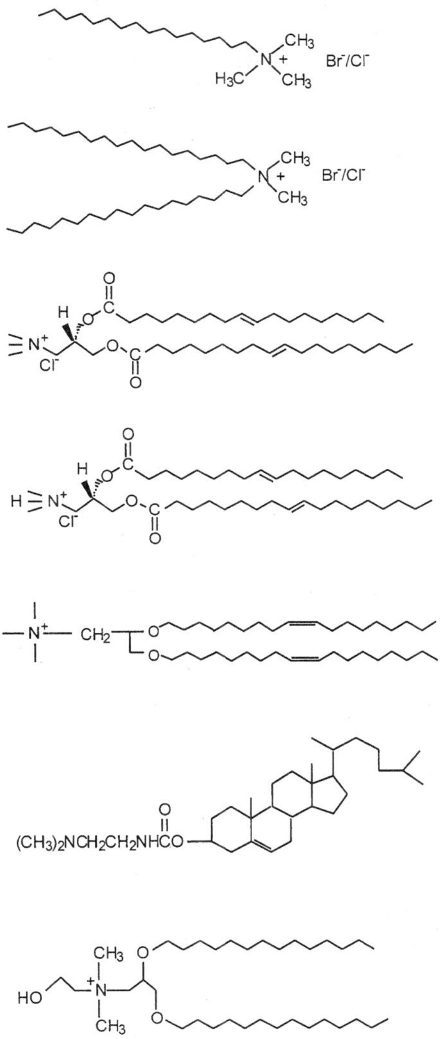

CTAB/C

DODAB/DODAC

DOTAP

DODAP

DOTMA

DC-Chol

DMRIE

FIGURE 4.31 Chemical structures of some cationic lipids investigated in relation to gene therapy. (Redrawn from Lasic, Adv. Drug Delivery Rev. 1996, 20, 221.)

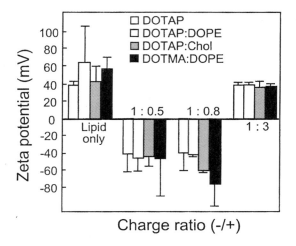

FIGURE 4.32 Zeta potential of plasmid/lipid complexes formed for different cationic lipids and colipids as a function of the plasmid/lipid ratio. (Redrawn from Rolland, Crit. Rev. Ther. Drug Carrier Syst. 1998, 15, 143.)

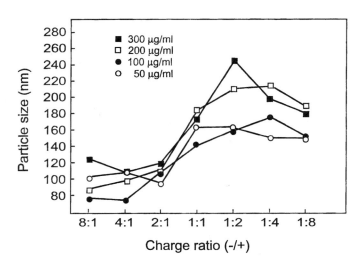

FIGURE 4.33 Effect of the DNA/lipid charge ratio on the size of the complexes formed at different DNA concentrations. (Redrawn from Tomlinson et al., J. Controlled Release 1996, 39, 357.)

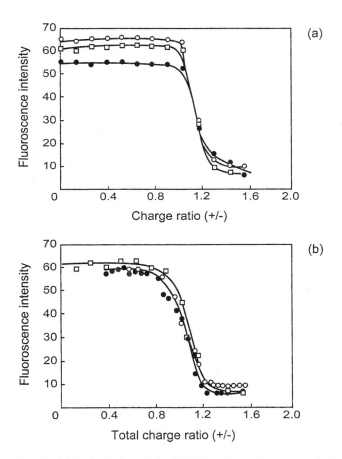

FIGURE 4.34   (a) Effect of the DNA length and liposome: DNA ratio on the fluorescence intensity. The length of the DNA (in base pairs) was 100–300 (filled circles), 500–8000 (open squares), and 23,000 (open circles). (b) The effect of poly(lysine) on the fluorescence of DNA-liposome complexes as a function of the total number of positive charges (poly(lysine) + DOTMA). Results are shown for DOTMA with no further additions (open squares), DOTMA + 1.25 · 10^{-5} M poly(lysine) (concentration in momoneric units; open circles), and DOTMA + 2.5 · 10^{-5} M monomeric lysine residues (concentration in monomeric units; filled circles), respectively. (Redrawn from Gershou et al., Biochemistry 1993, 32, 7143.)

somes. More specifically, DNA collapse occurs at a positive/negative charge ratio of about 1, irrespectively of the the DNA molecular weight (over a wide span) or the presence of other types of positive charges.

Furthermore, the collapse is given by the ratio between the total number of positive and negative charges. Thus, addition of poly(lysine) reduces the concentration of cationic liposome needed to induce collapse, but the number of positive charges needed to induce the collapse is constant, and corresponding to a charge ratio of about 1.

Complex formation between DNA and titrating liposomes may also occur and is of some interest in relation to gene therapy. In particular, endosomes normally acidify rapidly and transfer their content for enzymatic degradation. Considering this, strategies have been developed to reach release of the endosomal content. This can be achieved, e.g., by liposomes which are stable in neutral or alkaline pH, but become unstable at acidic pH. Through the instability of such systems on acidification of the endosomes, the DNA release to the cytosol can be increased.

It has been found that the transfection efficiency depends on the net charge of the DNA/liposome complex. Unfortunately, the dependence is not entirely straightforward, and different cell lines require different complex charge for optimal expression. Although considerable work has been performed with both positively and negatively charged liposome complexes, as well as with titrating ones, cationic liposome complexes have received the bulk attention in gene therapy. In particular, cationic liposomes have been found to result in significantly improved transfection in a range of cell lines compared to bare DNA (Figure 4.35). The transfection has also been observed to depend on a number of different parameters, such as the structure of the lipids used and the size of the liposomes (Figure 4.36).

Thus, it seems that shorter and unsaturated lipids, yielding more fluid bilayers, are beneficial for transfection, probably due to more efficient packing in the complexes for such systems. More unexpectedly, larger liposomes have been found to result in a better transfection than smaller ones. The origin of the latter effect is unclear at present.

Cationic lipid-based systems have also been found to be comparatively efficient for gene delivery in vivo, e.g., to pulmonary epithelial cells, endothelial cells after direct application to the endothelial surfaces or after intravenous administration, solid tumors after interstitial administration, and metastases after intravenous delivery. Furthermore, therapeutic cDNAs have been delivered by cationic liposomes in human gene therapy trials and no toxicity has been observed at low doses administered. An example that gene delivery may work also in vivo is given in Figure 4.37. Thus, nude mice bearing breast tumors were treated by intravenous injection of a p53 gene-expression system containing DOTMA:DOPE lipids, and a clear tumor regression was observed compared with the control groups.

There are also several potential problems with in vivo gene delivery medi-

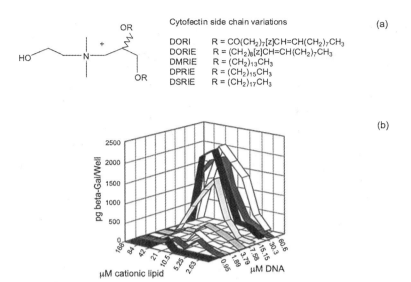

Cytofectin side chain variations (a)

DORI   R = CO(CH$_2$)$_7$[z]CH=CH(CH$_2$)$_7$CH$_3$
DORIE   R = (CH$_2$)$_8$[z]CH=CH(CH$_2$)$_7$CH$_3$
DMRIE   R = (CH$_2$)$_{13}$CH$_3$
DPRIE   R = (CH$_2$)$_{15}$CH$_3$
DSRIE   R = (CH$_2$)$_{17}$CH$_3$

(b)

FIGURE 4.35 (a) Chemical structure of cytofectin side chain variations. (b) Effect of the composition of complexes formed between DNA and (small) liposome (DORI/DOPE) on the transfection of efficiency. An increased level of beta-Gal corresponds to an increased transfection efficiency. (Redrawn from Felgner et al., J. Biol. Chem. 1994, 269, 2550.)

ated through complex formation with cationic liposomes, lipids, surfactants, or polyelectrolytes. For example, for the cellular uptake to be efficient the complexes should carry a net positive charge. On intravenous administration, however, the positively charged complex carrier encounters net negatively charged serum proteins, lipoproteins, and blood cells, with risk for flocculation and emboli formation. Furthermore, intravenously administered positively charged particles are cleared from circulation rapidly by the RES, which in itself precludes efficient DNA delivery to other tissues. Carriers administered through the airway, on the other hand, face problems related to the lung surfactants. In both cases, there is also a risk of the carriers not being able to maintain their positive charge until they reach their target, which will deteriorate their performance. Despite these obstacles, however, DNA administration through cationic liposome complexes has been found to be more efficient than naked DNA delivery.

4.4.5 Ocular Administration

The eye is protected by several efficient mechanisms, e.g., an epithelial layer which constitutes an efficient barrier to penetration, tear flow, and the blinking

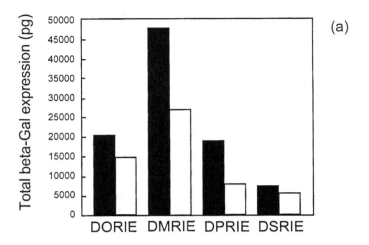

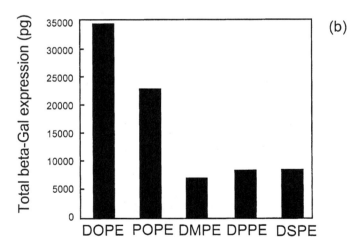

FIGURE **4.36** Effects of alkyl chain length and saturation for the cationic (a) and the zwitterionic (b) lipid on the transfection efficiency. In (a) results are shown for both small unilamellar liposomes (open bars) and large multilamellar liposomes (filled bars). (Redrawn from Felgner et al., J. Biol. Chem. 1994, 269, 2550.)

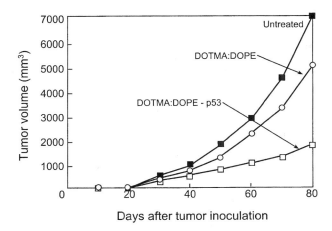

FIGURE 4.37 Effect on tumor volume for mice carrying breast cancer of gene delivery through DOTMA:DOPE/DNA complexes. Results are shown for mice injected with DOTMA:DOPE-p53 (open squares), DOTMA:DOPE (open circles), or were left untreated (filled squares). (Redrawn from Lesoon-Wood et al., Human Gene Ther. 1995, 6, 395.)

reflex. Together, these generate an efficient washing out system, and result in a generally poor drug penetration into deeper layers of the cornea. Liposomes and other types of colloidal drug carriers therefore offer at least some potential in relation to ocular drug delivery, since they can be used to generate a sustained release, and also a prolonged retention of the drug in intraocular cell populations. A central strategy of the use of liposomes in ocular drug delivery based on liposomes has been to improve the adhesion between the liposomes and the cornea. This can be achieved in different ways, including:

1. Ganglioside-containing liposomes together with wheat ger agglutinin, a lectin binding to both the cornea and gangliosides
2. Liposomes coated with antibodies to components in the corneal surface
3. Lipsomes coated with mucoadhesive polymers (see also Chapters 8 and 9)

4.4.6 Pulmonary Administration

Also in relation to pulmonary administration, liposomes may offer some opportunities as a regiospecific alternative to systemic administration, e.g., for treatment of allergies and asthma, for antibiotics to pulmonary infections, or in cancer therapy. The use of liposomes in this context is still relatively experimental. On the other hand, pulmonary administration of phospholipids has been well established for almost 40 years in relation to treatment of respiratory distress syndrom (RDS) in newborns.

Interestingly, there seems to be little dependence of the liposome size on its performance in relation to pulmonary administration, and both the pattern of deposition and the kinetics of removal have been found to be essentially identical for MLV and SUVs, which indicates that it is the aerosol droplet size rather than that of the liposome which determines deposition and clearance.

Through the use of liposomes, sparingly soluble drugs may be administered to the lung. Also, through the sustained drug release from the liposomes, peak plasma concentrations may be reduced or eliminated, which is beneficial since it reduces the occurrence of side effects. Also, a prolonged effect may be reached.

4.4.7 Triggered Release from Liposome Formulations

As with many other formulation types, responsive transitions are of interest also for liposome-based drug delivery systems. In particular, significant emphasis has been placed on temperature-sensitive liposome formulations. For example, such formulations may be very stable at low temperature during storage, but release incorporated drugs on a minor temperature increase. An application area where this may have potential is within directed chemotherapy. Thus, on applying external radio frequency phased arrays, the temperature in at least some cancer tissues (e.g., prostate and ovarian cancers) increases. Therefore, a localized release and drug targeting in chemotherapy is possible if the drug carrier can be made to accumulate in the tumor and the drug release triggered by a minor temperature increase. As discussed above, the release of incorporated drugs by liposomes is affected by the transitions in the lipid bilayers. Specifically, the release is increased as the melting transition is approached. By working with lipid mixtures, very abrupt release transitions may indeed be achieved (Figure 4.38).

4.5 OTHER TYPES OF DISPERSED LIQUID CRYSTALLINE PHASES

Although liposomes are without doubt the most frequently studied and used dispersed lipid system for drug delivery, there are also other such systems based on liquid crystalline phases (Figure 4.39). For example, formulations based on dispersed cubic liquid crystalline phases have potential in drug delivery, e.g., via the parenteral route, due to their capacity to solubilize both water-soluble and oil-soluble drugs, and also to immobilize bioactive proteins.

Such systems are typically prepared through high pressure homogenization of cubic liquid crystalline phases stable also in equilibrium with excess water. The dispersed cubic phase particles need to be stabilized against flocculation and coalescence, e.g., by a PEO-containing copolymer. Due to the small size that can

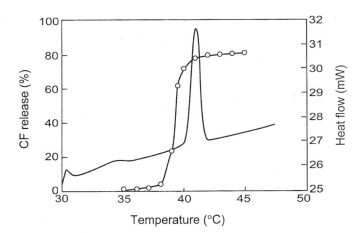

FIGURE 4.38 DSC scanning profile (solid line) and accumulated release (circles) of carboxyfluorescein (CF) by DPPC:MPPC liposomes as a function of temperature. (Redrawn from Anyarambhatla et al., J. Liposome Res. 1999, 9, 491.)

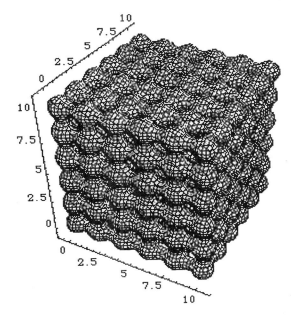

FIGURE 4.39 Schematic illustration of the structure of a dispersed cubic liquid crystalline phase ("cubosome"). (Redrawn from Larsson et al., Curr. Opinion Colloid Interface Sci. 2000, 5, 64.)

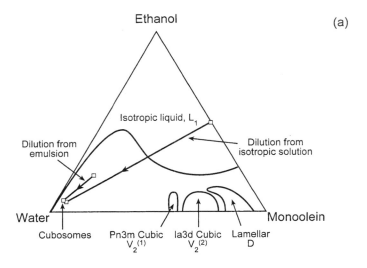

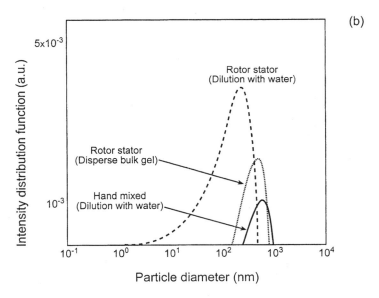

FIGURE 4.40 (a) Ternary phase diagram for the monoolein-ethanol-water system, with water dilution lines to form cubosomes from an isotropic solution and an emulsion system. (b) Particle size distribution of cubosome dispersions obtained with the dilution process and through dispersion of a bulk gel system. (Redrawn from Spicer et al., Langmuir 2001, 17, 5748.)

be reached ($\approx 100-300$ nm) and the PEO-based coatings, these particles are capable of bloodstream circulation for an considerable time. Therefore, such systems offer potential advantages relating to increased drug bioavailability and reduced toxic side effects in RES-related tissues.

Recently, preparation of cubosomes has been found to be possible also by simple mixing in the presence of a suitable hydrotrope, e.g., ethanol. Thus, by addition of water to a system of monoolein, ethanol (and water), both isotropic solutions and emulsions may be transformed to dispersed cubosome systems through homogenous nucleation (Figure 4.40). Furthermore, due to the low viscosity of the systems used with the latter approach, small particles may be generated with only marginal energy input.

BIBLIOGRAPHY

Cevc, G., Transfersomes, liposomes and other lipid suspensions on the skin: permeation enhancement, vesicle penetration, and transdermal drug delivery, Crit. Rev. Ther. Drug Carrier Syst. 13:257–388 (1996).

Gregoriadis, G., ed., Liposome Technology, vol. 3, CRC Press, Boca Raton, FL., 1984.

Gulati, M., M. Grover, S. Singh, M. Singh, Lipophilic drug derivatives in liposomes, Int. J. Pharm. 165:129–168 (1998).

Höhne, G., W. Hemminger, H. J. Flammersheim, Differential Scanning Calorimetry. An Introduction for Practitioners, Springer, Berlin, 1996.

Israelachvili, J., Intermolecular and Surface Forces, Academic Press, London, 1992.

Kreuter, J., ed., Colloidal Drug Delivery Systems, Drugs and the Pharmaceutical Sciences, vol. 66, Marcel Dekker, New York, 1994.

Lakowics, J. R., Principles of Fluorescence Spectroscopy, Plenum, New York, 1983.

Lasic, D., F. Martin, eds., Stealth Liposomes, CRC Press, Boca Raton, FL, 1995.

Lasic, D. D., N. S. Tempelton, Liposomes in gene therapy, Adv. Drug Delivery Rev. 20: 221–266 (1996).

Lee, R. J., L. Huang, Lipidic vector systems for gene transfer, Crit. Rev. Ther. Drug Carrier Syst. 14:173–206 (1997).

Malmsten, M., ed., Biopolymers at Interfaces, Surfactant Science Series vol. 75, Marcel Dekker, New York, 1998.

Patel, H. M., Serum opsonins and liposomes: their interaction and opsonophagocytosis, Crit. Rev. Ther. Drug Carrier Syst. 9:39–90 (1992).

Rand., R. P., V. A. Parsegian, Hydration forces between phospholipid bilayers, Biochim. Biophys. Acta 988:351–376 (1989).

Rolland, A. P., From genes to gene medicines: recent advances in nonviral gene delivery, Crit. Rev. Ther. Drug Carrier Syst. 15:143–198 (1998).

Rosoff, M., ed., Vesicles, Surfactant Science Series, vol. 62, Marcel Dekker, New York, 1996.

Small, D. M., The Physical Chemistry of Lipids, vol. 4, Plenum Press, 1986.

Tabata, Y., Y. Ikada, Phagocytosis of polymer microspheres by macrophages, Adv. Polym. Sci. 94:107–141 (1990).

Torchilin, V. P., Targeting of drugs and drug carriers within the cardiovascular system, Adv. Drug Delivery Rev. 17:75–101 (1995).

5

Microemulsions

5.1 BASICS OF MICROEMULSIONS

Microemulsions are systems consisting of water, oil, and surfactant(s), which constitute a single optically isotropic and thermodynamically stable liquid solution. Such systems are useful for drug delivery due to their capacity to solubilize both water-soluble and oil-soluble compounds, frequently in high amounts, their excellent stability, ease of preparation, optical clarity, as well as other administration-specific advantages.

5.1.1 Microemulsions and Emulsions Are Fundamentally Different

Despite their name, microemulsions are fundamentally different from emulsions, and should not be seen as mere emulsions with a small droplet size. This is not always realized within drug delivery, and care should therefore be taken to clarify whether or not true microemulsion systems are used and caution applied when reading the existing literature in the field. Since they are fundamentally different, there are a number of factors which differ microemulsions from emulsions:

1. Microemulsions are thermodynamically stable systems, and display indefinite stability in the absence of chemical degradation of any of its components. Emulsions, on the other hand, are merely kinetically sta-

bilized but thermodynamically unstable, which means that emulsions will eventually separate to macroscopically separated oil and water phases.

2. Due to their thermodynamic stability, microemulsions form spontaneously, and no work has to be added to prepare them. Emulsions, on the other hand, are not thermodynamically stable, and hence energy must be added to form them. As will be discussed in Chapter 6, this frequently involves the use of high-pressure homogenization.

3. Emulsions consist of relatively large droplets (typically 100 nm–10 µm in drug delivery), whereas microemulsions may consist of very small droplets (typically 10–100 nm), but also display a range of other structures.

4. As a result of this, microemulsions are transparent, whereas emulsions are milky in their appearance.

5. Due to the larger droplets in emulsion systems, the surface area is generally smaller in emulsions than in microemulsions, and consequently, less surfactant is generally needed to generate an emulsion than a microemulsion system.

5.1.2 Microemulsion Structure

Microemulsions can accomodate a number of different microstructures, depending on the nature of the surfactants, the system composition, temperature, and presence of cosurfactants and cosolutes. For example, at low oil concentrations (ϕ), micelles swollen with oil constitute the microemulsion, whereas at high oil concentrations, water-swollen reversed micelles appear. Between these extremes, there may be a gradual structural progression, with the occurence of bicontinuous structures at intermediate composition (Figure 5.1).

When the interfacial area of a system increases, there is an energetic penalty for this related to the surface tension. When the surface tension is high, generation of new surface is highly energetically unfavorable. Hence, the system minimizes the surface area, which eventually results in macroscopic phase separation. Only when the surface tension is very low, this term opposing the generation of a large surface area (such as that in a microemulsion) becomes dominated by the entropy gain in this process and microemulsions form. Hence, microemulsion formation is intimately related to low interfacial tension (Figure 5.2).

For many nonionic surfactant systems, a sufficiently low surface tension may be obtained for the surfactant/oil/water systems without any further additions. For ionic surfactants, on the other hand, the surface tension lowering capacity is insufficient, and a cosurfactant must be added in order to achieve a dense packing at the interface and thereby reach a sufficiently low interfacial tension for microemulsion formation to occur.

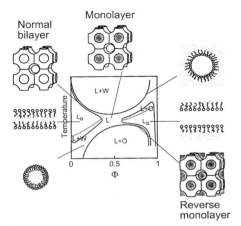

FIGURE 5.1 Schematic illustration on the gradual progression of the microstructure with the system composition for a microemulsion prepared from EO-containing nonionic surfactants. (Redrawn from Lindman et al., in Kumar et al., eds., Handbook of Microemulsion Science and Technology, Marcel Dekker, 1999.)

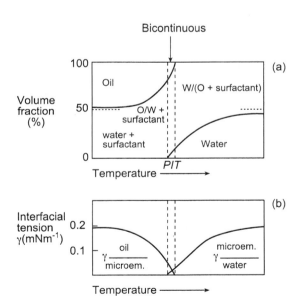

FIGURE 5.2 Relation between the oil-water surface tension and the occurrence of microemulsion in a typical nonionic surfactant system. (Redrawn from Saito et al., J. Colloid Interface Sci. 1970, 32, 642.)

5.1.3   Microemulsions Formed by Ionic Surfactants

Microemulsions formed by ionic surfactants were the first to be investigated, and are frequently prepared through titrating a intermediate-chain alcohol (a typical "cosurfactant") into the system until a clear solution is obtained (Figure 5.3).

The concentration and nature of the cosurfactant affects also the microstructures formed in the microemulsion system. For example, increasing the concentration of a long-chain cosurfactant results in a gradual transition from a swollen micellar solution via a bicontinuous structure to a system consisting of water-swollen reversed micelles. This is illustrated in Figure 5.4, in which the self-diffusion coefficient of water and oil is followed as a function of surfactant/alcohol ratio at fixed composition of the other components in the system. As can be seen, a low alcohol concentration yields a high water diffusion (just slightly lower than that of neat water) but a low oil diffusion. This clearly indicates that the system is water continuous and consisting of small swollen micelles (the size of which may be extracted from D_{oil} according to Eq. (9.1). At high alcohol concentrations, on the other hand, the situation is reversed, and the system consists of water-swollen micelles in oil. At intermediate alcohol concentrations, finally, fast diffusion of both water and oil molecules is observed, which means that the microemulsion is bicontinuous.

Thus, there is a progressive decrease in the curvature toward oil and at high alcohol concentrations an increasing curvature toward water with increasing

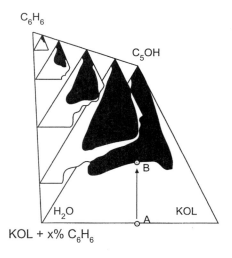

FIGURE 5.3 Generation of a microemulsion (dark area) in the potassium oleate (KOL)/water/benzene system may be achieved through titration of the system with *n*-pentanol from *A* to *B*. (Redrawn from Sjöblom et al., J. Colloid Interface Sci. 1978, 67, 16.)

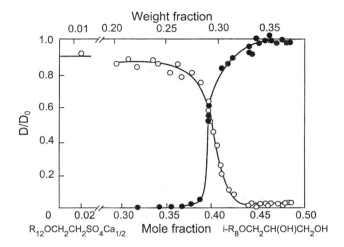

FIGURE 5.4 Relative self-diffusion coefficient (D/D_0) of water (open symbols) and oil (filled symbols) of the ratio between $R_{12}OCH_2CH_2SO_4Ca_{1/2}$ and $i\text{-}R_8OCH_2$-$CH(OH)CH_2OH$ in a system containing also 8 wt% $CaCl_2$ and decane. The system is tuned by the surfactant mixing ratio so that the system is water continuous at low $i\text{-}R_8$ and oil continuous at high $i\text{-}R_8$ fractions. (Redrawn from Lindman et al., J. Phys. Chem. 1988, 92, 4702.)

concentration of the long-chain alcohol. Naturally, this is analogous to the growth observed in micellar systems or the phase progression micellar → hexagonal → lamellar → reversed hexagonal → reversed micellar on addition of long-chain alcohols to ionic surfactants systems observed in micellar and liquid crystalline phases, respectively (see Chapters 2 and 3).

Also the nature of the cosurfactant greatly affects the microstructure of the microemulsions formed. This can be observed, e.g., by comparing the effect of the chain length of *n*-alcohols. As can be seen in Figure 5.5, increasing the length of the alcohol at a fixed composition results in a continuous decrease in the water self-diffusion, while the oil self-diffusion initially increases somewhat and then remains essentially constant. Hence, the longer the alcohol, the more small reversed structures are favored. Again, this is analogous to the general effects on the surfactant packing as discussed in Chapters 2 and 3.

Similarly, salt affects both the occurrence and microstructure of microemulsions in ionic microemulsion systems. In particular, the presence of salt promotes closer packing between the charged surfactant headgroups. Therefore, increasing the salt concentration in microemulsion systems formed by ionic surfactants results in a progression from water-continuous via bicontinuous to oil-continuous structures (Figure 5.6).

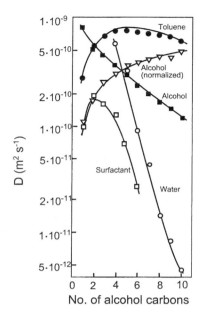

FIGURE 5.5 Self-diffusion of different components in a toluene-water-alcohol-SDS system as a function of the alcohol chain length. Open triangles refer to alcohol self-diffusion coefficients normalized with the bulk alcohol diffusion coefficient. (Redrawn from Lindman et al., Faraday Discuss. Chem. Soc. 1983, 76, 317.)

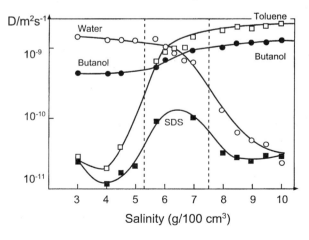

FIGURE 5.6 Self-diffusion of water, oil, surfactant, and cosurfactant for the system SDS-butanol-water-NaCl-toluene as a function of NaCl concentration. (Redrawn from Guering et al., Langmuir 1985, 1, 464.)

Figure 5.6 provides some information also about the diffusion properties of the surfactant and the cosurfactant. As can be seen, the surfactant diffusion is higher for the bicontinuous structure than for the water- and oil-continuous ones. This is expected, since for bicontinuous structures the surfactants can diffuse essentially freely in two dimensions, whereas for the disperse structures, the surfactant diffusion is limited by the diffusion of the droplets and the low surfactant concentration in the continuous phase. The diffusion of the cosurfactant, on the other hand, is less dependent of the microemulsion structure, and is fast for all salt compositions. This is due to this substance having a relatively good solubility in both the water and oil phases.

In the same way as cosurfactants are generally necessary for generating microemulsion systems in the case of ionic surfactants, their removal from such microemulsion systems causes destabilization of the latter. In particular, dilution with water of microemulsions formed by ionic surfactants in the presence of cosurfactant lowers the cosurfactant concentration and destabilizes the microemulsion, often resulting in a transition to an emulsion. This is important to keep in mind when using such systems in drug delivery, where the formulation is often diluted after administration as a result of the contact between the formulation and the body fluids.

5.1.4 Microemulsions Formed by Nonionic Surfactants

Nonionic surfactants are particularly interesting in relation to microemulsion formation. Thus, due to the absence of repulsive electrostatic interactions, the close packing of such surfactants in self-assembled structures and at interfaces favors a low surface tension, thereby allowing microemulsion formation also in the absence of cosurfactants. This also means that such microemulsion systems are often stable toward dilution, which is of obvious advantage in drug delivery applications. In the same way that salt-dependent effects have a generic influence on the structure of microemulsions formed by ionic surfactants, temperature plays a pivotal role for oligo(ethylene oxide)-containing microemulsions. In particular, due to a gradual dehydration of the oligo(ethylene oxide) chains with increasing temperature the polar head groups can pack more densely, resulting in, e.g., micellar growth and a progression toward structures less curved toward oil or more curved toward water (e.g., micellar → hexagonal → lamellar → reversed hexagonal → reversed micellar) with increasing temperature. Similarly, microemulsions formed by these systems go from normal micellar structures in water, over bicontinuous structures, to reversed micellar structures in oil. This can be clearly seen from the water self-diffusion, which decreases continuously from a value initially close to that in neat water with increasing temperature. The oil self-diffusion coefficient behaves in the opposite way (Figure 5.7).

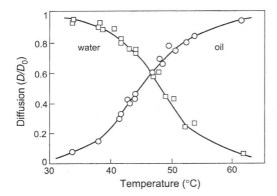

Figure 5.7 Self-diffusion of water and oil vs. temperature in the system $C_{12}E_5$-water-tetradecane. The system is tuned by temperature, and is water continuous at low temperature and oil continuous at high temperature. (Redrawn from Olsson et al., J. Phys. Chem. 1986, 90, 4083.)

In fact, for nonionic EO-based microemulsion systems, the combined effect of the oil phase and temperature may be observed in a nice way. As can be seen in Figure 5.8, increasing the oil content tends to favor reversed type of structures, which is a consequence simply of a larger oil volume needing to be accommodated in the system. Note, however, that little micellar growth occurs

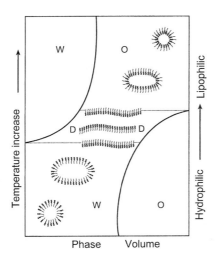

Figure 5.8 Schematic illustration of the combined effects of temperature and oil/water ratio on the phases and microstructures formed in nonionic microemulsion systems. (Redrawn from Shemoda, Progr. Colloid Polym. Sci. 1983, 68, 1.)

on increasing the content of the discontinuous phase, and therefore that o/w and w/o microemulsions are able to accommodate only a finite amount of oil and water, respectively, before phase separation occurs. Only in a rather narrow temperature range for a given surfactant system is the system able to accommodate a large range of oil/water ratios between 0 to 1. Such systems are referred to as being "balanced."

5.1.5 Incorporation of Drugs in Microemulsions

As with other types of surfactant and block copolymer systems, it is important to realize that the presence of a drug in a microemulsion may affect its stability and structure. For example, if the drug is soluble in water and charged, it behaves largely as a salt, and might therefore have a significant effect on the properties on microemulsions formed by ionic surfactants, whereas those formed by nonionic surfactants are less sensitive to the presence of the drug. For water-insoluble but oil-soluble drugs, on the other hand, the drug behaves essentially as an oil, thereby causing a progression of structures toward those less curved toward oil or more curved toward water for both ionic and nonionic surfactants. At higher concentration, phase separation may occur if the surfactant system is not balanced. For surface-active drugs, finally, the effect of the drug is determined by a delicate balance between different interactions. Nevertheless, addition of surface active drugs can be expected to have significant effect on the microemulsion stability and structure. An example of this is given in Figure 5.9 for sodium salicylate, which is found to stabilize the microemulsion for the particular system shown.

The amount of drug which can be incorporated into microemulsions depends on both the microemulsion structure and the properties of the drug. As discussed above, unless the microemulsion is completely balanced, an o/w microemulsion can only incorporate a certain fraction of oil or hydrophobic drug and a w/o microemulsion only a certain amount of water or a polar drug without phase separation. As an example of this, Figure 5.10 shows the maximum amount of the water-soluble drug hydrocortisone which can be incorporated in a w/o microemulsion formed by sodium stearate together with water, an *n*-alkane, and an *n*-alcohol. In particular, the maximum amount of hydrocortisone solubilized in the microemulsion decreases with an increasing length of the *n*-alcohol. Most likely, this is due to the decreased droplet size resulting from the presence of longer chain alcohols.

5.2 CHARACTERIZATION OF MICROEMULSIONS

5.2.1 Methods Based on Mass Transport

As with many other surfactant-containing systems, NMR constitutes a particularly interesting method for investigating microemulsion structures. As exempli-

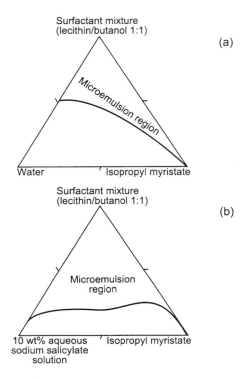

FIGURE 5.9 Pseudoternary phase diagrams at room temperature of quaternary systems containing lecithin, butanol, isopropyl myristate, and water (a) or a 10 wt% aqueous solution of sodium salicylate (b) at a lecithin/butanol ratio of 1/1. (Redrawn from Lawrence, Eur. J. Drug Metab. Pharmacokinet. 1994, 3, 257.)

fied above, NMR self-diffusion allows straightforward determination of whether the microemulsion consists of oil droplets in an aqueous continuum, of water droplets in an oil continuum, or a bicontinuous structure (Chapter 2). Moreover, from the oil and water self-diffusion in o/w and w/o systems, respectively, the droplet size (distribution) may be determined. Also, the self-diffusion of all components may be determined simultaneously, which is useful for understanding, e.g., the partitioning of the drug between the oil and the water phase, and hence for understanding drug release properties. Note, however, that a qualitative identification of w/o microemulsions can be done straightforwardly with as simple a method as conductivity measurements. Thus, for an o/w microemulsion, the conductivity is high, and comparable to that of the aqueous solution, whereas w/o microemulsions display a conductivity comparable to that of an oil (cf. Figure 6.8).

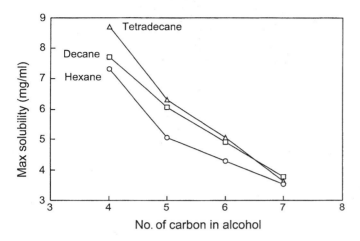

FIGURE 5.10 Maximum solubility of hydrocortisone in a microemulsion formed by sodium stearate/water/n-alkane/n-alcohol as a function of the chain length of the alcohol. The *n*-alkane used was hexane (circles), decane (squares), and tetradecane (triangles). (Redrawn from Jayakrishnan et al., J. Soc. Cosmet. Chem. 1983, 34, 335.)

5.2.2 Scattering Techniques

Due to the absence of long-range order in microemulsions, diffraction methods are not useful for microemulsion systems. Scattering of light, X-rays, and neutrons, on the other hand, is quite powerful for characterizing microemulsion structures. Parameters which may be determined with these techniques include, e.g.,

o/w (w/o)	Size of micelles
	Size of micellar core
	Thickness of palisade layer
	Micellar aggregation number
	Micellar water content (oil content)
	Micellar shape
Bicontinuous	Correlation length ξ (Figure 5.11)

Naturally, not all scattering techniques provide information on all these parameters. Also, some of the parameters above can only be obtained by so-called contrast matching, achieved, e.g., by balancing hydrogenated/deuterated component mixture (neutron scattering) in order to selectively observe a particular component or compartment in the system. Moreover, not all parameters may be determined simultaneously. For example, micellar size can generally only be determined assuming a particular micellar shape.

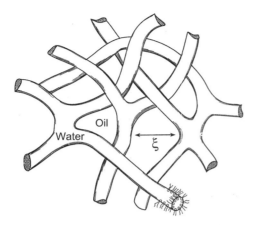

FIGURE 5.11 Schematic illustration of the physical meaning of the correlation length ξ in microemulsion systems. (Redrawn from Chen et al., J. Phys. Chem. 1986, 90, 842.)

5.3 DRUG RELEASE FROM MICROEMULSIONS

As discussed and exemplified above, structure has a major influence on the mass transport in microemulsion systems. This has implications also for the release of drugs incorporated in microemulsion systems. Specifically, for o/w microemulsions, the diffusion and hence the release of hydrophobic drugs is slow, whereas that of water-soluble drugs is high. For w/o microemulsions, on the other hand, the situation is the opposite.

Apart from the microemulsion structure, the drug release rate depends on the partitioning of the drug between the oil and water phases.* For this system, the release of steroid hormones of different lipophilicities from o/w microemulsions correlates closely to the partition coefficients of the hormones (Figure 5.13).

The effect of the drug oil/water partioning on the drug release rate therefore offers a possibility to control the drug release rate by changing the oil-water partitioning of the drug. Although the drug can be altered chemically in order to adjust its oil-water partitioning, there may also be simpler methods available. For example, charged amphiphilic drugs may be rendered largely oil-soluble but poorly water soluble by complexation with an oppositely charged excipient (fre-

---

* This is illustrated in Figures 5.12 and 5.13. Thus, on increasing the amount of butanol in a (o/w) microemulsion formed by Aerosol OT, isopropylmyristate, water, butanol, and betamethasone, the latter substance partitions increasingly toward the oil phase, which results in a decreased release rate, despite the droplet size decrease also caused by the increased butanol concentration.

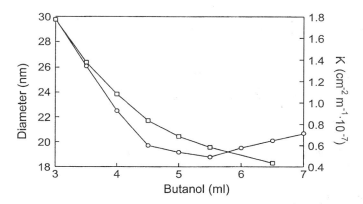

FIGURE 5.12 Effect of the concentration of butanol in a (o/w) microemulsion containing AOT, isopropyl myristate, water, and betamethasone, on the droplet diameter (circles) and permeation coefficient (*K*; squares) through a 1000 M_w cut-off membrane. (Redrawn from Trotta et al., Acta Pharm. Technol. 1990, 36, 226.)

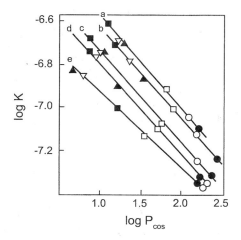

FIGURE 5.13 Correlation between the permeation coefficient *K* of steroid hormones of different lipophilicities from o/w microemulsions and their partition coefficients *P*. *a* = butanol, *b* = cyclopentanol, *c* = cyclohexanol, *d* = isobutanol, *e* = tert-amyl alcohol. Open triangles = hydrocortisone, filled triangles = prednisolone, filled squares = prednisone, open squares = betamethasone, open circles = hydrocortisone acetate, filled circles = prednisolone acetate. (Redrawn from Trotta et al., Acta Pharm. Technol. 1990, 36, 226.)

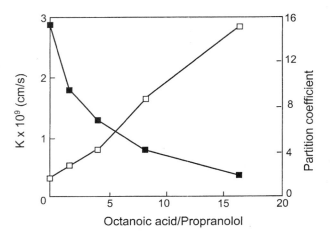

Octanoic acid/Propranolol

FIGURE 5.14 Isopropyl myristate/buffer partition coefficient (open squares) and permeability coefficient (K; filled squares) of propranolol over a hydrophilic membrane from Tween 60, isopropyl myristate, butanol, water microemulsions with varying octanoic acid/propranolol ratio. (Redrawn from Gasco et al., Int. J. Cosmet. Sci. 1988, 10, 263.)

quently called ion complexation). As an example of this, Figure 5.14 shows how ion-pair formation between propranolol and octanoic acid in o/w microemulsions effectively increases the lipophilicity of propranolol, and allows a sustained release of this drug.

The possibility to control the drug release rate by the microemulsion structure and composition, as well as by the drug partitioning, makes microemulsions of interest for sustained release applications. An example of this is given in Table 5.1.

5.4 MICROEMULSIONS IN DRUG DELIVERY

Microemulsions offer a range of advantages for drug delivery. Some of these are given in Table 5.2. There are numerous factors which in the general case may affect the absorption in vivo of a drug administered through a microemulsion formulation, e.g.,

- Microemulsion structure
- Partitioning of the drug between the water and oil phases
- Site or path of absorption
- Metabolism of the microemulsion oil
- Effect of the microemulsion on gastric emptying
- Possible absorption promotion caused by microemulsion excipients

TABLE 5.1 Half-Life Values of Technetium
Activity in Rabbits Injected with Technetium
in W/O Microemulsion or Aqueous Solution

Rabbit	Microemulsion	Aqueous solution
1	132	10.6
2	151	12.5
3	57*	17.9
4	46*	12.1
5	69*	9.8
6	122	8.2
7	189	9.2

* These animals showed biexponential decay; half-
lives reported are those of monoexponential func-
tions with the same intercept and the same blood
concentration vs. time integrals as those of the biexponential fit.
Source: From Bello et al., J. Pharm. Pharmacol.
1994, 46, 508.

So far, microemulsions have found use primarily in topical and oral administration, but also to some extent in other applications, such as buccal, occular,
and nasal drug delivery. On the other hand, the use of microemulsions in parenteral drug delivery is much less explored due to issues relating to the stability
of the microemulsion on dilution after intravenous administration, and toxicity
issues relating to the use of formulations containing high amounts of surfactants
in this administration route. This will be further discussed and exemplified below.

5.4.1 Microemulsions in Oral Administration

Due to rapid developments in protein engineering and to vast new knowledge
emerging on the human genome, peptide, protein, and other types of "biotechnological" drugs are becoming more important, a development which could be
expected to continue also in the future. Examples of such compounds include,
e.g., biomedical peptide hormones, synthetic peptides, enzyme substrates and
inhibitors. Ailments which may possibly be treated more efficiently with such
drugs include hypertension, mental disorders, autoimmune diseases, cancer, and
metabolic and cardiovascular diseases (Table 5.3).

Such drugs are generally formulated in a lyophilized form and administered
intravenously or through the nasal or pulmonary routes. In particular, intravenous
administration has been found to be efficient for administration of these types of
drugs. Other administration routes, on the other hand, frequently yield poor drug

TABLE **5.2** Pharmaceutical Advantages of Microemulsions

General advantages
Ease of preparation
Clarity
Stability
Ability to be filtered
Vehicle for drugs of different lipophilicities in the same system
Low viscosity (no pain on injection)
Specific advantages
Water-in-oil (w/o):
Protection of water soluble drugs
Sustained release of water soluble material
Increased bioavailability
Oil-in-water (o/w):
Increased solubility of lipophilic drugs
Sustained release of oil soluble material
Increased bioavailability
Bicontinuous:
Concentrated formulation of both oil and water soluble drugs

Source: From Lawrence, Eur. J. Drug Metab. Pharmacokinet. 1994, 3, 257.

bioavailability. Notably, peptide/protein absorption following oral administration may be very low indeed (Table 5.4).

The chemical degradation of the drug and inefficient absorption due to the large size of peptide/protein drugs generally pose the most substantial obstacles for a satisfactory bioavaliability after oral administration of such drugs (Figure 5.15). Thus, in order to be absorbed following oral administration, peptides and protein drugs must pass the physical absorption barrier of the gastrointestinal tract, consisting of mucus, apical and basal cell membranes and cell content, tight junctions, basement membrane, and the wall of the lymph and blood capillaries. Here, the size of protein and polypeptide drugs may cause problems regarding their oral absorption. Even more serious than the physical absorption barrier, however, is that of enzymatic activity in the intestinal tract. This enzymatic barrier is exceptionally well designed to digest peptides and proteins, and the susceptibility of the latter to enzymatic degradation is enhanced by oligopeptides containing several linkages, each of which may be susceptible to hydrolysis mediated by one or several peptidases (Table 5.5).

Ways to improve the oral bioavailability of peptide drugs include chemical modification (e.g., PEGylation), coadministration of absorption enhancers

TABLE 5.3 Some Examples of Proteins and Peptides and Their Possible
Function and Application

Peptide/protein	Function/application
Angiotensin II antagonist	Lowering of blood pressure
Atriopeptin	Regulation of cardiovascular function and electrolyte and fluid balance
Bradykinin	Improving peripheral circulation
Calcitonin gene-related factor	Vasodilatation
Cholecystokinin	Suppression of appetite
Colony stimulating factor	Stimulation of granulocyte differentiation
Delta sleep-inducing peptide (DSIP)	Improvement of disturbed sleep
β-Endorphin	Relief of pain
Gastrin antagonists	Reduction of gastric acid secretion
Growth hormone	Increase height in growth hormone deficient children
Histamine releasing factor	Control of histamine release from mast cells
Leutinizing hormone-releasing hormone	Induction of ovulation in women with hypo-thalamatic amenorrhea
Melanocyte inhibiting factor-I	Mood improvement in depressed patients
Melanocyte stimulating hormone	Improvement of attention span
Muramyl dipeptide	Stimulation of nonspecific resistance to bacterial infections
Nerve growth factor	Stimulation of nerve growth and repair
Neuropeptide Y	Control of feeding and drinking behavior
Neurotensin	Inhibition of gastric juice secretion
Somatostatin	Reduced bleeding of gastric ulcers
Tissue plasminogen activator	Dissolution of blood clots
Tumor necrosis factor	Control of polymorphonuclear function
Thyrotrophin releasing hormone	Prolonged infertility and lactation in women who are breast-feeding

Source: From Lee, Pharm. Int. 1986, 8, 208.

(e.g., EDTA, salicylates, surfactants, bile salts, and fatty acids), and coadministration of inhibitors to the peptide metabolism. Furthermore, since formulation
excipients can be used to improve on the unspecific uptake of drugs and since
drugs may be protected from biological and chemical degradation as discussed
also elsewhere in this volume, a proper choice of formulation offers some possibilities for improving the oral bioavailability of protein and peptide drugs.
Microemulsions have been found to constitute an interesting alternative in this
context.

As an example of how microemulsions can be successfully used in order

TABLE 5.4   Percent of Dose Absorbed from
Alternative Nonparenteral Routes of Administration

	Insulin ($M_w = 6000$)	Leuprolide ($M_w = 1210$)
Oral	0.05	0.05
Nasal	30	2–3
Buccal	0.5	—
Rectal	2.5	8
Vaginal	18	38
Subcutaneous	80	65

Source: From Lee, CRC Crit. Rev. Ther. Drug Carrier Syst.
1988, 5, 69.

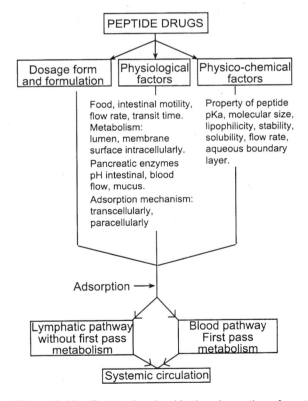

FIGURE 5.15   Factors involved in the absorption of peptide and protein drugs after
oral administration. (From Sarciaux et al., Int. J. Pharm. 1995, 120, 127.)

TABLE 5.5 Half-Life of Proteins/
Peptides in Illeal Homogenates

Protein/peptide	Half-life (min)
YGGFM	15.1 ± 2.0
YGGFL	20.8 ± 1.5
YAGFM	226.5 ± 1.5
Substance P	5.8 ± 0.2
Insulin	98.1 ± 6.4
Proinsulin	55.7 ± 7.0

Source: From Lee, CRC Crit. Rev. Ther.
Drug Carrier Syst. 1988, 5, 69.

to improve the bioavailability of protein and peptide drugs after administration to the gastrointestinal tract, Figures 5.16 and 5.17 show the plasma concentration of SK&F-106760, a water-soluble RGD fibrinogen receptor antagonist, as a function of time after intraduodenal administration. As can be seen, the plasma concentration of SK&F-106760 after administration from a microemulsion formula-

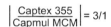

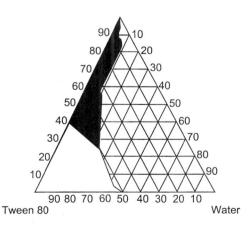

FIGURE 5.16 Partial phase diagram for the system oil (Captex 355/Capmul MCM)/ Tween 80/water at ambient temperature. The w/o microemulsions spans the shaded area. The system used for the evaluation of the absorption enhancement (Figure 5.17) was from the upper part of the dark field. (Redrawn from Constantinides et al., Pharm. Res. 1994, 11, 1385.)

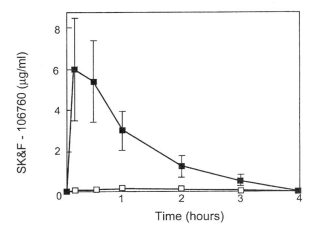

FIGURE 5.17 Plasma concentration of SK&F-106760 as a function of time after intraduodenal administration from an aqueous solution (open symbols) or a microemulsion (filled symbols). (Redrawn from Constantinides et al., Pharm. Res. 1994, 11, 1385.)

tion (stability area indicated in Figure 5.16) is significantly higher than that found for the corresponding aqueous solution over the entire time-span investigated, thus indicating a significantly higher bioavailability for the microemulsion formulation. Clearly, the microemulsion protects SK&F-106760 from degradation.

However, as will be discussed more extensively in Chapter 8 in relation to complex formation between surfactants and polymers, surfactants may bind to protein and peptide drugs, thereby causing conformational changes of the latter, and hence also risking to affect the protein and peptide biological activity. Care must therefore be taken to avoid biological activity loss when formulating peptide and protein drugs also in microemulsion systems.

Naturally, not only peptide and protein drugs can be sensitive to degradation in the gastrointestinal tract limiting their absorption. Instead, both ester-containing and other synthetic and ''biotechnological'' drugs may undergo extensive acid-catalyzed hydrolysis at the very low pH present in the stomach. Also, for such compounds, (w/o) microemulsions may offer an interesting alternative for oral drug delivery.

One area within oral drug delivery where microemulsions are of interest is administration of sparingly soluble hydrophobic drugs. Thus, it is commonly found that on oral administration of such substances a low and strongly varying uptake occurs. The latter depends significantly on a number of factors, e.g., gender, age, weight, state of feeding/fasting, and bile. This inter- and intrasubject variability poses considerable difficulties in a therapeutic situation, since the plasma concentration frequently varies considerably, and may result in insufficient bioavailability for the required drug action, or, if the dose is increased, in an occasional too high concentration, the latter increasing the risk for occurrence of detrimental side effects.

Cyclosporine (Figure 5.18) is a potent immunosuppressive agent which is used to prolong allograft survival in organ transplantation, and in the treatment of patients with certain autoimmune diseases. Following oral administration, the absorption of cyclosporine is incomplete, typically amounting to about 30% of the dose or less. The absorption is also highly variable, and affected by physiological and pharmaceutical factors such as bile, food, and drug delivery vehicle.

Unlike many other oligopeptides, cyclosporine is not extensively degraded by enzymatic action. Instead, its limited bioavailability following oral administration is due to its poor absorption, which in turn originates from the high molecular weight and lipophilicity of the substance. Therefore, the bioavailability of cyclosporine may be improved by coadministration of absorption enhancers, e.g., in the form of a crude emulsion. This results not only in an improvement of the

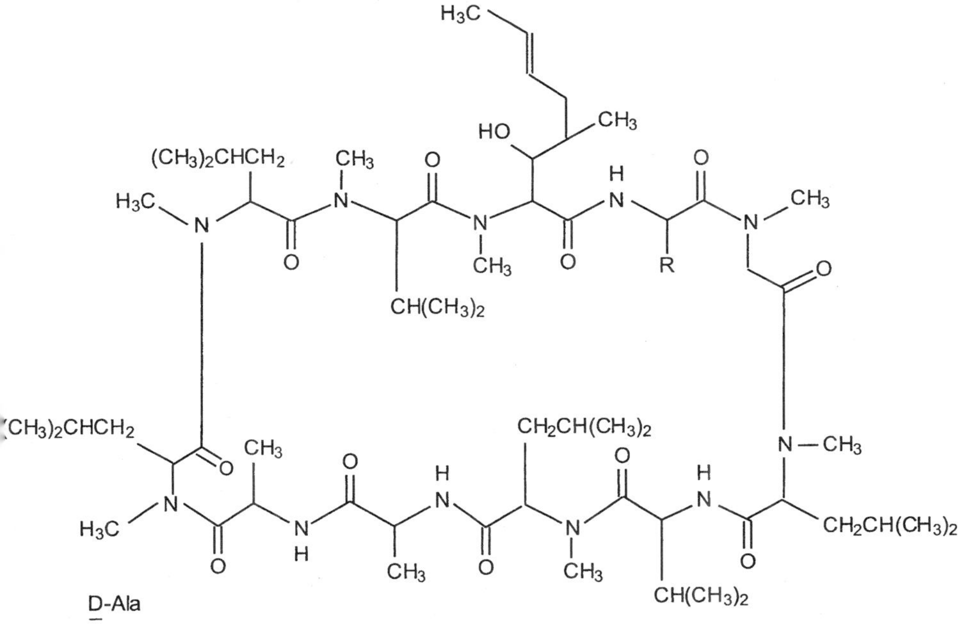

FIGURE 5.18 Molecular structure of cyclosporine.

cyclosporine bioavailability but also in a decreased variability. By reducing the droplet size of the emulsion formulation, it is possible to further enhance the intestinal absorption (Chapter 6).

Given the increased absorption with decreasing droplet size following oral administration of cyclosporine in emulsions, the use of microemulsions for this purpose should be advantageous. Indeed, by use of a microemulsion formulation the bioavailability of cyclosporine can be further improved compared with the emulsion formulation, at the same time the pharmacokinetic variability is reduced (see Figures 5.19 and 5.20, as well as Table 5.6).

5.4.2 Microemulsions for Topical Administration

The human skin is a vital and complex tissue, which simplistically can be seen as consisting of several layers. The outermost layer of of the skin, the epidermis, is also layered. Of particular interest to topical drug delivery is the outermost layer of the epidermis, the stratum corneum, which consists of keratin-rich dead cells embedded in a lipid matrix (Figure 5.21).

The most important function of the stratum corneum is to act as a barrier and to limit transdermal transport, with the overall aim to protect the body from chemical and biological attack and to to prevent dehydration. The lipids, which only constitute about 10% of the stratum corneum, seem to be particularly impor-

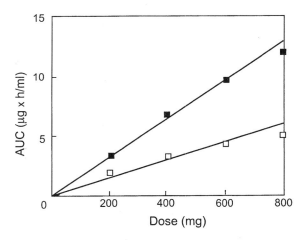

FIGURE 5.19   Relationship between cyclosporine bioavailability, given as AUC (integral of the blood concentration versus time curve), and dose after oral administration of a crude emulsion (open symbols) or a microemulsion formulation (filled symbols) to healthy volunteers. (Redrawn from Mueller et al., Pharm. Res. 1994, 11, 301.)

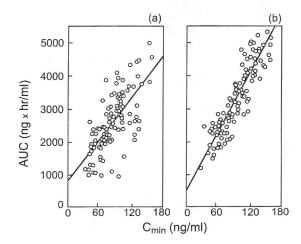

FIGURE 5.20 Correlation between the cyclosporine C_{min} (measured blood concentration 12 hours after administration) and AUC during steady-state oral treatment with an emulsion (a) and microemulsion (b) formulation. The solid lines are regression fits. (From Kovarik et al., Transplantation 1994, 58, 658.)

TABLE 5.6 Comparison of Intraindividual Variability of the Steady-State Pharmacokinetic Parameters of Cyclosporine in the Emulsion and Microemulsion Formulation

Parameter	Emulsion (%)	Microemulsion (%)
C_{min}	20	14
t_{max}	74	22
C_{max}	33	15
AUC	18	10
%PFT	27	14

C_{min} = measured blood concentration 12 h after administration.
t_{max} = time between administration and maximum blood concentration.
C_{max} = highest measured blood concentration.
AUC = area under the blood concentration versus time curve.
%PFT = Pitman-Morgan procedure comparing the variances of replicate determinations between formulations.
Source: From Kovarik et al., Transplantation 1994, 58, 658.

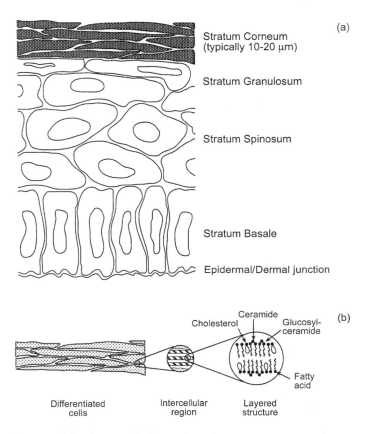

FIGURE 5.21   Schematic illustration of the epidermis and the stratum corneum.

tant for its function. These are arranged partly in layered structures, and it has therefore been inferred that it is the stucture of the lipid self-assemblies which governs the barrier properties. Consequently, surfactant-based formulations, which may interact with the lipids in the stratum corneum and alter their structure, offer a way to modify this protective barrier, and specifically to reach an enhanced drug penetration over the stratum corneum and result in an improved bioavailability following topical administration.

There are numerous examples where an improved bioavailability of topically administered drugs has been reached through the use of microemulsions. As an illustration of this, Figure 5.22 shows results on the transdermal penetration of scopolamine from a w/o microemulsion formulation. As can be seen, a significantly higher transport rate can be obtained for transdermally administered

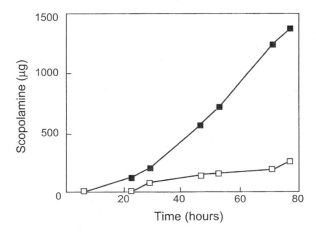

Figure 5.22   Transport of scopolamine through human skin from a lecithin-isopropyl palmitate-water microemulsion (filled squares) and from an aqueous buffer solution (open squares). (Redrawn from Willimann et al., J. Pharm. Sci. 1992, 81, 871.)

scopolamine for the microemulsion formulation than for an aqueous solution at the same concentration.

The origin of the advantageous effects of microemulsions for topical drug delivery is not entirely understood. However, since microemulsions are usually quite efficient in solubilizing hydrophobic as well as hydrophilic substances, it is likely that microemulsions can disrupt the lipid structures of stratum corneum. On the downside, this results in a potential risk of skin irritation, which may depend on both the solubilizing capacity of the surfactants and the structure formed at the skin after evaporation of water and other volatile components (e.g., whether a lamellar liquid crystalline phase or a reversed structure phase, is formed).

5.4.3   Other Administration Routes for Microemulsions

Buccal Administration

Drug delivery to the oral cavity is frequently based on a in situ thickening system, e.g., based on a phase transition in surfactant and block copolymer systems. Also here, microemulsions or micellar solutions with a hydrophobic drug incorporated in the micelles have found use as easily injectable systems, which on entering the oral cavity undergo a transition into a liquid crystalline phase. This is discussed in some detail in Chapter 3.

Parenteral Administration

Although microemulsions offer opportunities in a number of drug delivery applications, there are several potential difficulties relating to the use of microemulsions in parenteral administration. In particular, the high surfactant concentration generally present in such systems results in a risk for toxicity-related effects, which severly limit the type of surfactants that can be used in the formation of such systems. Furthermore, many microemulsions containing cosurfactants are not stable on dilution with water. On intravenous administration of such a system, therefore, there is a risk for phase separation, possibly resulting in emboli formation. Hence, safe intravenous use of such systems demands knowledge on what happens to the microemulsion on dilution with blood.

Nevertheless, microemulsions have indeed been found promising also for this administration route. As an illustration of this, Table 5.7 shows results with a bicontinuous microemulsion system composed of medium-chain triglyceride, soybean phosphatidylcholine, and poly(ethylene glycol)(660)-12-hydroxystearate (12-HSA-EO15). On dilution with water, this microemulsion is transformed into an emulsion phase, i.e., there is a spontaneous in situ emulsification. The emulsion droplets generated in this process are of a size acceptable for intravenous applications. Furthermore, it has been found that this particular microemulsion formulation can be administered up to 0.5 ml/kg of the microemulsion (oil weight fraction 50%) without significant detrimental effects on the acid-base balance, blood gases, plasma electrolytes, mean arterial blood pressure, heart rate, and time lag between depolarization of atrium and chamber. Therefore, it seems

TABLE 5.7 Mean Droplet Diameter and Polydispersity Index of O/W Emulsions Resulting from Dilution by Water of a Microemulsion Consisting of a Medium-Chain Triglyceride, Soybean Phosphatidylcholine, and Poly(ethylene glycol)(660)-12-hydroxystearate, Poly(ethylene glycol) 400, and Ethanol

Oil weight fraction	Diameter (nm)	Polydispersity index
0.06	187.9	0.54
0.21	65.8	0.32
0.38	67.8	0.23
0.60	105.3	0.08
0.72	132.5	0.19

Source: From von Corswant et al., J. Pharm. Sci. 1998, 87, 200.

that also for intravenous administration, microemulsion-based formulations may indeed have some potential.

BIBLIOGRAPHY

Attwood, D., in J. Kreuter, ed., Colloidal Drug Delivery Systems, Marcel Dekker, New York, 1994.

Bourrel, M., R. S. Schechter, eds., Microemulsions and Related Systems. Formulation, Solvency, and Physical Properties, Surfactant Science Series, vol. 30, Marcel Dekker, New York, 1988.

Drewe, J., R. Meier, J. Vonderscher, D. Kiss, U. Posanski, T. Kissel, K. Gyr, Enhancement of the oral absorption of cyclosporin in man, Br. J. Clin. Pharmac. 34:60–64 (1992).

Evans, D. F., H. Wennerström, The Colloidal Domain, Wiley, New York, 1999.

Jones, N. M., Surfactants in membrane solubilisation, Int. J. Pharm. 177:137–159 (1999).

Jönsson, B., B. Lindman, K. Holmberg, B. Kronberg, Surfactants and Polymers in Aqueous Solution, Wiley, New York, 1998.

Kovarik, J. M., E. A. Mueller, J. B. van Bree, W. Tetzloff, K. Kutz, Reduced inter- and intraindividual variability in cyclosporine pharmacokinetics form a microemulsion formulation, J. Pharm. Sci. 83:444–446 (1994).

Kovarik, J. M., E. A. Mueller, J. B. van Bree, S. S. Flückiger, H. Lange, B. Schmidt, W. H. Boesken, A. E. Lison, K. Kutz, Cyclosporine pharmacokinetics and variability from a microemulsion formulation—a multicenter investigation in kidney transplant patients, Transplantation 58:658–663 (1994).

Kumar, P., K. L. Mittal, eds., Handbook of Microemulsion Science and Technology, Marcel Dekker, New York, 1999.

Lee, V. H. L., Enzymatic barriers to peptide and protein absorption, CRC Crit. Rev. Ther. Drug Carrier Syst. 5:69–97 (1988).

Mueller, E. A., J. M. Kovarik, J. B. van Bree, W. Tetzloff, J. Grevel, K. Kutz, Improved dose linearity in cyclosporine pharmacokinetics from a microemulsion formulation, Pharm. Res. 11:301–304 (1994).

Shaw, D. O., ed., Micelles, Microemulsions and Monolayers, Marcel Dekker, New York, 1998.

Tenjarla, S., Microemulsions: An overview and pharmaceutical applications, Crit. Rev. Ther. Drug Carrier Syst. 16:461–521 (1999).

6

Emulsions

Despite their finite stability, emulsions have several advantages as drug delivery systems. For example, they offer opportunities for solubilizing relatively large amounts of hydrophobic substances, with advantages relating to, e.g., the effective drug solubility, the drug release rate, and the drug chemical stability. Furthermore, the amount surfactant required for generating and stabilizing emulsions is generally quite low, and relatively nontoxic surfactants, such as phospholipids and other polar lipids, as well as block copolymers, can be used as emulsifiers/stabilizers.

6.1 FORMATION OF EMULSIONS

Since oil and water do not mix, oil-water mixtures eventually separate into two macroscopic phases. Thus, contrary to microemulsions, emulsions are thermodynamically unstable systems. In order to form emulsions which are useful for drug delivery, their kinetic destabilization must generally be slowed down by the use of different surface active agents. These may also help forming the emulsion, and to reach a sufficiently small droplet size.

   The formation of emulsion systems is a complex process which involves generation and stabilization of new oil-water interface. In drug delivery, high-pressure homogenization is frequently used for generating new surface, and for producing emulsion droplets. Within high-pressure homogenization, the liquid mixture is passed through a chamber where turbulent motions are generated. This, in turn, generates shear forces, which "tear appart" any larger entities in the system, and result in droplet formation. With increasing pressure used in the homogenization process the shear forces increase, which results in the formation of smaller droplets (Figures 6.1 and 6.2). Of course, the effect of pressure depends also on the geometry of the homogenization chamber.

Furthermore, since the high-pressure homogenization is usually performed in a flow system, where the system passes through the high pressure chamber, the latter is only exposed to the shear forces for a limited time. Therefore, exposing the system to the shear forces for a prolonged time results in a more efficient homogenization. Practically, this is achieved by passing the system through the homogenization chamber a number of times. Consequently, with an

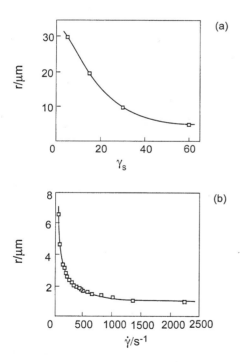

FIGURE 6.1   Dependence of the drop radius r on the shear strain amplitude γ_s (a) and steady shear rate $\dot{\gamma}$ (b). The o/w emulsion consisted of nonylphenol heptaethoxylate/water/PDMS at an oil volume fraction of 0.7. (Redrawn from Mason et al., Phys. Rev. Lett. 1996, 77, 3481 and Langmuir 1997, 13, 4600.)

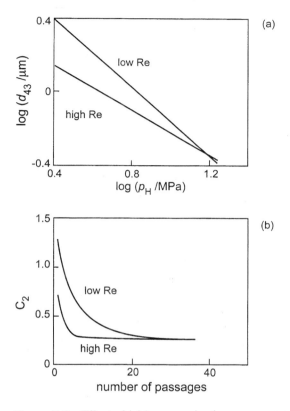

FIGURE 6.2 Effect of (a) homogenization pressure p_H on the emulsion droplet size d_{43} and (b) the number of passages on the width of the droplet size distribution c_2 of the emulsion formed. Results obtained with two high-pressure homogenizers are shown, one very small (low Re) and one large (high Re). (Redrawn from Walstra et al., in Binks, ed., Modern Aspects of Emulsion Science, The Royal Society of Chemistry, 1998.)

increasing number of passages, the droplet size generally decreases and becomes more uniform.

If the droplets generated in the homogenization process are not stabilized, they will almost momentarily coalesce to two macroscopic phases, since this reduces the free energy associated with the surface area. In order to stabilize emulsion droplets, surface active components such as surfactants, polymers or proteins are added. While the long-term stabilization puts certain requirements on these stabilizers, as discussed below and also in Chapter 9, the emulsification process as such requires relatively fast transport of the surface active component to newly generated surface. This, in turn, makes particularly low molecular weight surfactants useful as emulsifiers. The role of the surfactant in the emulsification process is therefore:

1. To reduce the interfacial tension and thereby promote droplet formation (the free energy increase of forming new surface is directly proportional to the interfacial tension)
2. To stabilize emulsion droplets from flocculation and coalescence

Surfactants generally display an adsorption at oil-water interfaces which is low at low concentrations, increases monotonously with increasing surfactant concentration, and levels off at the cmc. In parallel, the interfacial tension decreases monotonously with increasing surfactant concentration until it reaches the cmc, where it levels off. This concentration-dependent surfactant adsorption and interfacial tension reduction facilitates emulsification, as seen by a decreasing emulsion droplet size (or increasing the specific surface area A). In fact, there is a direct relation between the size of the emulsion droplets formed during emulsification, on one hand, and the oil-water interfacial tension in the presence of the emulsifier, on the other (Figure 6.3).

Note, however, that interfacial tension measurements generally relate to equilibrium conditions. In the emulsification process, on the other hand, the situation is highly dynamic. Therefore, not only the equilibrium adsorption and interfacial tension but also the adsorption kinetics and the dynamic surface tension behav-

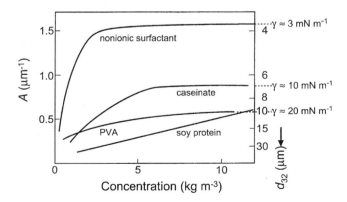

FIGURE 6.3 Specific droplet surface area A and average droplet size d_{32} as a function of emulsifier concentration at an oil volume fraction of 0.2. Plateau values of the interfacial tension are also given. (Redrawn from Walstra et al., in Dickinson et al., eds., Food Colloids: Proteins, Lipids and Polysaccharides, The Royal Society of Chemistry, 1997.)

ior are of importance for emulsification processes. In particular, sufficiently fast mass transport to newly formed oil-water interface and following surface tension reduction is required for reaching an efficient emulsification. This is the reason why proteins and high molecular weight polymers, which are frequently very good stabilizers of preformed emulsions, are generally not very efficient emulsifiers.

As an illustration of the latter, Figure 6.4 shows the effective "adsorption" isotherms for a protein stabilizer (β-casein) in emulsions and at a macroscopic oil-water interface. As can be seen, much higher concentrations are needed to reach a high adsorption for the emulsion system than for the corresponding macroscopic surface in the case of β-casein. The reason for this is the insufficient adsorption time for the protein in the emulsification process. For a low molecular weight emulsifier (SDS), on the other hand, identical adsorption isotherms are obtained for the emulsion and the macroscopic interface, showing that in this case the adsorption is sufficiently fast in order to reach surface saturation also in the emulsification process.

Due to the deformability of emulsion droplets in a shear field, and a finite mass transport even of low molecular weight surfactants, there is ample opportunity during the emulsification process for creation of surfactant concentration gradients at the oil-water interface. This, in turn, allows for a number of different processes to occur, essentially instantaneously (Figure 6.5).

Both in drug delivery and in other contexts, the term "spontaneous emulsification" is used for some systems. True spontaneous emulsification leads to the

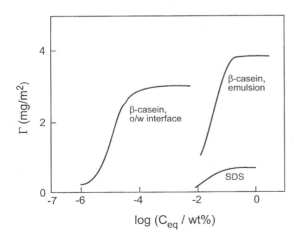

FIGURE 6.4 Adsorption of β-casein and SDS at a macroscopic interface and in an emulsion. (Redrawn from Walstra et al., in Binks, ed., Modern Aspects of Emulsion Science, The Royal Society of Chemistry, 1998.)

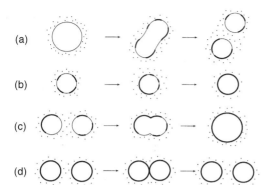

FIGURE 6.5 Schematic illustration of processes occuring during emulsification related to surfactant interfacial gradients. Processes illustrated are *a*: droplet breakage, *b*: gradient relaxation, *c*: coalescence, and *d*: droplet stabilization. (Redrawn from Walstra et al., in Dickinson et al., eds., Food Colloids: Proteins, Lipids and Polysaccharides, The Royal Society of Chemistry, 1997.)

formation of microemulsions, but this is generally not what is intended. Instead, such ''spontaneous emulsification'' generally results in droplets with a size typical for emulsion systems. The origin of sponatenous emulsification is the following: If two liquids (phase 1 and 2) are both good solvents for a surfactant, but the solubility in phase 2 is better than that in phase 1, but the surfactant initially is present only in phase 1, the difference in chemical potential of the surfactant in the two phases results in an unstable system. If the interfacial tension between the two phases is sufficiently low, the occurrence of minor turbulence may cause surfactant gradients, which in turn may lead to small droplets of phase 1 breaking off into phase 2 (Figure 6.6).

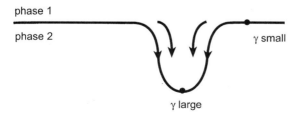

FIGURE 6.6 Schematic illustration of the mechanism of "spontaneous emulsification." Phase 1 originally contains the surfactant, which, however, is more soluble in phase 2. (Redrawn from Walstra et al., in Binks, ed., Modern Aspects of Emulsion Science, The Royal Society of Chemistry, 1998.)

6.2 STRUCTURE OF EMULSIONS

The type of emulsion formed (e.g., w/o or o/w) depends on a number of factors, including the surfactant, the oil and water volume fraction, temperature, salt concentration, and the presence of cosurfactants and other cosolutes. In particular, the "hydrophobicity" of the surfactant plays a major role in determining the type of emulsion formed. This is summarized in the so called Bancroft's rule, which says that the phase in which the emulsifier is most soluble will be the continuous phase after emulsification. From a practical perspective this means that extensively water-soluble surfactants (high HLB; see Chapter 3) favor formation of o/w emulsions, whereas hydrophobic surfactants which are readily soluble in the oil phase but not so in the aqueous phase (i.e., with a low HLB number) form w/o emulsions (Figure 6.7).

There are many ways to discriminate o/w and w/o emulsions. Particularly straightforward and not experimentally demanding is simply to measure the electrical conductivity in the system. Thus, while the conductivity in water-continuous emulsions is high even at quite high oil volume fractions, w/o emulsions display orders of magnitude lower conductivity even at high water content (Figure 6.8).

6.3 PHASE INVERSION OF EMULSIONS

An important feature of emulsions is the so called phase inversion displayed by such systems. By this we mean the transition from a water-continuous o/w emul-

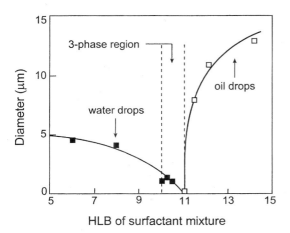

FIGURE 6.7 Effect of the HLB of the surfactant mixture (nonylphenol ethoxylates) on the emulsion structure as probed by droplet size measurements. (Redrawn from Brooks et al., Chem. Eng. Sci. 1994, 49, 1053.)

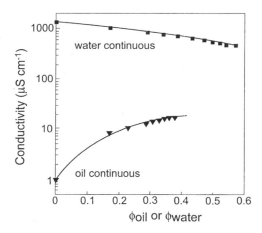

FIGURE 6.8 Conductivity of o/w and w/o emulsions as a function of volume fraction φ of the discontinuous phase. (Redrawn from Smith et al., Langmuir 1994, 10, 2516.)

sion to an oil-continuous w/o emulsion, or vice versa, on changing some parameter, such as the surfactant mixture composition, temperature, or the salt concentration. The dramatic effects this may have on transport-related properties (such as conductivity or drug release rate) is illustrated in Figure 6.9 for an emulsion

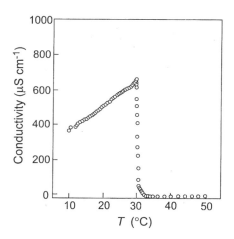

FIGURE 6.9 Effect of temperature on the conductivity for a heptane-water emulsion stabilized by $C_{12}E_5$. Note, that the system undergoes a transition from water continuous to oil continuous at 30°C. (Redrawn from Binks, Langmuir 1993, 9, 25.)

stabilized by $C_{12}E_5$ undergoing phase inversion from o/w to w/o at a critical temperature (the so called phase inversion temperature, PIT).

The phase inversion in emulsion systems is related to the packing of the surfactants at the interface. In analogy to micellar, liquid crystalline, and micro-emulsion systems, nonionic EO-containing surfactants favor cruvature toward the oil at low temperature, and toward water at elevated temperature. This, in turn, results in o/w emulsions at low temperature and w/o emulsions at elevated temperature. At a given intermediate temperature, planar interfaces are favored, resulting in a structural transition for emulsion systems. Naturally, this is completely analogous to the temperature-dependent surfactant packing in other types of surfactant structures (cf. Chapters 2, 3, and 5). Not entirely unexpected, the phase inversion temperature, with its high surfactant packing density, is also characterized by a very low oil-water interfacial tension (Figure 6.10).

The phase inversion conditions also depend on the composition of both the aqueous phase, the surfactant mixture used for emulsification, and the oil phase. For example, addition of moderate to high salt concentrations affects the solvency conditions for EO-containing nonionic surfactants (cf. Chapters 2 and 3). In a similar manner, addition of salt affects the phase inversion temperature. As is the case also for other nonionic surfactant systems, such salt effects are mainly lyotropic in nature and occur first at rather high salt concentrations (Figure 6.11).

Also, the nature of the oil affects the PIT in nonionic surfactant systems (Figure 6.12). The main origin of this is the relative solubility of the surfactant

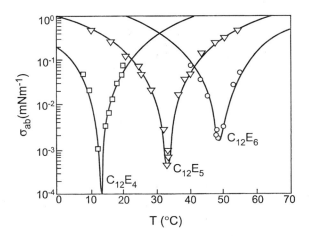

FIGURE 6.10 Temperature-dependent water-octane interfacial tension σ_{ab} at $c >$ cmc for a few $C_{12}E_n$ surfactants. (Redrawn from Sottmann et al., J. Chem. Phys. 1997, 106, 8606.)

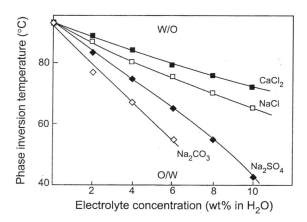

FIGURE 6.11 Effect of salt on the phase inversion temperature of a water-heptane emulsion stabilized by a nonylphenol surfactant. (Redrawn from Shinoda et al., J. Colloid Interface Sci. 1970, 32, 642.)

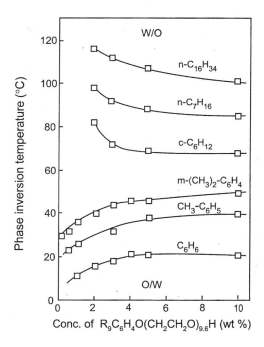

FIGURE 6.12 Effect of the hydrocarbon structure on the PIT shown by 1:1 oil: water emulsions stabilized by a nonylphenol ethoxylate surfactant. (Redrawn from Shinoda et al., J. Phys. Chem. 1964, 68, 3485.)

in the water and the oil phases. According to Bancroft's rule, for w/o emulsions to be favored (i.e, for the PIT to be low), the surfactant should be readily soluble in the oil phase, and in fact more soluble in the oil phase than in the water phase. This is illustrated in Figure 6.12, showing that in the case of aromatics, benzene, for example, in which the nonylphenol ethoxylate surfactant is readily soluble, displays a low PIT, whereas long-chain alkanes, such as hexadecane, in which the surfactant has a limited solubility, are characterized by a high PIT.

In a similar way that the structure of nonionic surfactants affects their self-assembly to form micelles, liquid crystalline phases, and microemulsions, it affects the PIT of emulsions. Specifically, with increasing length of the polar head group and/or decreasing size of the hydrophobic part, aggregates curved toward the oil become relatively more favored. An analogous behavior is observed in emulsion systems, in that o/w emulsions are relatively more favored over a larger temperature range for surfactants with a large polar head group and a small hydrophobic part (i.e., more hydrophilic surfactants), whereas w/o emulsions are favored by more hydrophobic surfactants. Expressed in the vocabulary generally used for emulsions, the higher the HLB, the higher the PIT, and vice versa (Figure 6.13).

Another type of temperature-dependent emulsions of interest in relation to drug delivery are those stabilized by phospholipids. The latter are efficient emulsifiers and stabilizers since their molecular structure generally favors close to planar packing (as in larger emulsion droplets), and since they exert hydration force stabilization of emulsion droplets. They are also of natural origin and well

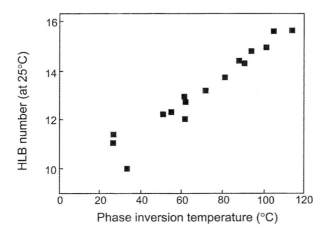

FIGURE 6.13 Correlation between HLB and PIT for water-cyclohexane emulsions stabilized with nonionic surfactants. (Redrawn from Shinoda et al., Emulsions and Solubilization, Wiley, 1986.)

tolerated in various drug delivery applications. Often, pharmaceutical emulsions are prepared from technical lecithins, the composition of which depends on the origin, but which generally is dominated by PC (Figure 1.9) followed by PE, PI, PA, and PS and lysophosphatides, the latter two in minor quantities. Also pure PC and fractions thereof are used sometimes for emulsification and emulsion stabilization.

An important aspect to consider for phospholipid emulsifiers is the chain melting temperature. As discussed also in Chapter 4, the hydrophobic chains are in a liquidlike state above the chain melting temperature, but "frozen" below this temperature. Since an efficient emulsification requires fast transport to the newly created interface and packing there, temperatures below the chain melting temperature are detrimental for emulsification. Therefore, emulsification should preferably be performed above the chain transition temperature. This means that the longer and more saturated the phospholipid, the higher the emulsification temperature required (Figure 6.14).

At high temperature, on the other hand, there may also be detrimental effects, e.g., relating to Ostwald ripening (see below), chemical degradation of compounds incorporated in the emulsion, etc. Partly for this reason, but also due to cost issues, phospholipids used for drug delivery are often technical lecithin mixtures. Since these contain a distribution of chain lengths and saturation, and also minor fractions of charged phospholipids, the chain melting temperature is generally considerably lower for such lecithins than for the pure phospholipid components.

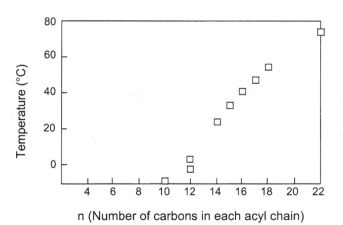

FIGURE 6.14 Effect of chain length on the main transition temperature for phosphatidylcholine. (Redrawn from Small, Handbook of Lipid Research, Plenum Press, 1986.)

6.4   RHEOLOGY OF EMULSIONS

The rheology of emulsion systems is of some general interest in drug delivery. In some applications, a high viscosity and shear resistance is desired (e.g., ointments and creams), whereas in others, e.g., injectable emulsions, a low viscosity is required for practical administration reasons and for reduction of pain for the patient. As with other types of disperse systems, the rheological properties of emulsion systems depend critically on the volume fraction of the disperse phase. However, the most abundant phase is not necessarily the continuous one. Instead, the emulsion structure is given largely by the relative solubility of the surfactant in the two phases. It is therefore possible to have, e.g., a water-continuous emulsion containing 90% oil and less than 10% water (Figure 6.15).

The viscosity of emulsions is relatively insensitive to the volume fraction of the disperse phase up to rather high volume fractions. Only at volume fractions of the order 0.3–0.5 does the viscosity increase more dramatically (Figure 6.16). The onset of the viscosity increase is a result of an increasing degree of "close packing" of the droplets, and hence depends on both the droplet size distribution

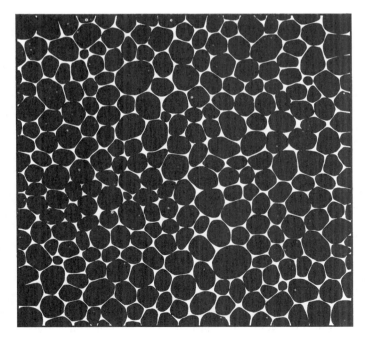

FIGURE 6.15 Schematic illustration of an emulsion where the volume fraction of the disperse phase is high.

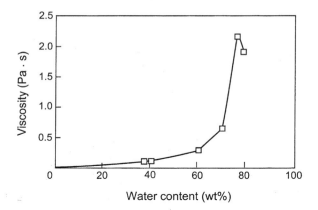

FIGURE 6.16 Viscosity of a w/o emulsion containing PEG7-hydrogenated castor oil/dicaprylyl ether/decyl oleate/MgSO$_4$ as a function of water content (i.e., water droplet volume fraction). (Redrawn from Förster et al., Cosmet. Toiletries. 1997, 112, 73.)

and on the interaction between the emulsion droplets. For example, for very poly-disperse droplets, increasing the droplet concentration without causing a major viscosity increase is facilitated. For droplets stabilized by thick polymer layers or through long-range electrostatic interactions, on the other hand, the viscosity increase with increasing droplet concentration is more pronounced.

Such "self-thickened" emulsion systems (e.g., w/o systems containing 65–80% water) are commonly used in cosmetic and topical drug delivery applications. Even more concentrated emulsions may be prepared, and for certain systems the volume fraction of the disperse phase may be as large as 0.99! Due to the gel-like consistency of such systems, they are frequently referred to as "emulsion gels." An attractive feature with such systems is that they are frequently transparent, which may offer opportunities in, e.g., periodontal anesthesia, and in dermal or occular drug delivery. Also, such systems are interesting for drug delivery due to their capacity to incorporate both water-soluble and oil-soluble drugs. With increasing volume fraction of the discontinuous phase, the release of substances incorporated in this increases. The diffusion and release of a compound from emulsion gels will also depend on its partitioning between the oil and the water phase. As an illustration of this, Figure 6.17 shows the effect of addition of salt on the partitioning of mandelic acid toward the oil phase, and on its diffusion rate. As can be seen, the ratio between the observed diffusion coefficient and the partition coefficient remains essentially constant over the salt concentration range, indicating that for this particular system, the diffusion is entirely determined by the partitioning between the phases.

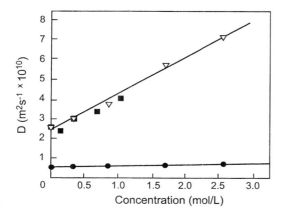

FIGURE 6.17 Effect of electrolyte concentration on the diffusion coefficient D of mandelic acid from gel emulsions consisting of water-decane-$C_{10}E_3$. Shown also is the diffusion coefficient normalized with the partition coefficient as a function of salt concentration (circles). Triangles and squares refer to NaCl and Na_2SO_4, respectively. (Redrawn from Caldero et al., Langmuir 1997, 13, 385.)

A promising feature is that emulsion gels may be used as in situ forming gel systems. Thus, as can be seen in Figure 6.18, the system water-decane-$C_{16}E_4$ with a water volume fraction of 99% and an oil/surfactant ratio of 1.5 displays a pronounced increase in elastic modulus on increasing the temperature from room temperature to body temperature. Quantitatively, however, the temperature-

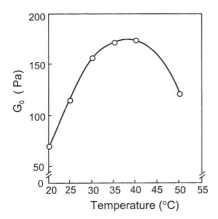

FIGURE 6.18 Elastic modulus G_0 as a function of temperature for the system water-decane-$C_{16}E_4$ with a water volume fraction of 99% and an oil/surfactant ratio of 1.5. (Redrawn from Pons et al., J. Phys. Chem. 1993, 97, 12320.)

induced thickening is much smaller than that displayed, e.g., by block copolymer (Chapter 3) and polysaccharide (Chapter 8) systems.

6.5 DESTABILIZATION OF EMULSIONS

In analogy to other disperse systems, emulsions are not thermodynamically stable, but instead undergo continuous destabilization until one macroscopic water phase and one macroscopic oil phase have been formed. The timescale for destabilization of emulsions depends critically on a number of factors, and several different destabilization mechanisms exist. In general, the kinetics of destabilization of emulsions is therefore more complex than that of destabilization of a polymer latex dispersion (Chapter 9). At least four different emulsion destabilization mechanisms may be identified, i.e., creaming, flocculation, coalescence, and Ostwald ripening (Figure 6.19). The relative importance of the first three of these depends primarily on the emulsion droplet size and the droplet concentration, with creaming favored for large droplets at low droplet concentrations, coalescence at high droplet concentration, and flocculation for small emulsion droplets at low droplet concentration.

Since creaming is a gravity effect similar to sedimentation, it depends on the density difference between the continuous phase and the droplets. Thus, if the droplets are heavier than the continuous phase, sedimentation will occur, whereas creaming will occur for droplets less dense than the continuous phase. Apart from the density difference, the creaming rate depends on the droplet size.

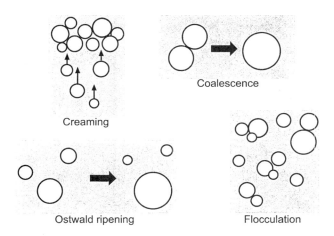

FIGURE 6.19 Schematic illustration of emulsion destabilization mechanisms.

With increasing droplet size, the buoyancy increases, thereby promoting cream-ing. Also, since the driving force for creaming is generally rather weak, it can be kinetically hindered by increasing the viscosity of the system, e.g., through a high droplet concentration or through addition of a thickening agent to the contin-uous phase (Figure 6.20).

Flocculation in emulsion systems is largely analogous to flocculation in other disperse systems, such as polymer latices. As discussed in some detail in Chapter 9, the main parameter of interest in this context is the interparticle (inter-droplet) interactions. As with polymer particles, electrostatic stabilization of emulsions is efficient at low droplet concentration and at low salt content. Addi-tion of salt, on the other hand, screens the electrostatic repulsion between the droplets, and promotes flocculation. This behavior is illustrated in Figure 6.21. Thus, as Ca^{2+} is added to Intralipid, a phospholipid-stabilized o/w emulsion used for parenteral nutrition, the droplet surface charge is reduced. At a certain Ca^{2+} concentration, the droplet electrostatic potential is zero, which results in fast flocculation of the emulsion. Increasing the Ca^{2+} concentration further results in charge reversal, i.e., at high Ca^{2+} concentration, the droplets are positively charged. They are then charge-stabilized again, and the flocculation rate therefore decreases.

Similar to polymer dispersions, emulsions are often further stabilized by adsorbed or otherwise surface-bound polymers, which generate a steric stabiliza-

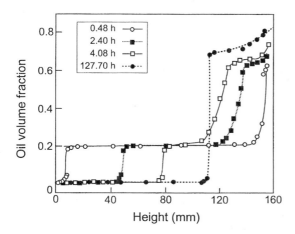

FIGURE 6.20 Creaming profiles at different times of 20 vol% heptane-hexadecane (9:1)-in-water emulsions stabilized by Brij 35 in the presence of hydroxyethyl cellu-lose in the aqueous phase. (Redrawn from Hibberd et al., Colloids Surf. 1988, 31, 347.)

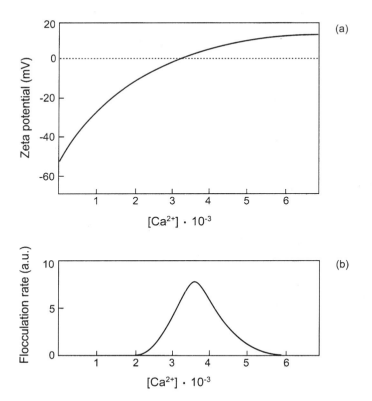

FIGURE 6.21 Effects of Ca^{2+} concentration on the droplet electrostatic potential (a) and the emulsion flocculation rate (b) for Intralipid emulsion. (Redrawn from Washington et al., in Sitges-Serra et al., eds., Clinical Progress in Nutrition Research, Karger, 1988.)

tion of the emulsions which is largely salt independent (Chapter 9). At moderate salt concentrations, however, electrostatic and/or hydration force interactions may be sufficient for reaching a sufficient emulsion stability.

For oil continuous systems such as w/o emulsions, the interdroplet interactions are different from those in o/w systems. Although electrostatic interactions are very long range due to the low dielectric constant of the oil phase, charges are energetically disfavored, and tend to be minimized, e.g., through extensive counterion binding or protonation/deprotonation. Therefore, w/o emulsions are generally not electrostatically stabilized. Instead, steric stabilization is frequently employed for such systems.

It is important to note, however, that just as for polymer lattices and other dispersions, the stability of emulsions against flocculation does not exclusively depend on the interdroplet interactions, but also on external fields, such as sedimentation/creaming, and shaking/shearing. Thus, in the presence of such external fields, which force the droplets to approach each other, the stability toward flocculation and coalescence is generally reduced. In fact, a commonly employed acceleration method for emulsion destabilization is to apply either random or regular shaking (Table 6.1). The stability of the emulsion is then determined by the interplay between interdroplet interactions and external fields.

When two droplets approach each other, as in flocculation, the water film between them becomes thinner due to drainage of the continuous phase. If the film ruptures, the two droplets can merge and become one, i.e., coalescence occurs. The probability for coalescence in emulsions therefore depends on the activation barrier for forming a hole in the film between droplets. The lower the activation energy, the more probable the coalescence. The activation energy for hole formation, in turn, depends on a number of factors. In particular, the spontaneous curvature of the surfactant molecules stabilizing the emulsions, as well as the surfactant film bending energy is of critical importance. For example, deemulsification may be caused by (1) reducing the absolute value of the monolayer spontaneous curvature (Figure 6.22), e.g., by addition of surfactant with the opposite spontaneous curvature, or by (2) reducing the monolayer bending elasticity, e.g., by addition of short chain alcohols.

Yet another destabilization mechanism for emulsion systems is so called Ostwald ripening. The origin of this effect is that the pressure inside droplets is higher the higher the surface curvature, i.e., the smaller the droplets. This, in turn, means that the solubility of an oil outside a small oil droplet is larger than that outside a larger droplet (and analogously for w/o emulsions). As a consequence of this, material contained within the small droplets will dissolve prefer-

TABLE 6.1 Mean Droplet Size (μm) of a Lecithin-Stabilized O/W Emulsion with 0.01 M Phosphate Buffer in the Aqueous Phase after Different Times of Shaking. The Emulsion Droplet Charge Decreases with Decreasing pH

Buffer	0 h	3 h	6 h	24 h	48 h
pH 9.3	0.37	0.37	0.37	0.37	0.37
pH 7.5	0.37	0.37	0.37	0.37	0.37
pH 5.7	0.37	0.38	0.43	0.54	phase sep.
pH 4.0	0.37	0.41	0.44	0.61	phase sep.
pH 2.5	0.37	0.86	2.02	phase sep.	phase sep.

Source: Data from Lindström et al., J. Disp. Sci. Technol. 1999, 20, 247.

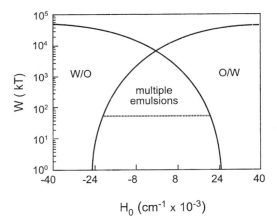

H_0 (cm^{-1} x 10^{-3})

Figure 6.22   Hole activation barrier W vs the monolayer spontaneous curvature H_0 for a phospholipid-stabilized emulsion. Note that in the vicinity of zero curvature, multiple emulsions are favored. (Redrawn from Kabalnov et al., Langmuir 1996, 12, 276.)

entially, diffuse through the continuous phase, and recondensate onto the larger droplets. Thus, the large droplets will grow larger while the small droplets will shrink until they eventually disappear. The kinetics by which this process occurs depends strongly on the solubility of the compounds contained in the droplets within the continuous phase. More precisely, the higher their solubility in the continuous phase, the faster the mass transport, and the faster the emulsion destabilization. As can be seen in Figure 6.23, the destabilization kinetics increases with decreasing oil chain length, and is also higher for alkenes than for alkanes. Both these effects follow the solubility of the oils in the aqueous phase.

Since the emulsion destablization through Ostwald ripening has nothing to do with droplet flocculation or coalescence, surfactant addition may have little or no effect on the emulsion destabilization kinetics (Figure 6.24). Note, however, that the role of the surfactant in Ostwald ripening may also be somewhat more complex than this at $c >$ cmc, since the solubilization in the aqueous phase and the oil transport from small droplets to large ones can occur through micelles. The destabilization kinetics in that case depends on the solubilization capacity of the micelles, the micelle concentration, and the size of the micelles, all determining the total oil mass transfer between small and large droplets.

Apart from working at surfactant concentrations just below the cmc and using sparingly soluble oils (o/w emulsions), another possibility to slow down

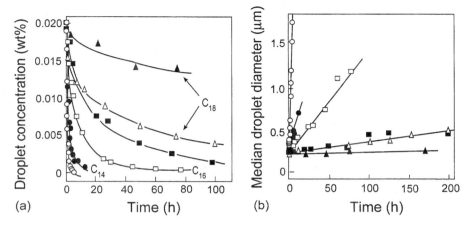

(a)   (b)

FIGURE 6.23 (a) Time dependence of the drop concentration for o/w emulsions containing 0.02 wt% hydrocarbon in a 2 wt% Tween 20 aqueous phase. (b) Time dependence of the median drop diameter for the same emulsions as in (a). Circles: C_{14}; squares: C_{16}; triangles: C_{18}; filled symbols: alkanes; open symbols: alkenes. (Redrawn from Weiss et al., Colloid Surf. A 1997, 121, 53, and Coupland et al., J. Food Sci. 1996, 61, 1114.)

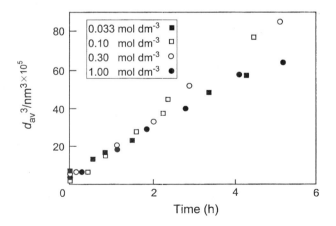

FIGURE 6.24 Variation of the average droplet diameter d_{av} with time for SDS-containing undecane-in-water emulsions undergoing Ostwald ripening for different SDS concentrations. Note that the droplet growth is essentially independent of SDS concentration. (Redrawn from Kabalnov, Langmuir 1994, 10, 680.)

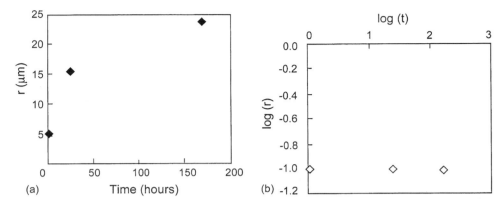

FIGURE **6.25** Droplet size *r* increase as a function of time in the absence (a) and presence (b) of a ripening inhibitor (Migliol 812) in o/w diamino ether emulsions stabilized by galactolipids. (Redrawn from Welin-Berger et al., Int. J. Pharm. 2000, 200, 249.)

Ostwald ripening is to add a second component to the oil phase, with a lower solubility in the water phase than that of the oil. Due to the solubility difference between the two oil components, the Ostwald ripening–related transport between small and large droplets will occur at different rates for the two oil components, which means that the smaller droplets will be successively enriched in the least water-soluble component, whereas the opposite applies for the larger droplets. This gradual concentration increase results in an increased chemical potential of the least soluble component in the smaller droplets, and of the more soluble component in the larger droplets, both of which counteract the curvature-driven transport from smaller to larger droplets. At a certain point, the ''back transport'' equals the Ostwald ripening, and no further overall destabilization of the emulsion through Ostwald ripening occurs (Figure 6.25).

6.6   MULTIPLE EMULSIONS

Multiple emulsions refer to emulsions where the dispersed phase contains inner droplets of the continuous phase. Such emulsions can either be of the water-in-oil-in-water (w/o/w) or oil-in-water-in-oil (o/w/o) type (Figure 6.26). Generally, both types of multiple emulsions are prepared through a double homogenization process, e.g., first preparing a w/o emulsion, and then dispersing this in an aqueous phase to reach a w/o/w emulsion, or the opposite procedure for preparing an o/w/o emulsion. However, multiple emulsions may also be prepared in a one-step procedure, and utilizing the PIT. As shown, e.g., in Figure 6.22, multiple

Normal simple emulsions

W/O 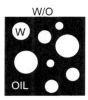 O/W

Multiple or double emulsions

$O_1/W/O_2$ 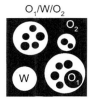 $W_1/O/W_2$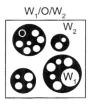

FIGURE 6.26 Schematic illustration of w/o/w and o/w/o multiple emulsions. (Redrawn from Nielloud et al., eds., Pharmaceutical Emulsions and Suspensions, Marcel Dekker, 2000.)

emulsions are favored close to zero curvature of the surfactant monolayer, i.e., close to the PIT. Frequently, however, multiple emulsions are quite unstable, and rapidly separate into o/w or w/o emulsions.

6.7 EMULSIONS IN DRUG DELIVERY

Emulsions, and particularly o/w emulsions, offer several advantages as drug delivery systems. In particular, due to their relatively large droplet size, the hydrophobic volume is relatively large in comparison to the o/w surface area. This means that relatively large amounts of hydrophobic active ingredients may be incorporated in o/w emulsions, with advantages relating to, e.g., the effective drug solubility, and the drug release rate and chemical stability. Furthermore, since the specific surface area is not very large, the amount of surfactants required for generating and stabilizing emulsions is comparatively low, and relatively nontoxic surfactants, such as phospholipids and other polar lipids, can be used as stabilizers.

The oils used for pharmaceutical emulsions are generally of natural origin. In some cases, i.e., when the drug is a liquid ''oil,'' the drug itself may constitute the oil phase of the emulsion with no other added oil components. More frequently, however, the drug is solubilized in the oil phase (for o/w emulsion for-

TABLE 6.2   Oils Commonly Used in
Pharmaceutical Emulsions

Natural oils	Synthetic/semisynthetic materials
Cottonseed	Triolein
Soybean	Ethyl oleate
Safflower seed	Dibutyl sebacate
Sesame	Iso-amyl salicylate
Cod liver	
Linseed	
Coconut	
Corn	
Olive	

Source: From Boyett et al., in Lieberman et al., eds.,
Pharmaceutical Dosage Forms, Vol. 2, Marcel Dekker, 1989.

mulations of hydrophobic drugs). Oils commonly used for this include, e.g., soybean and safflower oil. Irrespective of the origin of the oil, however, these are
generally multicomponent mixtures (Tables 6.2 and 6.3.).

The quality of an oil processed from a potentially variable source must
be closely controlled in order to minimize oxidation, remove ''unsaponifiable''
materials (such as waxes and steroidal components), and check for possible presence of aflatoxins, herbicides, pesticides, which may be inadvertent contamina-
tions. In general, high-quality food grade oils are likely sources for the preparation of injectable emulsions or emulsions for oral administration. For dermal use,
the quality requirements are generally less rigorous.

TABLE 6.3   Distribution of Fatty Acids in Cottonseed,
Soybean and Safflower Oils

Fatty acid	Cottonseed	Soybean	Safflower
Palmitic (C16:0)	21	12	7
Stearic (C18:0)	2	4	3
Oleic (C18:1)	29	24	13
Linoleic (C18:2)	45	51	77
γ-Linolenic (C18:3)	2	9	—

Source: From Boyett et al., in Lieberman et al., eds., Pharmaceutical
Dosage Forms, Vol. 2, Marcel Dekker, 1989.

Commonly used emulsifiers in drug delivery are either pure phospholipid fractions or lecithin mixtures, obtained from animal (egg yolk) and vegetable (soybean) sources. Apart from being relatively efficient emulsifiers and providing quite good physicochemical stability to the emulsion, these are rather stable toward hydrolysis and oxidation. Furthermore, they are metabolized in the same way as fats, rather than excreted via the kidneys as are many synthetic surfactants.

Due to their natural origin, lecithins are multicomponent mixtures, which may also contain compounds unsuitable, e.g., for intravenous injection. They must therefore be purified (e.g., chromatographically) before use in injectable emulsions. However, some purified lecithins are insufficient emulsifiers, and additives are therefore commonly used for such systems to improve emulsion stability. Examples of such additives include PEO-containing surfactants and block copolymers. Improved stability may also be obtained by a slight hydrolysis of lecithin, achieved, e.g., by addition of a small amount of NaOH.

Since emulsified oil exerts a limited osmotic effect, additives to the aqueous phase are sometimes necessary in order to achieve isotonic conditions. Examples of such additives include electrolytes (e.g., NaCl), reducing sugars (e.g., glucose), glycerin, and others (sorbitol, xylitol, etc.).

6.7.1 Emulsions in Parenteral Drug Delivery

Given the numerous destabilization mechanisms of emulsions, their frequently broad droplet size distribution, and the need for small emulsion droplets and absence of large ones, the use of emulsions in intravenous applications is rather challenging. These and other aspects result in a number of requirements for the safe and efficient use of injectable emulsions (Table 6.4).

First, the emulsions should be prepared with a sufficiently small droplet size and with a sufficiently narrow droplet size distribution. If the droplets are larger than a certain size, typically a few micrometers in diameter, they can "get stuck" in narrow blood vessels, e.g., in the lung, thereby causing emboli (Figure 6.27).

Once prepared, the emulsions should typically be stable for at least 2 years of storage at room temperature without considerable droplet size growth or formation of large droplets. Emulsions for intravenous use should also be sufficiently stable against shear-induced flocculation or coalescence. Apart from coalescence, these requirements on colloidal stability are not different from those on other injectable colloidal dispersions. However, due to the possibility of both coalescence and Oswald ripening in emulsion systems, the latter are generally more difficult to stabilize than, e.g., polymer latex dispersions.

Another practical issue of some complexity in injectable emulsion formulations is that of sterility. In particular, heat sterilization is frequently not possible due to a combination of limited chemical stability of the emulsion components

TABLE 6.4   Requirements for Injectable Emulsions

Physicochemical

1. Physically stable (should not flocculate at high electrolyte concentrations)
2. Particle size less than 2 μm (in order to avoid thrombosis)
3. Sterilizable
4. Chemically stable (decomposition affects both drug effectivity and toxicity)

Biological

1. Low incidence of side effects (toxicity)
2. Nonantigenic ('immunologically acceptable')
3. All components metabolized or excreted (no substances may accumulate in the body)

Practical

1. Stable to temperature extremes
2. Reasonable cost

Source: From Boyett et al., in Lieberman et al., eds., Pharmaceutical Dosage Forms, Vol. 2, Marcel Dekker, 1989.

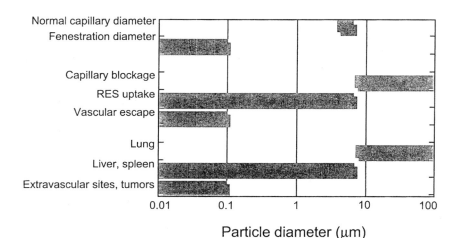

Particle diameter (μm)

FIGURE 6.27   Relationship between droplet size, physiological processes, and biodistribution of intravenously administered emulsion droplets. (Redrawn from Buszello et al., in Nielloud et al., eds., Pharmaceutical Emulsions and Suspensions, Marcel Dekker, 2000.)

and increased emulsion destabilization through Oswald ripening at elevated temperature. Also, similar to other dispersed formulations, emulsions cannot be sterile filtered when the droplet size is of the order of a couple of hundred nanometers or larger. Ethylene oxide or radiation sterilization are both possible alternatives, however, as is sterilization of the emulsion components followed by aseptic manufacturing.

Despite the numerous problems with emulsion formulation stability, and the high requirements on any formulation to be used in intravenous drug delivery, o/w emulsions have indeed found use within this area (Table 6.5).

Even without active drug ingredients, o/w emulsions have found use in a couple of important biomedical applications. For example, parenteral administration of o/w emulsions has been used for nutrition of patients who cannot retain fluid or who are in acute need of such treatment. In these nutritional formulations, soybean, cottonseed, or safflower oil is typically emulsified with a phospholipid (mixture) in an aqueous solution containing also, e.g., carbohydrates. Furthermore, o/w emulsions have been used as blood substitute formulations. These are perfluorochemical emulsions with a typical droplet size of about 100–200 nm, which provide oxygen-carrying capacity through dissolution of oxygen in the oil droplets. Also, in the development of vaccines it is frequently found that purified immunogens do not provoke a strong immune response by themselves, but rather require the simultaneous presence of immune response promoters, or so called adjuvants. It is well known that adjuvants influence both the

---

TABLE 6.5 Examples of Uses of Emulsions as Injectable Formulation

1. Nutrition
   - Emulsions are concentrated sources of calories (higher than, e.g., proteins and hydrocarbons), exerting only a small negative osmotic effect.
   - Emulsions are able to provide essential fatty acids, which other nutrition sources are not.
2. Drug delivery
   - Emulsions allow incorporation of hydrophobic drugs in large quantities in the droplet interior.
   - The drug is not in direct contact with body fluids and tissues.
   - A controlled and sustained release/uptake of the drug may be achieved.
   - By surface modification of the droplets, some targeting to different tissues may be achieved.
   - Emulsions may provide chemical stabilization, e.g., for drugs which rapidly hydrolyze in aqueous solution.
3. Diagnostics
4. Vaccines (Emulsions may provide adjuvant effects.)
5. Blood substitute (fluorocarbon emulsions)

duration and the intensity of the immune response, as well as the actual type of immune response. In analogy to some other colloidal systems, o/w emulsions have been found to display adjuvant activity, and are therefore used in immunization applications.

Due to their capacity to solubilize large quantities of hydrophobic drugs, and the rather low surfactant concentration required, o/w emulsions are interesting in relation to intravenous drug delivery. As with other types of colloidal drug carriers, such as liposomes or polymer particles, the fate of emulsion droplets following intravenous administration is largely determined by the interaction between the emulsion droplets and RES. Similar to liposomes, o/w emulsion droplets to be administered intravenously are frequently surface modified in order to display low serum protein adsorption, and hence result in a prolonged bloodstream circulation and a more even tissue distribution (Chapter 4). In particular, adsorption of EO-containing surfactants or block copolymers has been found to be efficient in this context, although care must be taken in selecting the surfactant/block copolymer system so that extensive desorption does not occur due to the dilution of the formulation following intravenous administration. With these precautions, however, a prolonged bloodstream circulation after intravenous administration can be obtained also for emulsion systems (Figure 6.28).

Another advantage with these surface modifications is that they result in an additional emulsion stabilization mechanism, steric stabilization, which prevents the emulsion from flocculating at the high electrolyte concentration present under physiological conditions.

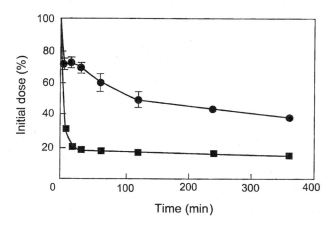

FIGURE 6.28 Blood clearance of ^{123}I-labeled emulsions stabilized by egg lecithin (squares) and Poloxamine 908 (circles) intravenously administered to rabbit. (Redrawn from Illum et al., Int. J. Pharm. 1989, 54, 41.)

Due to the finite physicochemical stability of emulsions, another possibility in relation to parenteral administration is to use microemulsions as precursors, generating o/w emulsions on dilution with aqueous solution following intravenous administration. As discussed in Chapter 5, microemulsions may be prepared such that on dilution with water, they form o/w emulsions, with a sufficiently small droplet size to avoid emboli formation. In fact, it has been found to be possible to administer up to at least 0.5 ml/kg of microemulsion with an oil weight fraction of 50% without significant detrimental effects on the acid-base balance, blood gases, plasma electrolytes, mean arterial blood pressure, heart rate, and time lag between depolarization of atrium and chamber.

6.7.2 Emulsions in Oral Drug Delivery

Emulsion formulations are relevant also for the oral administration route. Overall, the requirements on emulsion chemical and physical stability, as well as concerns regarding the purity of the raw materials used, are qualitatively similar to those in intravenous administration. Generally, however, both stability requirements and toxicity issues are somewhat less critical for this administration route.

As with intravenous administration, the use of emulsions in oral administration mainly originates from various drug delivery advantages, such as an effectively increased solubility of sparingly water-soluble drugs and decreased hydrolysis due to the low pH in the stomach. Emulsions are also commonly used in oral administration for taste masking. This is the case particularly for hydrophobic substances encapsulated in the droplets of o/w emulsions. Yet another specialized use of emulsions in oral drug delivery is in laxatives.

The absorption from o/w emulsion formulations in the gastrointestinal tract depends on a number of factors, including, e.g.,

1. Drug dissolution rate
2. The o/w partition coefficient of the drug
3. Flow of bile juice
4. Membrane permeability

As discussed also in Chapter 5, sparingly soluble hydrophobic drugs frequently display a poor bioavailability following oral administration. There are several reasons for this, including, e.g.,

1. Slow diffusion-controlled uptake due to low water solubility
2. Degradation of the drug in the gastrointestinal tract
3. Physical absorption barriers due to the charge and size of the drug

Furthermore, oral administration of hydrophobic drugs frequently results in a strong intra- and intersubject uptake variability, which precludes efficient

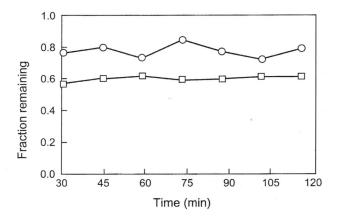

Figure 6.29 Fraction of cyclosporine remaining vs. time after intestinal perfusion in rats. Results are shown for both homogenized (droplet size 2.0 μm; squares) and stirred (droplet size 4.0 μm; circles) emulsions. In both cases, the cyclosporine concentration was 0.08 mg/ml. (Redrawn from Tarr et al., Pharm. Res. 1989, 6, 40.)

administration of the required dose in a safe and reproducible manner. Through the use of o/w emulsions as drug carrier systems, this variability following oral administration of hydrophobic drugs may be reduced. The improved uptake of hydrophobic drugs following oral administration by the use of o/w emulsions is illustrated in Figure 6.29 for cyclosporine, an oligopeptide drug used as an immunosuppressive agent in order to prolong allograft survival in organ transplantation and in the treatment of patients with certain autoimmune diseases. Interestingly, the intestinal absorption for this drug can be increased by reducing the droplet size, suggesting that the oil droplets, analogously to, e.g., biodegradable polymer particles used in oral vaccination (Chapter 9), are taken up in a size-dependent manner.

Not surprisingly, o/w microemulsions, with their very small "oil" droplets, have been found to be even more efficient than emulsions for the oral administration of cyclosporine (Chapter 5).

Also of interest in oral drug delivery are the so-called self-emulsifying emulsion. As discussed above, truly self-emulsifying emulsion systems would be microemulsions, but this is generally not what is referred to when using the term in pharmaceutical literature. Instead, "self-emulsification" is a result of differential surfactant solubility in the two phases, coupled to surfactant concentration gradients at the oil-water interface, and minor turbulence. Such "self-emulsifying drug delivery systems" have received particular attention as a means to increase the oral bioavailability of poorly absorbed drugs. The main reason

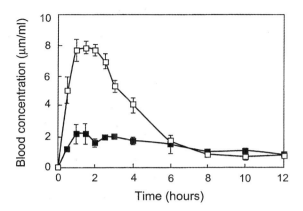

FIGURE 6.30 Average whole-blood concentration vs. time following intraduodenal administration of a penclomedicine in o/w mineral oil emulsion (open symbols) or mineral oil (filled symbols). (Redrawn from Myers et al., Int. J. Pharm. 1992, 78, 217.)

for this is that such systems combine the advantages of oil-based formulations, which are easier to formulate and stabilize than emulsions, with the better physiological effect of o/w emulsions compared to an oil phase formulation (Figure 6.30).

6.7.3 Emulsions in Dermal Drug Delivery

Like liposomes (Chapter 4) and microemulsions (Chapter 5), both o/w and w/o emulsions are of interest in dermal drug delivery. The emulsion formulations used in dermal drug delivery are frequently quite similar to those used in cosmetic products, but with a different ''active compound.'' O/W emulsions are characterized by an ''aqueous feel'' and, more importantly, by ease of removal by simple washing with water. Since the continuous water phase is in contact with air after administration, there is a continuous evaporation of water, as well as of other volatile components. As a result of this, there is a drift in the composition of the applied formulation, which must be taken into consideration in its design. W/O emulsions, on the other hand, often have a softening effect, and may result in an enhanced drug uptake. As with microemulsions and liposomes, the uptake from dermally administered emulsions is a complicated issue, which depends not only on the partition of the drug between the oil and water phases, the concentration of the drug, and the droplet size and concentration, but also on the interaction between the surfactants used for stabilizing the emulsion and the stratum corneum lipids.

TABLE 6.6 Examples of Emulsifiers Used in
Dermal Drug Delivery and Cosmetic Applications

Nonionic ethoxylates	Sucrose esters
Orthophosphoric acid esters	Glycerine esters
Protein condensates	Block copolymers
Amine oxides	Silicones
Phytosteroids	Beeswax

A number of different surfactants are used in both dermal drug delivery systems and cosmetic applications (Table 6.6). Ethoxylated surfactants play a particular role as emulsifier for emulsions for dermal drug delivery and cosmetic applications. Due to their uncharged nature, these are compatible with both cationic and anionic surfactants, and are also largely insensitive to pH and salt. An additional advantage is that this type nonionic surfactant have low skin sensitation, e.g., due to weak interactions with skin proteins. A disadvantage of these surfactants, however, is the presence of low amounts of dioxane originating from a side reaction in the ethoxylation process, as well as the formation of aldehydes as a result of partial oxidative degradation of the PEO chain after exposure to oxygen and light. During the last few years in particular, alternatives to EO-based nonionic surfactants have been developed. In particular, sugar-based surfactants have been found to be promising here.

Somewhat related to emulsions are ointments and creams. These semisolid formulation types undergo a transition from solidlike to liquidlike behavior under pressure, which allows easy administration to the skin, and an efficient localization after administration. In general, "ointments" refer to formulations which remain on the surface of the skin and display skin protection and occlusion, whereas "creams" refer to formulations which are able to penetrate the skin to at least some extent. Ointments are generally water-poor, or even water-free systems, whereas creams often are o/w or w/o emulsions (Figure 6.31).

6.8 EMULSIONS AS PRECURSORS FOR SLN

An interesting use of o/w emulsions in drug delivery is to use them as precursors for preparing solid lipid nanoparticles (SLN). There are several ways of preparing SLN, e.g.,

1. Preparation of an o/w emulsion containing the lipid and the drug dissolved in a volatile solvent, followed by evaporation of the solvent, and solidification of the lipid matrix (Figure 6.32)

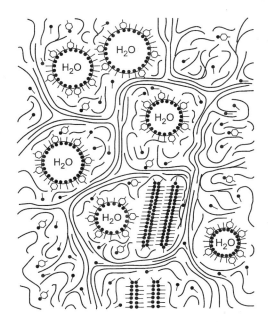

FIGURE 6.31   Schematic illustration of the structure of a w/o cream, consisting of both crystalline and amorphous domains, emulsion droplets, liquid crystalline phases, and free emulsifiers. (Redrawn from Junginger, in Kreuter, ed., Colloidal Drug Delivery Systems, Marcel Dekker, 1994.)

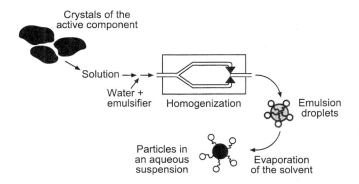

FIGURE 6.32   Schematic illustration of preparation of SLN through emulsification of the lipid mixture in an organic solvent, followed by the evaporation of the latter, and solidification of the lipid mixture. (Redrawn from Sjöström et al., J. Pharm. Sci. 1993, 82, 584.)

2. Preparation of an o/w emulsion by high-pressure homogenization at elevated temperature, followed by cooling and solidification of the lipids droplets
3. Spray cooling of a molten lipid/emulsifier mixture
4. Sonication of molten lipid

Spray cooling of a molten lipid/emulsifier mixture, although seemingly simple, is generally limited to larger particle sizes (of the order of several micrometers), and hence SLN prepared through this process generally less suitable for intravenous administration. Dissolution of the lipid/drug mixture in a volatile organic solvent, on the other hand, may result in quite small SLN, but a concern with this approach is residual solvent which may preclude use of SLN prepared in this manner in intravenous administration. It is therefore of major importance that the solvent is thoroughly evaporated and monitored (Figure 6.33).

Since SLN are prepared from emulsions, one would expect their size to

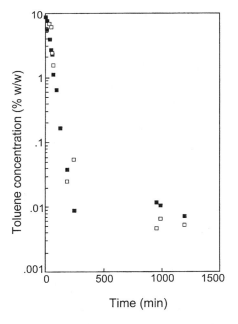

Time (min)

FIGURE 6.33 Concentration of toluene in a SLN dispersion as a function of evaporation time. The SLN consisted of cholesteryl acetate stabilized by PEO-(20)-sorbitan monooleate (5 or 10%; open and filled symbols, respectively), and were prepared through emulsification of cholesteryl acetate in toluene. (Redrawn from Sjöström et al., J. Disp. Sci. Technol. 1994, 15, 89.)

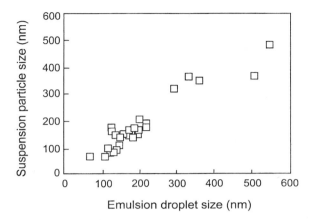

FIGURE 6.34 Correlation between the size of SLN and the corresponding precursor emulsion. The SLN were prepared by dissolving cholesteryl acetate in cyclohexane followed by emulsification of this oil phase in water in the presence of surfactant. Each point corresponds to one surfactant (mixture) composition. (Redrawn from Sjöström et al., J. Pharm. Sci. 1993, 82, 584.)

depend on the size of the precursor emulsion. In fact, at least in some cases, the particle size after solidification has been found to be essentially identical to that of the emulsion droplets (Figure 6.34).

SLN with a particle size essentially identical to that of the precursor emulsion is expected for SLN prepared through homogenization of the lipid mixture in the absence of solvent at elevated temperature, due to the small volume change on decreasing the temperature over a limited temperature range (in the absence of crystallization-induced large-scale morphological changes of the particles). For SLN prepared through use of a solvent, the finding of the SLN having a comparable particle size is, on the other hand, unexpected, and indicates that the particles prepared by this approach are hollow.

From Figure 6.34 it can further be noted that the emulsifier has a dramatic influence of the size of the resulting SLN. Thus, for identical conditions, and for otherwise identical composition, the nature of the surfactant largely determines both the emulsion droplet and the SLN particle size.

The degree of crystallinity is another parameter of interest for SLN systems. For a crystallizing lipid (mixture), one would expect crystallization to occur as SLN form, irrespective of whether the SLN formation occurs through cooling of a dispersed lipid mixture or evaporation of a solvent containing the lipid(s). However, the formation of SLN is a kinetic process, and at high lipid concentrations (e.g., in the melt or at low solvent concentrations), crystallization may be kinet-

TABLE 6.7 Thermoanalytical Data for Bulk Glycerides and Their Colloidal Dispersions

	Bulk	Disp. (fresh)	Disp. (stored)
Hard fat			
Melting point (β_i; °C)	38–39	12–13	31–33
Melting point (β'; °C)	32–33		
Melting point (α; °C)	20–22		
$T_{recryst}$ (°C)	28–29	8–10	
Tripalmitate			
Melting point (β_i; °C)	65–67	54–56	56–59
Melting point (β'; °C)	56–58		
Melting point (α; °C)	44–45	39–40	
$T_{recryst}$ (°C)	41–42	20–21	

α, β_i, and β' refer to different polymorphs.
Source: From Siekmann et al., Colloids Surf. B 1994, 3, 159.

ically hindered. As a result of this, it is generally found that the degree of crystallinity in SLN is lower than that for a corresponding macroscopic lipid sample. With increasing storage temperature, however, the dispersed material becomes more similar to the macroscopic sample, indicating that crystallization occurs slowly during storage (Table 6.7).

Furthermore, the crystallization in SLN may be more complex than that of the bulk glyceride systems. For example, the crystallization behavior of SLN may depend on, e.g., the SLN particle size, the nature of the emulsifier used, and the presence of a drug (Figure 6.35). With increasing temperature SLN typically become less stable, in analogy to the frequently poorer physicochemical stability displayed by emulsions (Figure 6.36).

From a practical drug delivery perspective, SLN systems are attractive for several reasons:

1. They allow a high load of hydrophobic drugs (in analogy to o/w emulsions).
2. Hydrolytic degradation is limited (in analogy to o/w emulsions).
3. The drug release rate can be controlled by the particle size and composition.
4. They combine the advantages of polymeric nanoparticles (in that they provide a solid matrix for controlled release) and o/w emulsions (in that they consist of physiological compounds and that they can straightforwardly be produced industrially on a large scale), but simultaneously avoid the disadvantages of these systems, such as the use of

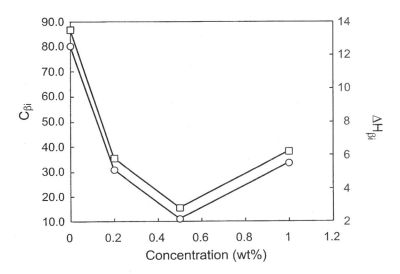

Figure 6.35 Effect of the concentration of ubidecarenone on the heat of fusion of the β$_r$-polymorph (ΔH$_{βi}$; circles) and the concentration of fat present in the β$_i$ form (C$_{βi}$; squares) for SLN prepared from hard fat, lecithin and sodium glycocholate. (Redrawn from Siekmann et al., Colloids Surf. B 1994, 3, 159.)

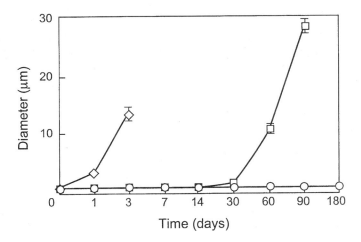

Figure 6.36 Typical result of the influence of storage temperature on the stability of SLN. Results are shown for 8°C (circles), 20°C (squares), and 50°C (diamonds). (Redrawn from Freitas et al., Int. J. Pharm. 1998, 168, 221.)

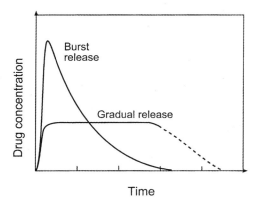

Figure 6.37 Schematic illustration of the burst release frequently observed with o/w emulsions, and the more gradual drug release from SLN.

solvents for the preparation of polymer particles and the burst release frequently observed for emulsion systems (Figure 6.37).

SLN formulations have been found to be of interest, e.g., in anticancer therapy. Due to the adverse side effects of several anticancer drugs, burst release is preferably avoided. Due to this, and the hydrophobic nature of several anticancer drugs, and particularly interchalating ones, SLN provide a formulation possibility. It has been found that the cytotoxicity of SLN in the absence of incorporated drugs is very low, which is beneficial for their use in vivo. Contrary to this, the cytotoxicity of SLN containing incorporated anticancer agents has been found to be substantial. In fact, for several drugs, SLN formulations have been found to be significantly more efficient than the free drug in solution, which indicates that particle-mediated uptake (e.g., phagocytosis) is of major importance here (Table 6.8).

Table 6.8 Inhibitory Concentration of Doxorubicin and Paclitaxel Producing 50% of Cell Inhibition or Death

	IC_{50}(HL60 cells; ng/ml)	IC_{50}(MCF-7 cells; ng/ml)
Doxorubicin (solution)	45.5	10.9
Doxorubicin (SLN)	0.9	1.0
Paclitaxel (solution)	11.1	102.0
Paclitaxel (SLN)	16.7	1.16

Source: From Miglietta et al., Int. J. Pharm. 2000, 210, 61.

Apart from displaying a higher efficiency, SLN also result in a decreased exposure of irrelevant tissue to the active substance, which should reduce side effects and allow a higher dosage.

BIBLIOGRAPHY

Becher, P., Encyclopedia of Emulsion Technology, vol. 1, Marcel Dekker, New York, 1983.

Becher, P., Encyclopedia of Emulsion Technology, vol. 2, Marcel Dekker, New York, 1985.

Binks, B. P., ed., Modern Aspects of Emulsion Science, The Royal Society of Chemistry, 1998.

Boyett, J. B., C. W. Davis, Injectable emulsions and suspensions, in H. A. Lieberman, M. M. Rieger, and G. S. Banker, eds., Pharmaceutical Dosage Forms: Disperse Systems, vol. 2, Marcel Dekker, New York, 1989.

Evans, D. F., H. Wennerström, The Colloidal Domain, Wiley, New York, 1999.

Johnston, I.D.A., ed., Current Perspectives in the Use of Lipid Emulsions, Marcel Dekker, New York, 1983.

Jönsson, B., B. Lindman, K. Holmberg, B. Kronberg, Surfactants and Polymers in Aqueous Solution, Wiley, New York, 1998.

Junginger, H. E., in J. Kreuter, ed., Colloidal Drug Delivery Systems, Drugs and the Pharmaceutical Sciences, vol. 66, Marcel Dekker, New York, 1994.

Kreuter, J., in J. Kreuter, ed., Colloidal Drug Delivery Systems, Drugs and the Pharmaceutical Sciences, vol. 66, Marcel Dekker, New York, 1994.

Nielloud, F., G. Marti-Mestres, eds., Pharmaceutical Emulsions and Suspensions, Drugs and the Pharmaceutical Sciences, Marcel Dekker, 2000.

Shinoda, K., S. Friberg, Emulsions and Solubilization, Wiley, New York, 1986.

Sjöblom, J., ed., Emulsions and Emulsion Stability, Surfactant Science Series, vol. 61, Marcel Dekker, New York, 1996.

7

Aerosols, Bubbles, and Foams

Due to the affinity of many surfactants, polymers, and proteins for the air-water interface, air can be readily dispersed in water (foams) and water can be dispersed in air (aerosols). While such systems have not found the widespread use in drug delivery applications as, e.g., emulsions, they are still interesting to consider in the present context, partly due to the similarities and differences between foams/aerosols and emulsions, and partly due to some practical applications of aerosol and microbubble formulations in drug delivery.

7.1 AEROSOLS

Aerosols refer to systems where liquid drops are dispersed in a gas, in the context of pharmaceutical applications generally air. Although aerosols may seem comparable to emulsions in many ways, air as the continuous medium makes them different from emulsions in many ways. For example, even for ''concentrated aerosols'' the viscosity of the continuous phase is orders of magnitude smaller than that for any liquid. Due to this, the stability of aerosols cannot straightforwardly be controlled, e.g., by addition of a surface active component.

Aerosols may be generated either by breaking up condensed material (liquid), e.g., under high pressure, or by condensing gas. The most common methods to disperse liquids mechanically include:

1. Air nebulizers
2. Spinning discs
3. Ultrasonic nebulizers
4. Vibrating orifice generators

Preparation of aerosols by nucleation, on the other hand, is based on the generation of supersaturation, which under suitable conditions may result in formation of relatively monodisperse droplets. In particular, the use of so-called propellants results in rapid evaporation and a following cooling-down effect. This, in turn, causes supersaturation and hence aerosol droplet formation.

Once formed, the stability of aerosols largely depends on the collision frequency of the droplets and on relative velocity differences between droplets. The latter may arise from different mechanisms, i.e.,

1. Thermal motion of gas molecules
2. Gravitational settling (different settling velocities for differently sized droplets)
3. Turbulence (acceleration of droplets by turbulent convection)
4. Motions induced by acoustic oscillations

To some extent, this is not entirely different from emulsions or dispersions, but in the case of aerosols, the collision impact is generally higher due to more rapid thermal motion and lower viscosity of the continuous medium. Also, in contrast to emulsions, the stability of aerosols is rather sensitive to pressure (Figure 7.1).

Aerosols are frequently not very stable systems, and particularly at high

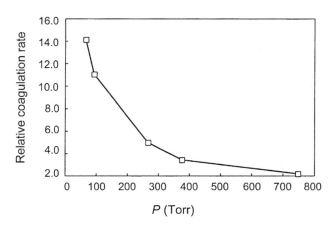

FIGURE 7.1 Coagulation rate for diethylhexyl sebacate in helium at different pressures P. (Redrawn from Wagner et al., in Kerker, ed., Colloid and Interface Science, Academic Press, 1976.)

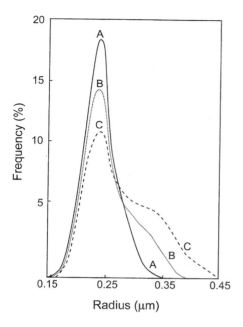

FIGURE 7.2 Typical evolution of the size distribution of a coagulating aerosol. Curves *A*, *B*, and *C* represent the size distribution after 0 s, after 33 s, and after 90 s, respectively. (Redrawn from Nicolaon et al., J. Colloid Interface Sci. 1972, 38, 460.)

droplet number concentrations, the coagulation half-life may be of the order of seconds or minutes (Figure 7.2).

In the presence of charged surfactants, these will adsorb at the air-water interface, which should result in a charging of the droplets, and which in principle should stabilize the droplets against coalescence. Due to the low dielectric constant of air, such electrostatic interactions should also be long-range, and therefore charged surfactants should act as stabilizers also for aerosols. However, the low dielectric constant of air also makes the presence of a charge close to the interface energetically unfavorable. This counteracts dissociation of the surfactant and its counterion, whereby the interdroplet electrostatic interaction is reduced. Together with the larger importance of thermal motion in aerosol systems, this means that controlling the stability of aerosols through surfactant addition is less straightforward than stabilizing, e.g., o/w emulsions.

7.2 BUBBLES AND FOAMS

A foam is a dispersion of a gas in a liquid or a solid. While solid foams are important in their own right, e.g., in the context of concrete foams or metal foams for lightweight construction material, pharmaceutical applications largely involve a gas (typically air) dispersed in a liquid (typically an aqueous solution). For a foam to form, surface-active components, such as surfactants, polymers, proteins, or colloidal particles, must stabilize the air-water interface. With an increasing concentration of the surface active component, the foamability increases. At the cmc, however, the improved formability due to an increasing surfactant concentration reaches saturation as a consequence of the essentially constant surfactant adsorption above the cmc (Figure 7.3).

Once formed, there are numerous mechanisms operating to destabilize the foam:

1. Gravity
2. Drainage of plateau regions due to pressure differences between the plateau regions and the junctions
3. Diffusion of gas from small bubbles to larger ones due to different pressure in different size bubbles (Figure 7.4; cf. Ostwald ripening; Chapter 6)
4. Attractive van der Waals interaction over the liquid films

There are several ways to stabilize a foam. First, since curvature-induced pressure differences cause the liquid to be transported from the plateau regions to the junctions, the presence of colloidal particles or droplets in the liquid can

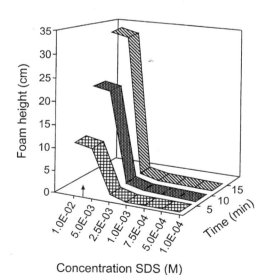

FIGURE 7.3 Effect of SDS concentration on the foam height at different foaming times. The cmc is indicated by an arrow. (Redrawn from Djuve et al., Colloids Surf. 2001, 186, 189.)

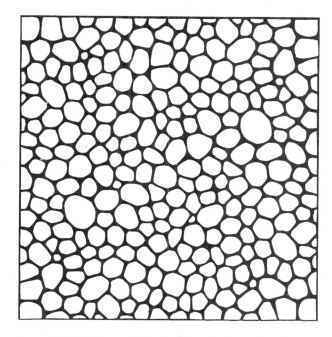

FIGURE 7.4 Schematic illustration of a foam structure.

effectively "block" the junctions, and hence improve the foam stability. More frequently, however, foams are stabilized by choosing surfactants which effectively stabilize the plateau regions through dense packing at the air-water interface, and by causing the surface elasticity to increase.

When selecting surfactants for achieving or avoiding foaming, the preferred packing of the surfactant molecules at the air-water interface should be considered. Specifically, good foamability and foam stability is obtained for surfactants packing at the interface with a small spontaneous curvature. For surfactants which are too hydrophilic, the packing density of the surfactant at the interface is low, and hence insufficient reduction in surface tension and insufficient surface elasticity results in poor foam formation and stability. For very hydrophobic surfactants, on the other hand, the surfactant favors packing in structures curved toward water, which, in turn, favors film rupture, thereby destabilizing the foam (Figure 7.5).

Therefore, for efficient foam formation and stability, the surfactant should prefer packing in structures of low curvature toward both air and water. For nonionic surfactants, this can be achieved, e.g., by tuning the length of the alkyl chain or the EO-chain in a similar way as, e.g., emulsion and microemulsion structure is controlled (Chapters 5 and 6) (Figure 7.6).

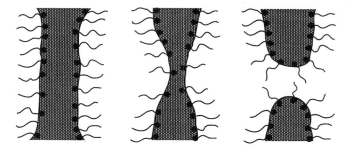

FIGURE 7.5 Schematic illustration of thermal film rupture in relation to surfactant packing at the air-water interface. Rupture is facilitated at high cpp, where the surfactant prefers structures curved toward water (Chapter 3). (Redrawn from Jönsson et al., Surfactants and Polymers in Aqueous Solution, Wiley, 1998.)

From a practical perspective, hydrophobic surfactants can be used also for destabilizing foams when the latter are not desired. Thus, addition also of relatively minor concentrations of a hydrophobic EO-PO-EO copolymer or EO-containing surfactant may be quite effective in reducing or eliminating foam formation.

For other types of surfactants, the interfacial packing can be controlled in similar ways as it is for liquid crystalline phases or microemulsions, e.g., through

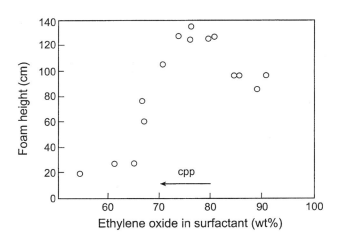

FIGURE 7.6 Effect of the length of the EO-chain of nonionic surfactants on their capacity to stabilize foams. (Redrawn from Jönsson et al., Surfactants and Polymers in Aqueous Solution, Wiley, 1998.)

the charge or electrostatic screening (i.e., pH and salt concentration), addition of consurfactants, and temperature (Chapters 3 to 5).

7.3 PHARMACEUTICAL APPLICATIONS OF AEROSOLS

Aerosols are of interest in drug delivery through the airways, particularly for the delivery of therapeutic proteins and peptides. The advantages with this approach compared with other administration routes include, e.g., that (1) the bloodstream can be reached from the alveolar epithelium without penetration enhancers, which facilitates a good bioavailability and (2) respiratory diseases can be treated by direct action at the site of interest.

Aerosol droplets/particles deposit in the airways by either gravitational sedimentation, interial impaction, or diffusion. Since particles greater than about 5 μm in diameter deposit primarily in the upper airways, while an efficient drug uptake requires that the droplets/particles reach the lower airways, and since submicron particles are generaly exhaled, most aerosol particles are of the size range 0.5–5 μm.

It has been shown that the pulmonary absorption of macromolecules decreases with increasing molecular weight of the macromolecule (Figure 7.7). Furthermore, the kinetics of absorption decreases significantly with increasing molecular weight (Figure 7.8).

Nevertheless, for a range of smaller macromolecules, e.g., hormones, a

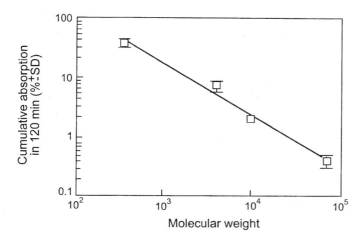

FIGURE 7.7 Correlation between pulmonary absorption in rats, expressed as percentage of the initial dose, and the drug molecular weight. (Redrawn from Morita et al., Biol. Pharm. Bull. 1993, 16, 259.)

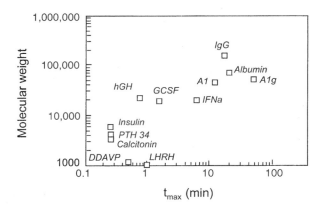

FIGURE 7.8 Relationship between the time to maximum serum concentration t_{max} after pulmonary delivery and molecular weight for a number of peptides and proteins. (Redrawn from Patton et al., J. Controlled Release 1994, 28, 79.)

significant absorption has been found. For example, compared with intravenous administration, the oral bioavailability of leuprolide, a potent luteinizing hormone-releasing hormone with a molecular weight of 1.2 kDa, is less than 0.05%, and the transdermal and nasal bioavailabilities less than 2%. On the other hand, the bioavailability after inhalation is much higher (up to 18%).

Furthermore, although the pulmonary absorption of macromolecules decreases with increasing molecular weight, pulmonary administration is not limited to small molecules. Instead, a number of larger polypeptides and proteins, e.g., growth hormone (22 kDa), α-interferon (18 kDa), and α_1-antitrypsin (51 kDa), have been found to be absorbed in the lung.

An interesting aspect of pulmonary drug delivery is that the presence of surfactants in the formulation has a marked influence on the drug absorption. In particular, various surfactants have been found to act as absorption enhancers. Although the understanding on the mechanism behind this is incomplete at present, it has been found that oleic acid, linoleic acid, palmitoleic acid, sodium oleate, and POE oleyl ether all display a significant absorption enhancement effect (Figure 7.9).

7.4 PHARMACEUTICAL APPLICATIONS OF BUBBLES AND FOAMS

Unlike emulsions, foams have not received widespread use as a drug delivery vehicle. In particular, the applications which have been identified generally involve introduction into a body cavity, as in vaginal or rectal drug delivery. The

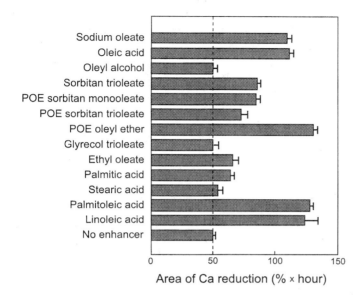

FIGURE 7.9 Enhancement of the pharmacological effect (higher area of Ca reduction is equivalent to a higher pharmacological effect) of salmon calcitonin following intratracheal administration with 0.5% fatty acid or surfactant in rats. (Redrawn from Kobayashi et al., Pharm. Res. 1994, 11, 1239.)

main advantage with foam formulations is their ability to fill up a given volume, which may facilitate contact between the formulation (and the drug) and all the surface which needs to be in contact with the drug (formulation). In general, since the foam is generated on administration, and since very stable foams are not required, the foam formulation composition is generally not very critical from a physicochemical perspective, although toxicity aspects are comparable to those of other surfactant-based formulation systems. Examples of drugs used together with foam delivery systems include:

1. Antimicrobial drugs
2. Steroidal antiinflammatorial drugs
3. Spermicides

In the general case, however, foam formation is disadvantageous in drug delivery, and is preferably avoided, e.g., by choice of surfactant or addition of a small amount of ethanol.

Somewhat related to the use of foams in drug delivery is the use of "microbubbles" in medical diagnostics. In particular, air-filled microspheres stabilized

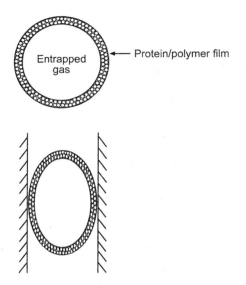

Deformation in capillaries

Figure 7.10   Schematic illustration of protein/polymer–stabilized microbubbles used as contrast enhancers in ultrasonic diagnostics.

by proteins, polymers, or phospholipids have found use as contrast enhancers in ultrasonic diagnostics. The origin of this is the low density and high elasticity of these bubbles. Free gas bubbles, however, are not stable in aqueous solution, and therefore a stabilizer is needed (Figure 7.10).

Such microbubbles can be prepared by simple sonication of a protein (typically albumin) or polymer solution, which generates bubbles of the micrometer range. Possibly due to their deformability, it has been found that even microbubbles in the size range 10 μm can be administered intravenously without causing any apparent detrimental effects relating to emboli formation. Such microbubbles have also been found to be quite stable (Figure 7.11).

A complicating factor with these systems is that air has a fairly good solubility in the aqueous solution. Together with the small molecular size of nitrogen and oxygen and their relatively good solubility also in the stabilizing protein film, the air "encapsulated" in the air bubbles can diffuse out to the surrounding aqueous solution. This can be followed, e.g., by following the microbubble size vs. temperature. As can be seen in Figure 7.12, decreasing the temperature below a certain value results in a decrease in the bubble size. This is caused by undersaturation of the air in the aqueous solution at the lower temperature, which causes

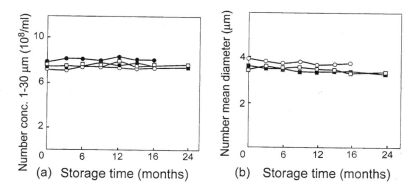

FIGURE 7.11 Effect of storage time on the stability of albumin stabilized microbubbles as determined by the bubble number concentration (a) and bubble diameter (b). Multiple samples are shown. (Redrawn from Christensen et al., Biotechnol. Appl. Biochem. 1994, 19, 307.)

the "encapsulated" air to diffuse out, thereby resulting in a volume and size reduction.

The amount of air encapsulated in such microbubbles depends on the concentration of surface active protein/polymer. More precisely, the higher the protein/polymer concentration, the larger the air volume which can be solubilized in microbubbles (Figure 7.13).

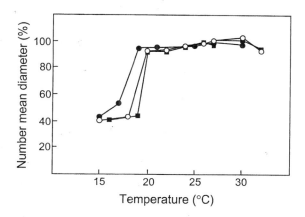

FIGURE 7.12 Effect of temperature on the diameter of three preparations of protein-stabilized air bubbles for ultrasonic contrast enhancement. (Redrawn from Sontum et al., J. Pharm. Biomed. Anal. 1994, 12, 1233.)

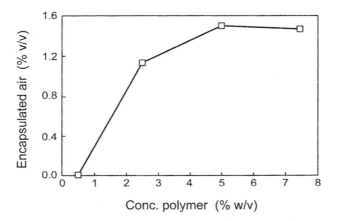

FIGURE 7.13   Effect of the polymer concentration used for stabilizing microbubbles, on the amount of air encapsulated. (Redrawn from Bjerknes et al., Int. J. Pharm. 1997, 158, 129.)

The ultrasonic contrast effect obtained depends strongly on the microbubble size. In particular, neither very small nor very large bubbles are efficient contrast enhancers, but rather an intermediate bubble diameter of about 10 μm is optimal (Figure 7.14). The reason for this is that small bubbles have insufficient capacity to interact with the ultrasonic field due to small volume. Very large bubbles, on the other hand, get stuck in small capillaries.

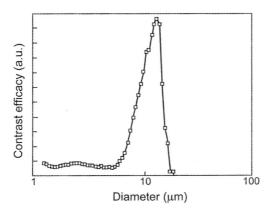

FIGURE 7.14   Contrast efficiency per microsphere from analysis of backscatter enhancement vs. the microbubble size. (Redrawn from Sontum et al., Invest. Radiol. 1997, 32, 627.)

BIBLIOGRAPHY

Bjerknes, K., P. C. Sontum, G. Smistad, I. Agerkvist, Preparation of polymeric microbubbles: formulation studies and product characterisation, Int. J. Pharm. 158:129–136 (1997).

Christiansen, C., H. Kryvi, P. C. Sontum, T. Skotland, Physical and biochemical characterization of Albunex, a new ultrasound contrast agent consisting of air-filled albumin microspheres suspended in a solution of human albumin, Biotechnol. Appl. Biochem. 19:307–320 (1994).

Hidy, G. M., J. R. Brock, The Dynamics of Aerocolloidal Systems, Pergamon Press, Oxford, 1970.

Johnson, K. A., Preparation of peptide and protein powders for inhalation, Adv. Drug Delivery Rev. 26:3–15 (1997).

Jönsson, B., B. Lindman, K. Holmberg, B. Kronberg, Surfactants and Polymers in Aqueous Solution, Wiley, New York, 1998.

Okumura, K., S. Iwakawa, T. Yoshida, T. Seki, F. Komada, Intratracheal delivery of insulin. Absorption from solution and aerosol by rat lung, Int. J. Pharm. 88:63–73 (1992).

Prud'homme, R. K., S. A. Khan, eds., Foams: Theory, Measurements, and Applications, Surfactant Science Series, vol. 57, Marcel Dekker, New York, 1996.

Vold, R. D., M. J. Vold, Colloid and Interface Chemistry, Addison-Wesley, London, 1983.

Yu, J., Y. W. Chien, Pulmonary Drug Delivery: Physiologic and Mechanistic Aspects, Crit. Rev. Ther. Drug Carrier Syst. 14:395–453 (1997).

8

Polymer Solutions and Gels

8.1 POLYMER SOLUTIONS

Polymers are used extensively in drug delivery, e.g., for rheology control, control of drug release rate, stabilization of colloidal drug carriers, and solubilization of sparingly soluble drugs. Many of the properties used in drug delivery rely on the chain-like nature of polymers. It is therefore natural to start any discussion about the use of polymers in drug delivery by considering the chainlike properties of polymers.

8.1.1 Polymer Conformation

The conformation of a single chain in a solvent may vary considerably between systems. The three conformational extremes are the random coil, the stiff rod, and the hard sphere (Figure 8.1). Naturally, intermediates between these extremes exist, including partly hydrated coils, oblate- or prolate-shaped polymers and wormlike chains of varying flexibility and solvation.

   Of particular importance for the use of polymer solutions and gels in drug delivery is the coil conformation. The flexible nature of the chain is of fundamental importance for essentially all properties of such structures. For ideal such systems, the average conformation (shape) may be characterized by the radius of gyration R_g, which describes the size of the polymer coil, and depends on the

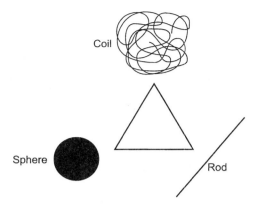

FIGURE 8.1 Schematic illustration of the shape/conformation extremes available for polymers.

number N and length l of freely jointed segments (e.g., monomeric units) making up the chain. Under ideal conditions, R_g scales with N as $R_g \sim N^{1/2}$. This should be compared to $R_{g,\text{sphere}} \sim N^{1/3}$ and $R_{g,\text{rod}} \sim N^1$; i.e., the size of the coil increases faster with the molecular weight than for hard sphere molecules (e.g., globular proteins), but more slowly than for stiff rods (e.g., nucleic acids or other highly charged polyelectrolytes at low excess electrolyte concentrations).

The size and shape of polymer molecules depend on a number of factors, in particular, intramolecular and intermolecular interactions. In the general system, these include van der Waals, electrostatic, hydrophobic, hydration, and other interactions. For example, if the polymer contains electric charges, the polymer tends to expand due to intramolecular electrostatic repulsive interactions, with consequences for, e.g., viscosity. This intramolecular effect also has consequences for the sensitivity of the polymer solution to electrolyte concentration and pH. For uncharged polymers, on the other hand, polymer-polymer and solvent-solvent interactions are usually more attractive than the polymer-solvent interaction. This results in an effective polymer-polymer attraction, which tends to contract the polymer molecules. At so-called θ-conditions, this interaction-driven contraction cancels the excluded volume effect. Such conditions, at which infinitely long polymers phase separate, may be found for all (uncharged) polymers by varying the solvent composition, temperature, or other parameters.

8.1.2 Thermodynamics of Polymer Solutions

In order to understand the thermodynamics of polymer solutions, it is essential to consider the free energy associated with mixing of polymer and solvent, and to estimate the entropy and enthalpy of mixing. From such considerations, it is found that the entropy change on mixing is always positive, which means that the entropy always favours mixing. However, the larger the polymer (i.e., the higher its molecular weight), the smaller the entropy gain of mixing per segment. For very large polymers, the magnitude of the mixing entropy is small, and essentially independent of the molecular weight (Figure 8.2).

In most uncharged polymer systems, polymer-polymer and solvent-solvent interactions are more favorable than the polymer-solvent interactions, and therefore the enthalpy of mixing generally opposes mixing. Instead, the driving force for mixing is provided solely by the mixing entropy, and the increased possibilities for adapting more configurations in the solution compared to the polymer melt.

This balance between entropy and enthalpy determines the phase behavior of polymer solutions. For example, since the entropy contribution is weighted by temperature T, the importance of this term increases with increasing temperature. This, in turn, means that most polymers become more soluble with increasing temperature, but phase-separate at sufficiently low temperature. Furthermore, due to the mixing entropy per segment decreasing with an increasing molecular weight. Thus, polymers become less soluble with increasing molecular weight (Figure 8.3).

For certain systems, however, and notably aqueous solutions of PEO and PPO, PEO derivatives (polymers and surfactants), and PEO-containing cellulose ethers, the solubility decreases with increasing temperature. Since entropy favors mixing to an increasing extent with increasing temperature, this means that a

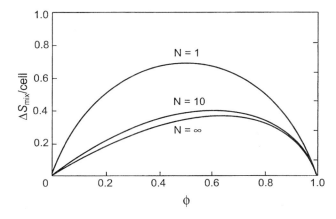

Figure 8.2 Magnitude of mixing entropy ΔS_{mix} as a function of polymer concentration ϕ and degree of polymerization N.

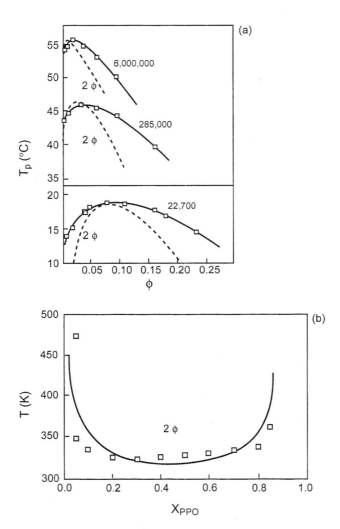

FIGURE 8.3   (a) Typical phase behavior of a polymer system (polyisobutylene in diisobutyl ketone). Solid lines are drawn through the experimental points, while the dashed lines are results obtained from calculations with the Flory-Huggins model. Note that phase separation (noted 2φ) occurs on lowering the temperature, and that the lower the polymer molecular weight, the lower the temperature required to cause phase separation. (b) Reversed phase behavior displayed by poly(propylene oxide) (PPO) in water. Note that phase separation in this case occurs at elevated temperature. (Redrawn from Flory, Principles of Polymer Chemistry, Cornell University Press, 1953 (a), and Linse, Macromolecules 1993, 26, 4437 (b).)

temperature-dependent enthalpic driving force decreases the polymer solubility with increasing temperature for these systems. There are several suggested mechanisms for this, including temperature-dependent conformational changes, hydrogen bonding, and water structure effects.

For ternary systems of polymer 1/polymer 2/solvent, phase separation is the rule rather than the exception. The reason for this is that for long polymer chains, the mixing entropy per segment is small, and even a weak attraction between the two polymers is sufficient to cause phase separation. In so-called segregative phase separation, each of the phases is enriched in one of the polymers and depleted in the other. In associative phase separation, on the other hand, one phase is rich in both of the polymers, whereas the other is depleted of both polymers (Figure 8.4). The latter occurs when there is an attraction between the two polymers, such as for polyelectrolytes of different charge.

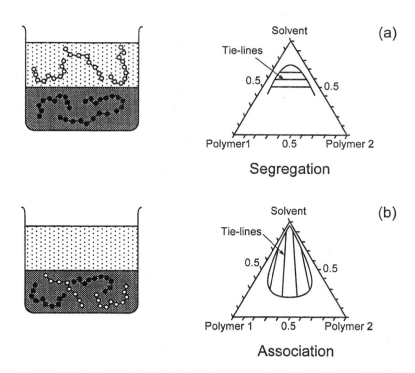

FIGURE 8.4 Schematic illustration of segregative (a), and associative (b) phase separation in binary polymer systems, together with typical phase diagrams for the two cases. (Redrawn from Piculell et al., Adv. Colloid Interface Sci. 1992, 41, 149.)

8.1.3   Polyelectrolytes

A polyelectrolyte is a salt between a charged polymer (polyion) and its counterions. In an aqueous solution, the counterions distribute according to the balance between entropically driven dissociation of counterions from the polyion, and a Coulumb attraction between the counterions and the polyion (Figure 8.5). The balance is determined by the charge density of the polyion, the valency of the counter ion, the polarity (dielectric constant) of the solvent, the polyelectrolyte concentration, and the concentration and valency of added salt. More precisely, the distribution is more inhomogeneous the higher the polyion charge density and counterion valency.

Due to the entropically driven counterion dissociation, the polyelectrolyte possesses a charge, and will therefore stretch as a result of intramolecular electrostatic interactions. Thus, the ''size'' of a polyelectrolyte is largher than that of an uncharged polymer, although depending on, e,g., polyelectrolyte and salt concentration, and for titrating polyelectrolytes also on pH (Figure 8.6).

The counterion dissociation also affects the solubility of polyelectrolytes dramatically. As discussed above, the solubility of a polymer is much smaller

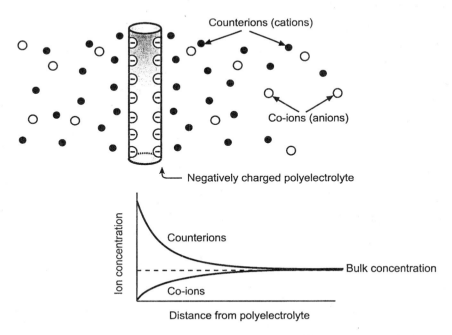

FIGURE 8.5   Schematic illustration of the distribution of ions around a polyelectrolyte chain.

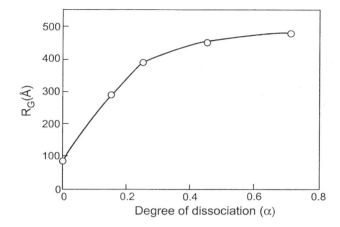

FIGURE 8.6 Effect of the polyelectrolyte (polymethacrylic acid) charge (increasing with increasing degree of dissociation α on the molecular stretching as given by the radius of gyration R_g. (Redrawn from Jönsson et al., Surfactants and Polymers in Aqueous Solution, Wiley, 1998.)

than that of the corresponding monomer for entropic reasons. For polyelectrolytes the counterion entropy of mixing is large. In fact, due to the small size and large number of counterions, the entropy related to the counterions is more important than, e.g., the chain mixing entropy for polyelectrolyte systems. This large entropy contribution favors mixing, and results in an increased solubility of polyelectrolytes. Therefore, a polymer may be made soluble (in polar solvents) by introducing charges. For example, polystyrene is very poorly soluble in water whereas polystyrene sulfonate is readily soluble. In fact, the entropy due to the counterions is the main reasons for the solubility of many important hydrophobic and/or stiff biopolymers, such as polypeptides and nucleic acids.

The phase behavior of multicomponent polymer mixtures is strongly affected by the presence of charges on the polymers. For binary polymer systems of opposite charge, there is generally an electrolyte-dependent associative phase separation, resulting in one concentrated phase containing the polymers, and one dilute phase depleted in the polymers (Figure 8.4). For systems with two uncharged polymers, segregative phase separation is the rule. For a system containing one polyelectrolyte and one uncharged polymer, however, the miscibility is much larger than for two uncharged polymers (or two oppositely charged polyelectrolytes). The reason for this is that the counterion entropy is dramatically reduced on phase separation in such systems due to the electroneutrality condition that all counterions must be located in the same phase as the polyion. At salt addition, this effect is reduced, and segregative phase separation may be ob-

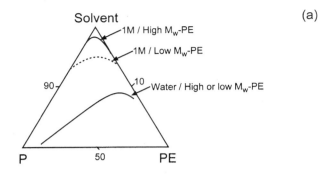

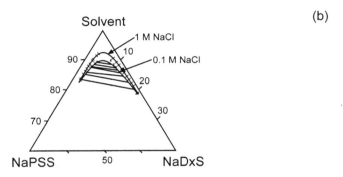

FIGURE 8.7 Typical phase diagrams for a polymer (P), polyelectrolyte (PE), water system at different electrolyte concentration and polyelectrolyte molecular weight (a) and a PE-PE-water system (polystyrene sulfonate-dextran sulfate) at different electrolyte concentration (b). (Adapted from Piculell et al., Adv. Colloid Interface Sci. 1992, 41, 149.)

served. For two similarly charged polyelectrolytes, finally, segregative behavior is expected, since both phases can contain counterions, and since no restrictions in the movement of the latter between the phases exist. Furthermore, the salt dependence for such systems is weaker (Figure 8.7).

8.2   POLYMER-SURFACTANT INTERACTIONS

Particularly over the last two decades, it has become increasingly clear that mixed polymer/surfactant systems display aggregation behaviour between the polymer and the surfactant. Since surfactants and polymers are frequently used together

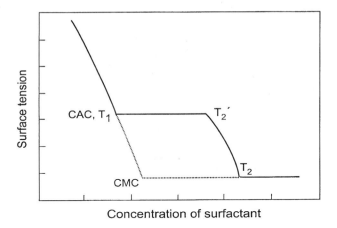

FIGURE 8.8 Schematic illustration of the effect of the surfactant concentration on the surface tension in the absence (dotted line) and presence (solid line) of polymer in solution. cac and T_1 represent the onset of surfactant-polymer association, whereas T_2' represents the polymer saturation and T_2 the formation of free surfactant micelles. (Redrawn from Goddard, in Goddard et al., eds., Interactions of Surfactants with Polymers and Proteins, CRC Press, 1993.)

in technical formulations, such aggregation also has important implications for numerous applications. This is the case also in drug delivery.

The first systematic observations of the effects of polymer-surfactant aggregation in solution were based on surface tension measurements. Thus, in the absence of polymer, the surface tension of surfactant solutions shows a monotonous decrease with increasing surfactant concentration, until the cmc, where the surface tension abruptly levels off and becomes essentially constant (Figure 8.8). On addition of polymer, on the other hand, a completely different behavior is observed. At low surfactant concentrations, the surface tension decreases in a similar way as in the absence of polymer, although for moderately surface active polymers the absolute value of the surface tension in the presence of the polymer is often lower than in the absence of polymer due to the adsorption of the polymer at the air-water interface. At a particular surfactant concentration (cac or T_1), however, the surface tension dependence of the surfactant concentration levels off, and only at higher surfactant concentrations does it decrease again to a second break point T_2.

The origin of this behavior is the following: At low surfactant concentrations, no surfactant self-assembly occurs ($c < cmc$), and the surface tension decreases monotonically with increasing surfactant concentration due to concentration-driven increasing adsorption at the air-water interface. In the absence of polymer, this proceeds until the cmc, above which the chemical potential of the individual nonmicellized surfactant molecules is approximately constant, and hence so is the adsorption and the surface tension. In the presence of polymer, on the other hand, addition of surfactant results in a decreased surface tension until cac, where aggregation occurs between the polymer and the surfactant. Addition of more surfactant at this point only results in increased polymer/surfactant aggregation while the concentration of the nonaggregated free surfactant molecules is largely constant. Hence, the surface tension lowering effect of the surfactant is reduced or eliminated in this region. At some point, however, the polymer is saturated with surfactant, and addition of more surfactant results in an increase in the free surfactant concentration, and hence in a surface tension reduction, until the free surfactant concentration equals the cmc, where free micelles are formed, and the surface tension becomes essentially independent of the surfactant concentration.

Given the saturation of the aggregation at sufficiently high surfactant concentrations, increasing the polymer concentration will result in a higher total surfactant concentration required to reach the cmc, and to cause the surface tension to approach that at the cmc (Figure 8.9).

The aggregates formed by many polymer-surfactant systems, notably those

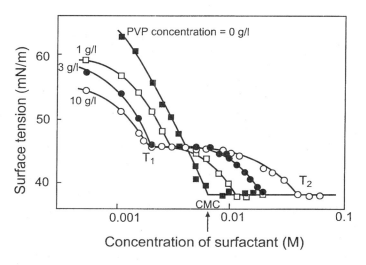

FIGURE 8.9 Surface tension as a function of SDS concentration in the absence and presence of polyvinyl pyrolidone (PVP) of different concentrations. (Redrawn from Goddard, in Goddard et al., eds., Interactions of Surfactants with Polymers and Proteins, CRC Press, 1993.)

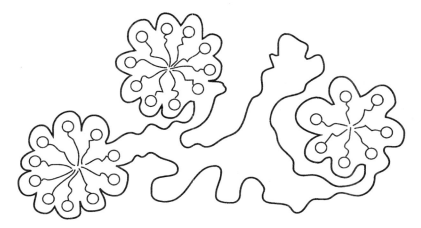

FIGURE 8.10 Schematic illustration of polymer-surfactant aggregates. (Redrawn from Nagarajan et al., Polym. Prepr. Am. Chem. Soc. Div. Polym. Chem. 1982, 23, 41.)

consisting of a nonionic polymer and an ionic surfactant, consist of "micellar-like" surfactant aggregates bound to and connected by the polymer (Figure 8.10).

Due to the formation of micellarlike structures, polymer-surfactant aggregation generally follows the same trend as surfactant self-assembly in the absence of polymer. For example, as discussed in Chapter 2, surfactant self-assembly is facilitated by increasing the length of the hydrophobic group. Similarly, increasing the alkyl chain length of the surfactant results in an earlier onset of the mixed micelle formation or surfactant binding at the polymer (Figure 8.11).

An important effect of polymer-surfactant complexation is that it may alter the phase behavior of the polymer and the surfactant. For example, mixtures of oppositely charged polymer-surfactant pairs may give rise to associative phase behavior, where the attractive electrostatic interaction between the polymer and the surfactant causes separation of much of the surfactant and polymer in a concentrated phase, which is an equilibrium with a more dilute phase (Figure 8.12).

As can be seen in Figure 8.12, mixing anionic sodium hyaluronate and the cationic surfactant $C_{14}TAB$ results in the formation of one phase rich in both the polymer and the surfactant, and one dilute phase, containing mostly water. Maximal phase separation occurs around charge neutrality, i.e., where the number of charges of the polymer and of the surfactant compensate each other. In other words, maximum phase separation occurs when the aggregate formed are essentially uncharged.

With increasing salt concentration, the phase separation region shrinks and

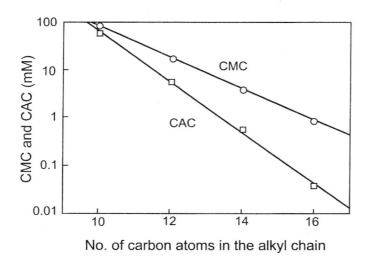

FIGURE 8.11 Comparison of the effect of the alkyl chain length on micellization (cmc; circles) and surfactant-polymer association (cac; squares) for alkyltrimethylammonium bromides and sodium hyaluronate. (Redrawn from Thalberg et al., J. Phys. Chem. 1989, 93, 1478.)

finally disappears, which is a consequence of electrostatic screening. At very high salt concentrations, finally, phase separation occurs once more, but in this case the phase separation is segregative, i.e., one phase is rich in the polymer and the other rich in surfactant. The latter phase separation is mainly driven by differences in nonelectrostatic polymer-polymer, polymer-surfactant, and surfactant-surfactant interactions, and is analogous to the phase separation in uncharged two-polymer systems (see above).

8.3 POLYMER GELS

The term ''gel'' is frequently used in pharmaceutical research and development to describe ''thick'' or ''nonflowing'' systems. This means that different gel systems may have drastically different structure and composition. More often than not, however, gels used in drug delivery contain water-soluble polymers. While some polymeric gel systems are suitable for molecular solubilization of sparingly soluble drugs due to the presence of hydrophobic domains, others are not capable of this due to the absence of such domains. However, although the solubilization capacity may be an important aspect in some drug delivery systems, it is frequently other aspects, e.g., the rheological properties or their consequences (e.g.,

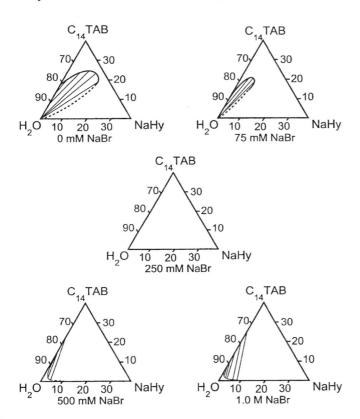

FIGURE 8.12 Pseudo three-component phase diagrams for the system sodium hyaluronate (NaHy)-C$_{14}$TAB-water system at different electrolyte concentrations. (Redrawn from Thalberg et al., in Mittal et al., eds., Surfactants in Solution, Plenum Press, 1991.)

relating to the drug release rate, bioadhesion, etc.), which make these gel systems interesting for drug delivery.

8.3.1 Chemically Cross-Linked Gels

In many respects, covalently cross-linked gels are the simplest ones for drug delivery, since they can be permanently fixed by use of stable chemical bonds, since the properties of the gel (e.g., swelling) can be straightforwardly controlled by the choice of chemistry used for the cross-linking, and since the gels do not disintegrate as a result of dilution, shearing, or drug release.

A parameter of importance in drug delivery applications is the degree of swelling of the gel. This is determined by the balance between entropic and enthalpic contributions in the same way as the conformation of a single polymer molecule. Thus, in a good solvent, polymer gels are highly swollen with solvent, whereas on decreasing the solvency the polymer-solvent contacts become increasingly unfavorable, and hence the gel contracts. The extent of which the gel can contract depends on the cross-link density. Thus, for a polymer solution (i.e., in the absence of cross-links), the polymer solution eventually phase separates at sufficiently poor solvency conditions. For a cross-linked system, on the other hand, macroscopic phase separation is hindered by the cross-links, and the higher the cross-linking density, the smaller the gel contraction in poor solvents (Figure 8.13). Similarly, in very good conditions, the gel swelling is limited by the cross-linking, and the higher the cross-linking density the smaller the swelling.

Analogous to the polyelectrolyte swelling in aqueous solution, introduction of charges affects the swelling of cross-linked polymer gels. In particular, the degree of swelling increases with the charging of the polymer network. This can be seen, e.g., by gradually increasing the content of charged groups in the synthe-

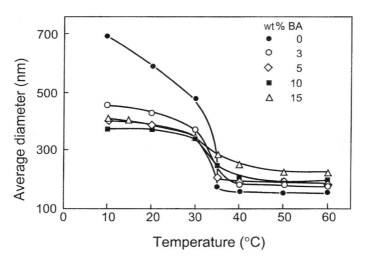

Figure 8.13 Effect of solvency and cross-linking density on the swelling/deswelling of chemically cross-linked gel particles. Data are shown for polyNIPAM, which displays a transition from good to poor solvency in aqueous solution with increasing temperature, as a function of the concentration of cross-linker (methylene-bis-acrylamide; BA) used. Note the solvency-driven collapse on increasing temperature, and that the contraction decreases with increasing cross-linking density. (Redrawn from McPhee et al., J. Colloid Interface Sci. 1993, 156, 24.)

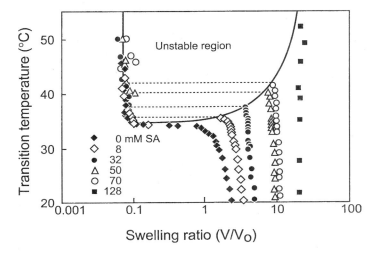

FIGURE 8.14 Swelling ratio of copolymer gels of polyNIPAM containing varying fractions of sodium acrylate (SA). The total monomer concentration used was 700 mM throughout. (Redrawn from Hirotsu et al., J. Chem. Phys. 1987, 87, 1392.)

sis in the gel, or by using a titratable group at fixed content and then varying pH (Figure 8.14).

Since ionic surfactants bind to nonionic polymers, as discussed above, another way to effectively introduce charges to a nonionic polymer gel is to add ionic surfactants. Since such charging depends on the cooperative binding of the surfactant to the polymer backbone, the gel swelling depends on parameters controlling the surfactant binding. This is illustrated in Figure 8.15, showing the transition temperature for polyNIPA gels in the presence of ionic surfactants. When the alkyl chain length of the surfactant increases, the binding affinity to the polymer increases, which effectively increases the "polymer charge density" and hence results in an increase in the temperature-dependent deswelling transition.

The degree of swelling directly affects the release of substances incorporated into a cross-linked gel. Thus, with increasing swelling, the diffusion of the incorporated molecules increases as a result of the decreasing polymer concentration (Figure 8.16).

8.3.2 Gels Formed by Polysaccharides

An important class of gel-forming polymers are the polysaccharides. Gel formation in aqueous polysaccharide systems is generally induced by helix formation,

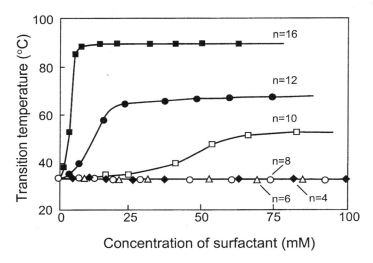

FIGURE 8.15 Deswelling transition temperature for polyNIPA gels as a function of
the concentration of alkyl sulfonate surfactants of various alkyl chain length. (Redrawn from Sakai et al., Langmuir 1995, 11, 2493.)

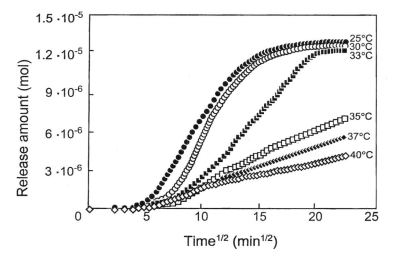

FIGURE 8.16 Release of sodium benzoate from polyNIPAAM gels as a function
of temperature. The lower consolute temperature for this polymer system is 33°C.
Note that the gel collapse at $T > 33°C$ results in a drastic decrease in the drug
release rate. (Redrawn from Makino et al., Colloids Surf. B 2001, 20, 341.)

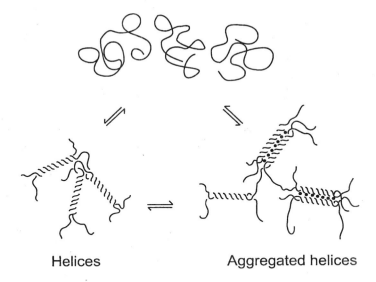

Helices   Aggregated helices

FIGURE 8.17 Schematic illustration of cross-linking initiated by helix formation. (Redrawn from Clark et al., Adv. Polym. Sci. 1987, 83, 57.)

sometimes followed by aggregation of helices (Figure 8.17). Since the helix formation involves a transition from a coil-like isotropic conformation to an optically active conformation, the coil-helix transition and the gelation can be followed, e.g., by optical rotation or circular dichroism (Figure 8.18).

As can be seen in Figure 8.18, helices formed by polysaccharides (and hence also polysaccharide gels) melt on increasing the temperature again. This is due to the increasing importance of the entropy of the system with increasing temperature, which results in ordered structures being less favorable. Polysaccharide systems therefore display temperature-reversible gelation. Often, however, there is a substantial hysteresis between gel melting on heating and gel formation on cooling.

For systems where helix aggregation occurs, there is a close correlation between the gel formation and phase separation. In fact, had it not been for the interconnecting disordered regions, the multihelix aggregates would separate from the aqueous solution. This can be seen, e.g., when working with short helix-forming polysaccharides. Thus, while high molecular polysaccharides form gels rather than phase separate, the reverse is true for low to intermediate molecular weight polysaccharides.

Electrolytes play an important role for the gelation in polysaccharide systems. The effects of electrolytes in such systems may be subdivided into lyotropic

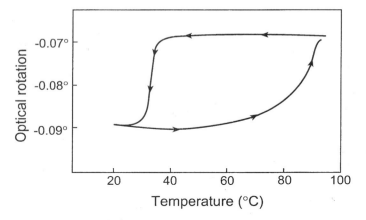

FIGURE 8.18 Typical optical rotation curve for gelation of agarose. Note the effect of helix formation on decreasing temperature, as well as the substantial hysteresis between heating and cooling. (Redrawn from Dea et al., J. Mol. Biol. 1972, 68, 153.)

effects, general electrostatic effects, and specific ion-binding effects. Regarding the first class of effects, it has been found that at quite high electrolyte concentrations (a few tenths of a molar), certain electrolytes tend to increase the macromolecular "solubility" (e.g., depressing helix formation), particularly for uncharged polysaccharides. These electrolytes (or more generally, solutes) are generally referred to as salting-in electrolytes (solutes). Other electrolytes act in the opposite way, and are referred to as salting-out electrolytes (Figure 8.19).

The origin of the lyotropic effects is still being debated, and models based on water structuring and interfacial effects are still being investigated. However, it has been found that salting-in electrolytes or solutes (which oppose helix formation) are enriched close to interfaces (oil/water, macromolecule/water). Although this enrichment is quite small, it is sufficient to lower the interfacial tension, and thus favor a large interfacial area (e.g., precluding self-association). Salting-out electrolytes (solutes), on the other hand, are depleted from the interfacial zone, thus causing the opposite effect.

For charged polysaccharides, general electrostatic effects are of major importance for any kind of physicochemical behaviour, and hence also for the coil-helix transition and for gelation. Specifically, since electrostatic repulsive interactions oppose helix formation, addition of electrolyte increases the relative stability of the ordered conformation (i.e., the helix), and hence promotes helix formation. Also, since divalent counterions are more efficient regarding electrostatic screening, they promote helix formation more strongly than monovalent ones (Figure 8.20).

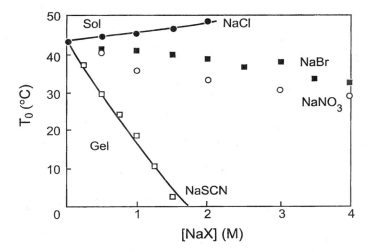

FIGURE 8.19 Effects of different anions on the gelation temperature T_0 for agarose. (Redrawn from Piculell et al., Progr. Colloid Polym. Sci. 1990, 82, 198.)

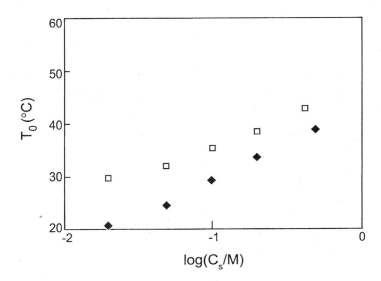

FIGURE 8.20 Onset of the coil-helix transition T_0 of furcellaran in the presence of NaCl (filled diamonds) and $CaCl_2$ (open squares) of different concentration c_s. (Redrawn from Zhang et al., Biopolymers 1991, 31, 1727.)

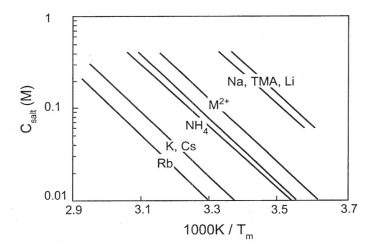

Figure 8.21 Cation specificity of the coil-helix transition T_m of κ-carragenan. Above each line, the system is in a helix state. (Redrawn from Rochas et al., Biopolymers 1980, 19, 1675.)

In a number of polysaccharide systems, not only general electrostatic and nonspecific lyotropic electrolyte effects are present, but also specific ion-binding effects are of importance. The origin of these ion-specific effects varies between different systems, but often they concern cations rather than anions (Figure 8.21).

From the prespective of drug release, it should be noted that polysaccharide gels are frequently formed at quite low polymer concentrations (≈wt%). This means that although the viscosity of the system may be very high, both water and small water-soluble solutes are largely free to diffuse within the polymer gel without major hinderance. Only for high molecular weight substances is the diffusion significantly reduced in the gel compared to in aqueous solution. Therefore, only for the latter type of system will a sustained release of a noninteracting drug from a gel formulation based solely on noninteracting polysaccharides be obtained (Figure 8.22).*

Furthermore, since polysaccharide gels do not contain any hydrophobic domains, they are not very suitable for solubilizing hydrophobic drugs and other solutes. However, if the drug can be made water soluble, e.g., by titrating it to a pH where it is charged, it can readily be incorporated in to such gels. The release of such substances from the gel may also be controlled by the electrolyte

---

* Note, however, that diffusion in the absence of convection is a slow process in itself, and that the drug release rate can be further sustained by an attractive polymer-drug interaction.

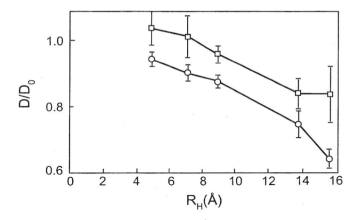

FIGURE 8.22 Effect of the size of a solute (monodisperse PEOs of different molecular weight, and therefore also hydrodynamic radius, R_H) on their self-diffusion D/D_0 in a κ-carragenan gel in the presence of 10 mM KCl (circles) and 100 mM KCl (squares). Note that with increasing size of the diffusing polymer, the diffusion rate decreases due to increased obstructions, but also that for all polymers investigated, the diffusion in the gel is quite fast. At the higher KCl concentration, the gel network contains larger "pores," and hence the PEO diffusion is faster. (Redrawn from Johansson et al., Macromolecules 1991, 24, 6019.)

concentration, presence of divalent counterions, and pH in much the same way as for covalently cross-linked polymer gels.

8.3.3   Gels Formed by Block Copolymers

One type of "gel" which has been extensively investigated in relation to drug delivery is that formed by certain PEO-PPO-PEO block copolymers. These systems are particularly interesting since even a concentrated polymer solution is quite low-viscous at low temperature, whereas a very abrupt "gelation" occurs on increasing the temperature. Although these systems are usually referred to as gels in the pharmaceutical literature, they are generally liquid crystalline phases or (partially) disordered liquid crystalline phases (Chapter 3).

8.3.4   Gels Formed by Polymer-Surfactant Mixtures

The complex formation between polymers and surfactants can result also in gel formation. Considering the bead-necklace structure in Figure 8.10, it is hardly surprising that surfactant-polymer aggregate formation may result in a viscosity increase for a range of such systems.

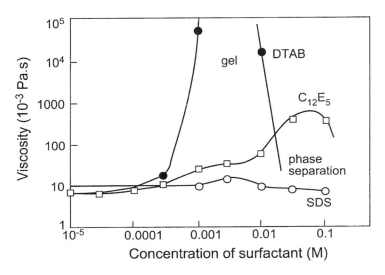

FIGURE 8.23   Effect of surfactant concentration on the viscosity of an aqueous solution of hydrophobe-modified polyacrylate. (Redrawn from Magny et al., Prog. Colloid Polym. Sci. 1992, 89, 118.)

In particular, hydrophobe-modified polymers, notably hydrophobically modified polyelectrolytes, may display dramatic thickening effects on addition of ionic surfactants. Thus, at very low surfactant concentrations, the viscosity of such polymer solutions is quite low, but depending on factors such as the polymer concentration and molecular weight, as well as on the length, number, and nature of the hydrophobic blocks. On addition of ionic surfactant of the opposite charge to the polyelectrolyte, there is a drastic increase in the viscosity. Surfactants with a similar charge as the polyelectrolyte, on the other hand, have a marginal effect on the viscosity. At high surfactant concentrations, finally, there is a decrease in the viscosity once more (Figure 8.23).

Further information on the origin of this behaviour can be obtained from fluorescence quenching experiments, in which the number of hydrophobic tails per hydrophobic domain can be determined. As can be seen in Figure 8.24, hydrophobe-modified EHEC displays such a thickening behavior with SDS. Parallel measurements of the number of polymer hydrophobic tails per hydrophobic domain show that at low surfactant concentrations this number is significantly higher than 1, indicating that the micelles act as cross-links in the system. As the surfactant concentration increases, however, the number of polymer hydrophobic tags in each hydrophobic domain decreases towards 1. Thus, the re-

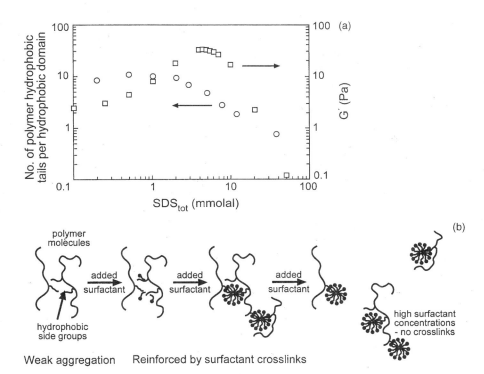

FIGURE 8.24   (a) Average number of polymer hydrophobic tails in the hydrophobic zones (circles) and the storage modulus G' of the h-EHEC solution (squares) as a function of SDS concentration. (b) Schematic illustration of the effects of surfactant binding to hydrophobe-modified polymers. (Redrawn from Thuresson et al., J. Phys. Chem. 1996, 100, 4909 (a), and Jönsson et al., 'Surfactants and Polymers in Aqueous Solution', Wiley, 1998 (b).)

duced elasticity at high surfactant concentration is correlated to a decreased degree of polymer "cross-linking" (Figure 8.24).

Together with surfactants cellulose ethers form systems of interest to rheology control in drug delivery. As illustrated in Figure 8.25, one notable feature of such polymers is their reversible gelation on increasing the temperature in the presence of certain ionic surfactants. The onset of gelation occurs at a temperature close to the cloud point in the absence of surfactant, and at a surfactant concentration substantially above the cmc (Figure 8.25).

As will be discussed further below, such systems offer opportunities in drug delivery due to possibilities for in situ gelation, and simultaneous capacity of solubilization of oil soluble substances (e.g., hydrophobic or amphiphilic drugs).

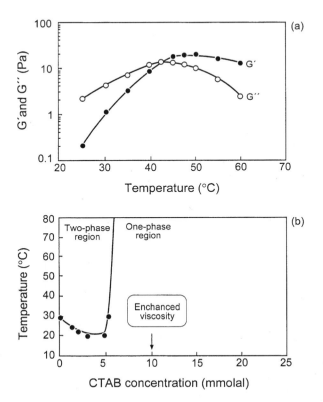

FIGURE 8.25   (a) Temperature-induced gelation of EHEC-CTAB solutions (1 wt%
EHEC, 0.36 wt% CTAB), monitored by the transition from $G'' > G'$ at low temperature (G' and G'' being the storage and loss moduli, respectively) to $G'' < G'$ at
high temperature. (b) Occurrence of the temperature-induced gelation in EHEC-
CTAB systems. (Redrawn from Carlsson et al., Colloids Surf. 1990, 47, 147.)

8.4   CHARACTERIZATION OF POLYMER SOLUTIONS
AND GELS

A family of methods used extensively for characterizing polymer solutions and
gels is that based on monitoring the viscosity and rheology of such systems.
Depending on the system, different rheological methods are used, and different
information obtained. In the present context, we will exemplify this by considering three cases: dilute polymer solutions, semidilute polymer solutions, and polymer gels.

    For dilute polymer solutions, determination of the intrinsic viscosity may
be used in order to obtain information about the molecular conformation of poly-

mers. This is achieved by measuring the zero-shear viscosity by an Ostwald viscometer as a function of polymer concentration, and extrapolating the viscosity to zero polymer concentration (Figure 8.26).

As an illustration of viscosity information about the polymer molecular shape, Figure 8.27 shows the viscosity of a polyelectrolyte solution as a function of salt and polymer concentration. The extrapolated zero polyelectrolyte concentration viscosity increases with a decreasing salt concentration, which shows that the polymer stretches out in low salt concentrations as a result of intramolecular electrostatic interactions.

Furthermore, the viscosity decreases drastically with the polyelectrolyte concentration at zero excess electrolyte, whereas the polymer concentration dependence at the higher salt concentrations is rather minor. This behavior follows from the electrostatic screening by the polyelectrolyte itself. Thus, similarly to low molecular weight salts, polyelectrolytes screen electrostatic interactions. Increasing the polyelectrolyte concentration therefore results in a contraction and

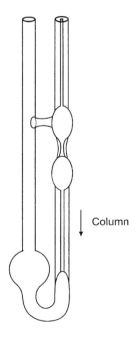

Column

FIGURE 8.26 Schematic illustration of an Ostwald viscometer. The time required for a polymer solution to pass the column relative to that of a liquid of known viscosity (normally the solvent in the absence of polymer) together with the known viscosity for the latter system yields the viscosity of the polymer solution. (Redrawn from Hiemenz, Principles of Colloid and Surface Chemistry, Marcel Dekker, 1986.)

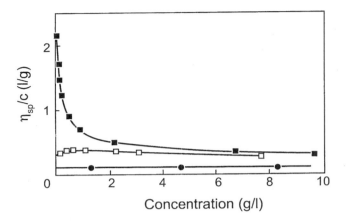

FIGURE 8.27 Effect of polymer concentration on the reduced viscosity η_{sp}/c of polyvinyl pyridinium bromide in water and electrolyte solutions. The salt used was KBr at a concentration of 0 M (filled squares), 0.001 M (open squares), or 0.0335 M (filled circles). (Redrawn from Fouss, Disc. Faraday Soc. 1951, 11, 127.)

a viscosity decrease. At high salt concentration, on the other hand, the additional screening provided by the relatively low concentration of polyelectrolyte is limited.

For more concentrated (semidilute) polymer solutions, rheological information is usually obtained through shear experiments, where a polymer solution between two solid bodies is sheared at a controlled rate, and the viscosity determined from the shear stress (Figure 8.28).

In the simplest case, the shear stress depends linearly on the shear rate, and the viscosity is independent of the shear rate. Such systems are called "new-

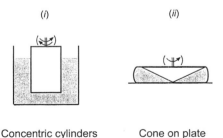

(i)   *(ii)*

Concentric cylinders   Cone on plate

FIGURE 8.28 Schematic illustration of two different experimental setups used for rheological experiments of polymer solutions.

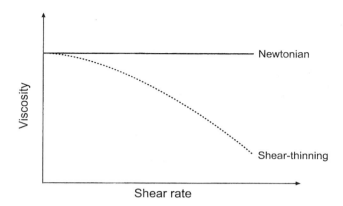

FIGURE 8.29 Schematic illustration of the effect of shear rate on the viscosity for a newtonian (solid line) and a shear-thinning (dotted line) polymer system.

tonian'' and are generally formed by low molecular weight nonassociating liquids. For many high molecular weight polymers, however, the molecules align in the shear fields, and as a consequence of this, the apparent viscosity decreases with the shear rate. Such systems are referred to as ''shear-thinning'' (Fig. 8.29).

Although some care should be applied when investigating shear-thinning polymer solutions through shear viscosity, such measurements can still be very useful for characterizing polymer solutions. For example, viscosity measurements can be used for determining the overlap concentration (c^*), at which the individual polymer coils start to overlap, and above which the polymer molecular weight is no longer of importance, but numerous properties instead determined by the polymer segment concentration or the entanglement density (Figure 8.30).

For gels formed by either covalent or physical cross-links, shear experiments will destroy the gel structure, and therefore provide rather limited information on such systems, which are better investigated by oscillatory measurements. In the latter, small deformations are executed to the polymer system in an oscillatory manner, and the phase and amplitude of the deformations followed (Figure 8.31).

If the phase angle between the applied deformation and the mechanical response is zero, the polymer system is completely elastic, whereas if the lag phase is 90°, the system is completely viscous. Real polymer solutions are generally neither perfectly elastic nor perfectly viscous, but rather something in between. In order to quantify the relative importance of the two responses, the relative magnitude of the elastic G' and loss G'' moduli are used, where G' and G'' are defined as the ratio of in-phase stress to strain and the ratio of 90° out-of-phase stress to strain, respectively. Thus, if G' is large and G'' is small, the

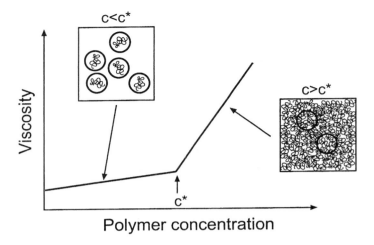

FIGURE 8.30 Schematic illustration of the effect of the polymer concentration on the viscosity of polymer solutions. c^* marks the overlap concentration, i.e., the transition from dilute to semidilute polymer solution. Note that the viscosity increases more strongly with polymer concentration at $c > c^*$.

system is largely elastic, whereas if $G'' \gg G'$ the system is largely viscous. Thus, the onset of gelation may operationally be defined as the conditions where $G' > G''$ (Figure 8.32).

Also, rheological data may be combined with mechanical theories in order to learn more about the structure of the gels. For example, the amplitude of G' in the limit of high oscillation frequency may be used for estimating the number of cross-links per unit volume, a valuable piece of information for understanding, e.g., polymer gel swelling.

8.5 RESPONSIVE POLYMER SYSTEMS

Due to the large number of segments typically present in a polymer molecule and the balance between entropic and enthalpic contributions, polymer systems often display a "responsive" nature, i.e., in response to external parameters they undergo abrupt transitions in their physical properties. Particularly for high molecular weight polymers, such transitions may be very dramatic, essentially of an "all or nothing" nature. As an illustration of this, Figure 8.33 shows the onset of temperature-induced phase separation of an aqueous polyNIPAM solution, which occurs over a temperature range of significantly less than 0.5°C.

The abrupt transition for polyNIPAM with elevated temperature concerns

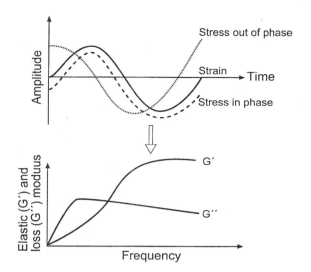

FIGURE 8.31 Schematic illustration of oscilloratory deformations of a polymer solution/gel, and of the mechanical response of the latter to the applied deformations. From information on the stress out of phase and in phase with the applied strain, information can be extracted in the form of an elastic (storage) modulus G' and a viscous (loss) modulus G''.

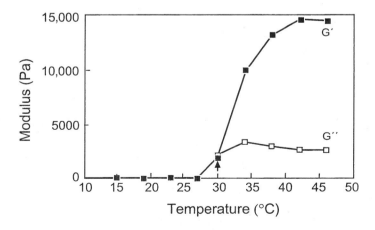

FIGURE 8.32 G' and G'' as a function of temperature for an aqueous Pluronic F127 system. The arrow indicates the onset of 'gelation.'

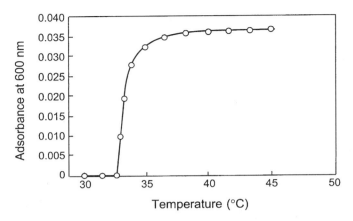

FIGURE 8.33 Absorbance of an aqueous polyNIPAM solution as a function of temperature.

not only the solubility but also a number of other physical parameters. For example, polyNIPAM gels undergo a collapse at the critical temperature, which is analogous to the phase separation for non-cross-linked polymer solutions (Figures 8.13 to 8.15). Also at interfaces, the decreased solvency at elevated temperatures results in analogous abrupt transitions. Thus, for adsorbed polyNIPAM the adsorbed layer collapses at the critical temperature and forms a concentrated ''surface phase'' of polymer (Figure 8.34).

The interfacial collapse, in turn, has consequences for surfaces and particles modified by polyNIPAM. For example, colloids stabilized by polyNIPAM undergo flocculation at the critical temperature as a consequence of the collapse of the adsorbed layers (Chapter 9).

This is just one example of a responsive polymer system. There are a number of other polymers undergoing reversed temperature-dependent solubility and analogous transitions with increasing temperature, including PEO, PPO, PEO/PPO copolymers, PEO-derivatives, cellulose ethers, PVA, etc. Moreover, all polymers which do not display a reversed temperature dependent solubility show the corresponding transitions with *decreasing* temperature. There are also ''switching parameters'' other than temperature. Thus, as discussed above in relation to gel swelling and polymer conformation, the salt concentration fulfills a similar role for polyelectrolyte systems. For titrating polyelectrolytes, pH is also of analogous importance, since it affects the polymer charge density. As discussed above, surfactants may also induce responsive transitions in polymer systems, as may other cosolutes, e.g., Ca^{2+} ions in alginate systems.

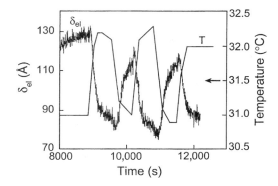

FIGURE 8.34 Effect of temperature on the adsorbed layer thickness δ_{el} of adsorbed polyNIPAM layers. The temperature was cycled around the transition temperature (indicated with an arrow) over time (solid line), and the effect on the adsorbed layer thickness monitored. (Redrawn from Carlsson et al., J. Colloid Interface Sci. 2001, 233, 320.)

8.6 POLYMER SOLUTIONS AND GELS IN DRUG DELIVERY

Within drug delivery, the term "gel" is frequently used rather generously for essentially any system displaying high viscosity. Structurally, gel systems may be very different, and include, e.g., polymer solutions, polymer/surfacant systems, and chemically cross-linked gels, but also liquid crystalline phases and concentrated disperse or polar lipid systems. Some care should therefore be taken to identify the type of "gelling" system in question in order to allow for their controlled use in pharmaceutical formulations.

8.6.1 Chemically Cross-Linked Gels

Chemically cross-linked gels are interesting primarily because of their robustness and because the cross-linking density may be controlled over wide ranges, the latter offering means to control, e.g., the gel swelling and drug release. In the context of oral drug delivery, gel systems responding to changes in pH or electrolyte concentration offer some opportunities, since swelling/deswelling transitions allow the exposure of the drug to the surrounding aqueous solution to be controlled, e.g., so that the drug is protected from the aqueous environment at low pH. In particular, polyacids are useful in this context, since they are protonated at the low pH in the stomach, resulting in a compact and somewhat dehydrated structure at these conditions. This, in turn, may lead to a low release rate and

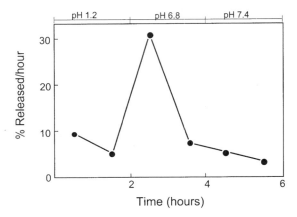

FIGURE 8.35 Fractional release rate of prednisolone from a hydrogel formed by cross-linked PEO and poly(methacrylic acid-co-methylmethacrylate) vs. time. The pH was changed in intervals during the experiment as indicated. (Redrawn from Carelli et al., Int. J. Pharm. 1999, 179, 73.)

some protection against acid catalyzed hydrolysis of the drug. On the other hand, the deprotonation at a higher pH, e.g., corresponding to that in the small intestine, causes the polymer system to swell as a result of intramolecular electrostatic interactions. This, in turn, facilitates the release of the drug in a region where it is absorbed more effectively, and where it is more stable against hydrolytic degradation (Figure 8.35).

Figure 8.35 shows results on the release of prednisolone from pH-sensitive hydrogels prepared from poly(methacrylic acid-co-methacrylate) and cross-linked PEO, showing that the prednisolone release depends on pH. Specifically, the results show that the higher degree of swelling, the faster the release of the drug. Similar results have been found for a range of pH-sensitive hydrogels and a range of drugs.

Another promising type of electrostatically responding system is that which depends on the electrolyte concentration. This can be illustrated by the release of nicotine from ion-exchange resins containing carboxyl groups. At pH 7.4, where nicotine is present in its positively charged form, and therefore electrostatically bound to the negatively charged ion-exchange resin, the release of nicotine increases with increasing ionic strength (Figure 8.36). This is expected, since increasing the ionic strength reduces the electrostatic attraction between nicotine and the resin, thus facilitating the release of the former.

Analogous effects may be obtained by temperature-responding cross-linked polymer gel systems. For polymers displaying reversed temperature solubility, this can be used to load the gels at low temperature, and to achieve a sustained

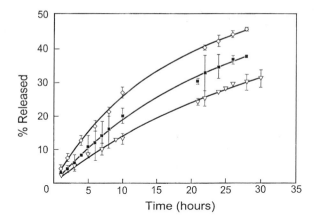

FIGURE 8.36 Release rate of nicotine from a negatively charged resin at pH 7.4 at an ionic strength of 0.11 M (triangles), 0.22 M (squares), and 0.44 M (diamonds). (Redrawn from Conaghey et al., Int. J. Pharm. 1998, 170, 215.)

release after administration (Figure 8.16). Furthermore, the swelling/deswelling of such gel systems may also affect the biological function of incorporated (protein) drugs. This can be illustrated by incorporating an enzyme in a responsive polymer gel particle and probing the enzyme activity. As can be seen in Figure 8.37, varying the temperature between a temperature just below and one just above the lower consolute temperature results in a reversible variation in the probed enzymatic activity.

Conversely, the properties of the drug influence the behavior of thermally responsive gel delivery systems. As an example of this, Figure 8.38 shows how the degree of swelling of thermally responsive hydrogels of N-isopropylacrylamide-containing hydrophobic comonomers is affected by the presence of ephedrine and ibuprofen. As can be seen, the hydrophilic drug ephedrine causes essentially no deswelling of these gels. On the other hand, addition of hydrophobic ibuprofen results in a gel collapse.

8.6.2 Gels Formed by Polysaccharides

Polysaccharide gels display many properties analogous to chemically cross-linked gels, e.g., relating to pH- or salt-dependent swelling for charged polymers, and the effect of this on the release of incorporated drugs. Also analogous to swollen chemically cross-linked gels, polysaccharide gels contain essentially no hydrophobic domains, and are therefore not very efficient in solubilizing uncharged hydrophobic drugs. As such, they can only solubilize either fully soluble

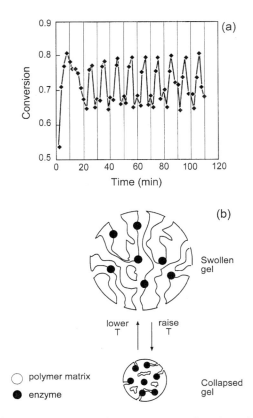

FIGURE 8.37 (a) Conversion as a function of time on performing a repeated 30–35°C cycle for β-galactosidase incorporated in polyNIPAM gel particles. (b) Schematic illustration of the effect of temperature on gel particles with incorporated enzyme. (Redrawn from Park et al., Appl. Biochem. Biotechnol. 1988, 19, 1.)

(hydrophilic) drugs, or dispersed drug (-containing) colloids. Nevertheless, a considerable drug loading can be reached by utilizing poor solvency contitions for the drug. This is illustrated in Figure 8.39 for the loading capacity of propranolol in gellan gum microgel particles by increasing pH to above the pK_a of propanolol prior to particle formation. Thus, by increasing pH prior to gel formation, thereby reducing the solubility of this drug, the drug loading of these particles can be significantly increased.

A useful type of polysaccharide gel in drug delivery is that formed by alginate and gellan gum. Thus, on addition of Ca^{2+} or other divalent cations,

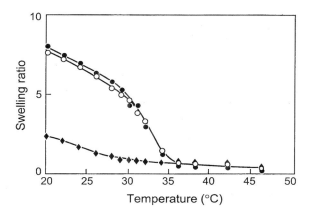

FIGURE 8.38 Effect of ibuprofen (filled diamonds) and ephedrin (filled circles) on the temperature-induced deswelling of polyNIPAAM gels. Shown also are results obtained in the absence of drugs (open circles). (Redrawn from Lowe et al., Polymer 1999, 40, 2595.)

gelation occurs through specific ion-binding and resulting conformational changes (Figure 8.40).

Although there are other cations which are more potent than Ca^{2+} in inducing gelation of alginate solutions (e.g., Ba^{2+} and Sr^{2+}), Ca^{2+} is usually used in drug delivery applications. The properties of Ca^{2+}-alginate gels depend on their

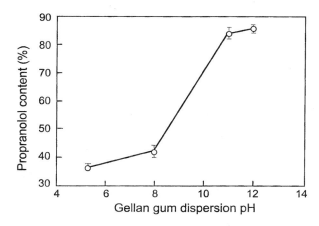

FIGURE 8.39 Effect of pH of the gellan gum dispersion on propranolol hydrochloride content. (Redrawn from Kedzierewicz et al., Int. J. Pharm. 1999, 178, 129.)

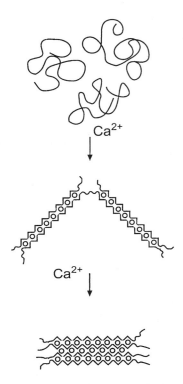

FIGURE 8.40 Schematic illustration of alginate network formation. Ca^{2+}-induced cross-linking involves lateral association between guluronate segments to form ordered junction zones, as well as helix aggregation. (Redrawn from Clark et al., Adv. Polym. Sci. 1987, 83, 57.)

composition, and in particular the Ca^{2+} concentration, which determines the 'cross-linking' density of the gels. In particular, with increasing Ca^{2+} concentration, the amount of drug which is incorporated is decreased as is the release kinetics (Figure 8.41).

An area where polysaccharide gels have potential is within colon drug delivery. The main reason for this is that the fermentation of polysaccharide carriers caused by microbial enzymes in the large interestine may be used, together with the inherent tendency for such systems to display sustained release of solubilized drugs, to obtain a localized drug release in the colon or the large intestine. Such localization is advantageous, e.g., for colon-localized indications, such as Crohn's disease, ulcerative colitis, spastic colon, constipation, and colon cancer. More-

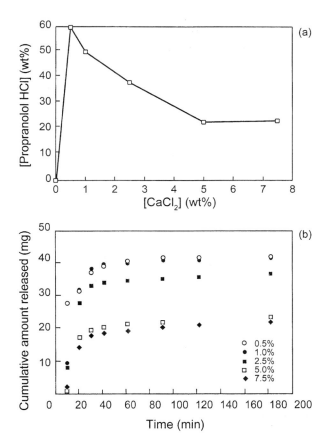

FIGURE 8.41 Effect of the Ca^{2+} concentration on the amount of propranolol HCl incorporated into (a) and released from (b) Ca^{2+}-alginate gels. (Redrawn from Lim et al., Drug Dev. Ind. Pharm. 1997, 23, 973.)

over, colon-localized administration is also promising for systemic absorption of, e.g., peptides and proteins, which are extensively degraded in the gastrointestinal tract. A number of polysaccharide systems have been investigated in this context, e.g., coatings by amylose, cyclodextrins, galactomannan or pectin, as well as matrices formed by, e.g., chondroitin sulfate, dextran, pectin, or galactomannan. Just to provide one illustrative example, Figure 8.42 shows results obtained on the release of indomethacin from a calcium pectate gel in the absence and presence of pectinolytic enzyme, known to be present in the colonic region.

As can be seen, essentially no release is observed in the absence of digestive

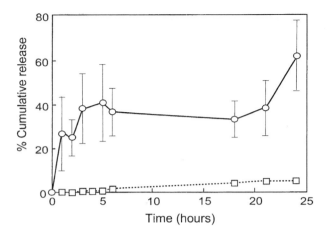

FIGURE 8.42 Cumulative release of indomethacin from a calcium pectate gel in citrate buffer in the presence (circles) and absence (squares) of pectinolytic enzyme. (Redrawn from Rubinstein et al., in Friend, ed., Oral Colon-Specific Drug Delivery, CRC Press, 1992.)

enzymes, whereas a significant release is observed in the presence of such enzymes. Therefore, the release to the colon may be controlled by the stability of the matrix to enzymatic degradation, and, more importantly, a specific targeting to the large intestine can be obtained by this approach.

8.6.3 Gels Formed by Block Copolymers

''Gels'' formed by certain PEO-PPO-PEO block copolymers are quite interesting for drug delivery since they form abruptly on increasing the temperature. However, although these systems are usually referred to as gels in the drug delivery literature, they are liquid crystalline phases or (partially) disordered liquid crystalline phases. They are therefore discussed in Chapter 3.

8.6.4 Polymer-Surfactant Mixtures

As discussed above, mixing polymers and surfactants frequently results in surfactant binding to the polymer backbone, as well as polymer-induced surfactant self-assembly. Apart from providing an effective transient cross-linking mechanism, such structures are interesting for drug delivery also since they contain hydropho-

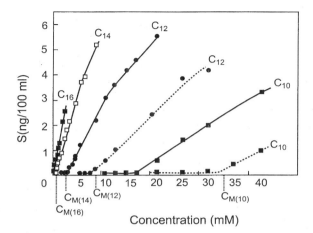

FIGURE 8.43 Solubilization of Orange OT *S* as a function of surfactant concentration in the presence (solid lines) and absence (dashed lines) of PVP for different surfactant alkyl chain length. cmc's (C_M's) for the different surfactants are also shown. (Redrawn from Lange et al., Kolloid Z.Z. Polym. 1971, 243, 101.)

bic domains which can solubilize hydrophobic drugs in a similar way as free surfactant micelles. This is illustrated in Figure 8.43.

The drug solubilization in such polymer-bound micelles can be controlled in similar ways as for free micelles, e.g., through the drug hydrophobicity and charge, by the head group of the surfactant, etc. For example, increasing the surfactant hydrophobic chain length promotes both polymer-induced micelle formation and micellization in solution. Since solubilization of hydrophobic solutes occurs only in the presence of micelles, this means that increasing the surfactant hydrophobic chain length results in an earlier onset surfactant concentration for solubilization both for the micellar solution and the polymer-surfactant systems (Figure 8.43.).

One type of polymer system which has been found to be interesting in the context of polymer-surfactant complexation is that of cellulose ethers and hydrophobe-modified cellulose ethers (Figure 8.25). For example, EHEC/surfactant systems form gels in the presence of timolol maleate and timolol chloride, the former a potent β-blocker. It has been found that timolol maleate can be incorporated in the thermogelling EHEC system at a concentration relevant to commercial eye drops, indicating a potential use of these systems in ocular drug delivery. The latter is also supported by a sustained release of the active ingredient displayed by the polymer/surfactant formulation in comparison to the aqueous solution (Figure 8.44).

By comparing formulations containing timolol maleate and timolol chloride as well as those with different surfactants, it can be inferred that for a gel to form at a low concentration of ionic surfactant, (1) the ionic drug should typically be a coion to the surfactant, (2) the counterions of the drug and the surfactant should be inorganic and with a low polarizability, and (3) the surfactant should have a low cmc but a Krafft temperature not higher than room temperature.

A notable feature of polymer-surfactant gels in drug delivery is the antibacterial properties of some surfactants, which may be used to create an added value of the formulation in some indications. As an illustration of this, Figure 8.45 shows results obtained with a local anesthetic formulation intended for the peridontal pocket consisting of lidocaine/prilocaine, EHEC, and myristoylcholine bromide. Due to the latter being a readily biodegradable and antibacterial cationic surfactant, this in situ–thickening formulation also acts to reduce inflammations, and is disintegrated as a result of biodegradation of the surfactant. As can be seen in Figure 8.45, at least moderate amounts of the active ingredients can be incorporated without detrimental effects on the gelation behavior.

As discussed in Chapter 4, complexation of DNA with cationic liposomes offers a way to improve the efficacy of gene transfection. Similarly, DNA complexation with cationic surfactants constitutes a way to improve the transfection. Due to the complexation with the oppositely charged surfactant the highly charged and therefore highly extended DNA is collapsed (Figure 8.46).

Furthermore, complexation reduces the net negative charge of the DNA. Since there is a repulsive interaction between the similarly charged cell surface and DNA the reduction of the net negative charge of the DNA is advantageous for transfection.

Naturally, not only liposomes and surfactants but also cationic polymers can be used for DNA compactation. Among many other cationic polyelectrolytes, poly(amino amine) cascade dendrimers have been investigated in relation to gene therapy. At charge neutrality large aggregates are formed and the transfection rate is relatively poor. With increasing concentration of cationic dendrimer, however, the size of the complexes formed decreases, and the complexes obtain a net positive charge (Figure 8.47), Both these effects are advantageous for transfection (Figure 8.48).

Polymer-surfactant complex formation has also been used as a therapeutic mechanism. Thus, the use of polymeric bile salt sequestrants for lowering the bile salt concentration is by now an established treatment for reducing high cholesterol levels. Thus, by binding the bile salt molecules to the polymeric sequestrant, the bile-mediated emulsification and fat uptake from the gastrointestinal tract may be decreased. In general, these polymeric sequestrants are cationic poly-

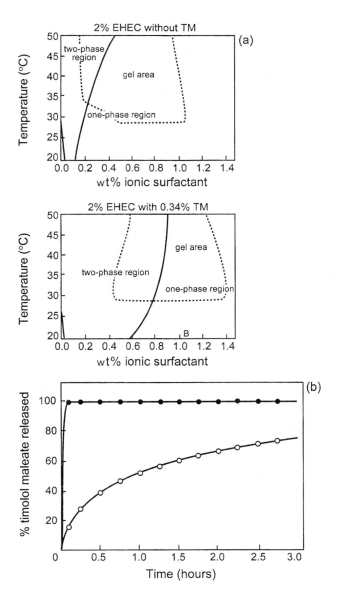

FIGURE 8.44 (a) Phase diagram of EHEC/alkyl betainate mixtures and the absence and presence of (0.34 wt%) timolol maleate (TM). (b) In vitro release profiles of timolol maleate from an EHEC/alkyl betainate gel formulation (open circles) and the corresponding aqueous solution in the absence of polymer (filled circles). (Redrawn from Lindell et al., Int. J. Pharm. 1993, 95, 219.)

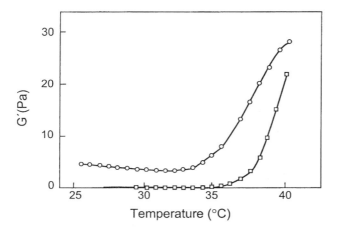

FIGURE 8.45 Elastic modulus *G′* of formulations containing EHEC (1 wt%) and myristoytlcholine bromide (3 mM) in the presence (circles) and absence (squares) of 0.5 wt% prilocaine/lidocaine (50/50), pH 9.2. (Redrawn from Scherlund et al., J. Colloid Interface Sci. 2000, 229, 365.)

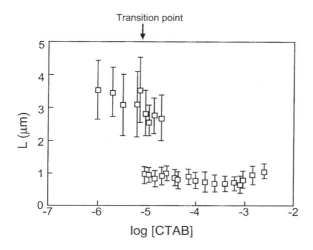

FIGURE 8.46 Long axis length *L* of T4DNA molecules vs. CTAB concentration. (Redrawn from Melnikov et al., J. Am. Chem. Soc. 1995, 117, 2401.)

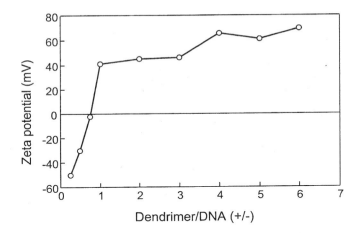

FIGURE 8.47   Zeta potential of plasmid/cationic dendrimer complexes as a function of dendrimer/DNA ratio. (Redrawn from Tomlinson et al., J. Controlled Release 1996, 39, 357.)

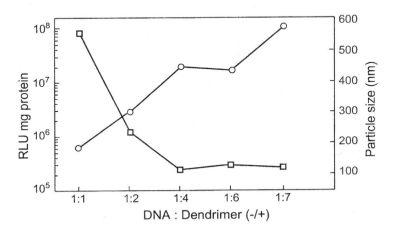

FIGURE 8.48   Effect of DNA/dendrimer ratio on particle size (squares) and transfection efficacy (circles; increasing RLU means increased transfection efficiency) of plasmid/dendrimer complexes. (Redrawn from Mumper et al., Proceed. Intl. Symp. Control Rel. Bioact. Mater. 1995, 22, 178.)

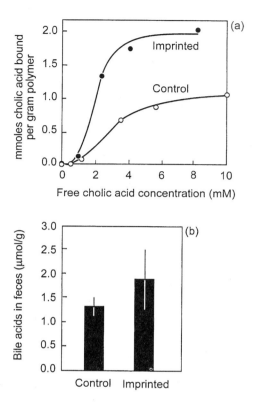

FIGURE 8.49 (a) Bile salt binding isotherm for a cross-linked imprinted poly (ammonium) salt (filled circles). For comparison, also data from a non-imprinted control polymer are shown (open circles). (b) Result of the in vivo bile salt excretion after treatment with the imprinted cross-linked poly(ammonium) salt in (a) compared to the control. (Redrawn from Huval et al., Macromolecules 2001, 34, 1548.)

electrolytes bearing ammonium groups, and the sequesting therefore based largely on electrostatically driven binding between the negatively charged bile salt surfactants and the positively charged polymer. Naturally, a critical factor related to the function of these polymers as sequestrants is their binding capacity for bile salts, since an efficient sequestrant should bind large amount of bile salt. One type of polymeric sequestrants which has been found to be promising for this reason is the imprinted poly(allylamine) polymer (Figure 8.49).

BIBLIOGRAPHY

Alexandridis, P., B. Lindman, eds., Amphiphilic Block Copolymers: Self-Assembly and Applications, Elsevier, Amsterdam, 2000.

Clark, A. H., S. B. Ross-Murphy, Structural and mechanical properties of bipolymer gels, Adv. Polym. Sci. 83:57–192 (1987).

Collyer, A. A., D. W. Clegg, eds., Rheological Measurement, Chapman & Hall, London, 1998.

Flory, P. J., Principles of Polymer Chemistry, Cornell University Press, 1953.

Garnett, M. C., Gene-delivery systems using cationic polymers, Crit. Rev. Ther. Drug Carrier Syst. 16:147–207 (1999).

Goddard, E. D., K. P. Ananthabadmanabhan, eds., Interactions of Surfactants with Polymers and Proteins, CRC Press, Boca Raton, 1993.

Hovgaard, L., H. Brøndsted. Current applications of polysaccharides in colon targeting, Crit. Rev. Ther. Drug Carrier Syst. 13:185–223 (1996).

Kwak, J.C.T., ed., Polymer-Surfactant Systems, Surfactant Science Series, vol. 77, Marcel Dekker, New York, 1998.

Morris, V. J., P. J. Wilde, Interactions of food biopolymers, Curr. Opinion Colloid Interface Sci. 2:567–572 (1997).

Park, K., W.S.W. Shalaby, Biodegradable Hydrogels for Drug Delivery, Technomic, 1993.

Piculell, L., Gelling polysaccharides, Curr. Opinion Colloid Interface Sci. 3:643–650 (1998).

Rubinstein, A., A. Sintov, Biodegradable polymeric matrices with potential specificity to the large intestine, in D. R. Friend, ed., Oral Colon-Specific Drug Delivery, CRC Press, Boca Raton, 1992.

Schild, H. G., Poly(N-isopropylacrylamide): experiment, theory and application, Prog. Polym. Sci. 17, 163–249 (1992).

Yuk, S. H., Y. H. Bae, Phase transition polymers for drug delivery, Crit. Rev. Ther. Drug Carrier Syst. 16:385–423 (1999).

9

Polymer Particles

9.1 INTERACTION BETWEEN PARTICLES

Most dispersed systems are thermodynamically unstable, and will therefore floc-culate and eventually display macroscopic phase separation. Such behavior has major influence on the performance of colloidal dispersions, and hence also for their application in drug delivery applications. In order to understand the stability of such colloidal systems, it is essential to have basic knowledge regarding the forces between the particles. Depending on the system, these forces may contain numerous contributions. Almost invariably, a van der Waals interaction is present in colloidal systems, generally contributing to an attractive interparticle interac-tion. Simply speaking, the larger the difference in refractive index between the particles and the ambient solution, the more attractive the van der Waals interac-tion. This means, e.g., that the van der Waals interaction between dense polymer particles is more attractive than that between solvent-swollen gel particles (Fig-ure 9.1).

For most disperse polymer particle systems, the van der Waals attraction is balanced by electrostatic interactions. In the case of simpler colloidal systems with only one type of particles, the similar charge of the particles generates a repulsive electrostatic interaction between the particles, which increases with the charge density. The range of the interaction decreases with increasing salt concen-tration (Figure 9.2).

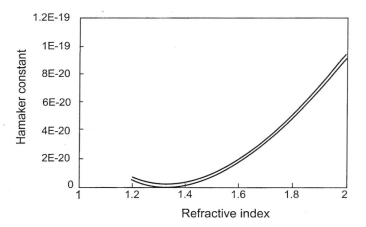

FIGURE 9.1 Effect of refractive index difference between polymer particles/ surfaces and the solvent on the van der Waals attraction. The larger the Hamaker constant, the more attractive the interaction. In the calculations, the refractive index of the solvent was taken to be 1.34 (i.e., that of water), and the refractive index of the particles/surfaces varied.

Within the so-called DLVO theory, the total particle-particle interaction is given by the combination of the attractive van der Waals and the repulsive electrostatic interactions (Figure 9.3).

In particular, the combined interparticle interaction curve displays a secondary maximum, followed by a primary minimum, and a final repulsion at small distances of separation. This means that for two particles to approach each other to the primary minimum, which corresponds to flocculation of the dispersion, they have to pass the secondary repulsive interaction barrier. The probability for the latter depends on the relative magnitude of the thermal motion of the particles and the height of the barrier. Eventually, however, all particles will pass the barrier, and therefore such dispersions are not thermodynamically stable, but merely kinetically stable over a given time frame.

Since the range of the electrostatic interaction decreases with increasing concentration of excess electrolyte the repulsive electrostatic interaction contribution becomes relatively less important with increasing salt concentration. In particular, the repulsive secondary maximum in the interparticle interaction curve decreases and eventually vanishes (Figure 9.4).

This means that with increasing salt concentration it becomes increasingly easy for two particles to approach each other sufficiently close to become locked in the primary minimum, and hence for dispersion flocculation to occur (Figure 9.5). With increasing valency of the counterions, the electrostatic screening is

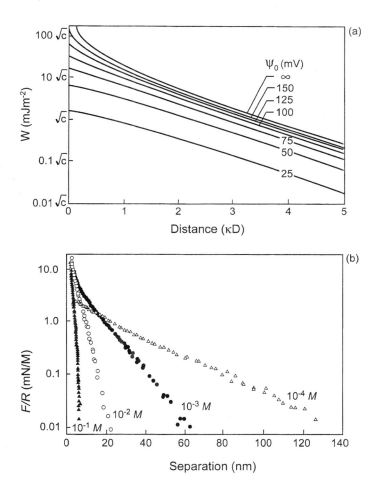

FIGURE 9.2   Typical results on the effect of (a) the electrostatic potential ψ_0 and (b) the salt concentration on the electrostatic repulsion (W or F/R) between similarly charged surfaces/particles. κ, D, and c refer to the Debye length (the decay length of the electrostatic interactions), the distance, and the electrolyte concentration, respectively. (Redrawn from Israelachvili, Intermolecular and Surface Forces, Academic Press, 1994 (a), and Shubin et al., J. Colloid Interface Sci. 1993, 155, 108.)

enhanced, and hence electrostatically stabilized dispersions are more easily flocculated. In general, therefore, electrostatic stabilization of colloidal systems is inefficient at high electrolyte concentration (present, e.g., in blood).

Given the electrolyte-induced flocculation of electrostatically stabilized colloidal dispersions, there is a need for alternative stabilization mechanisms for

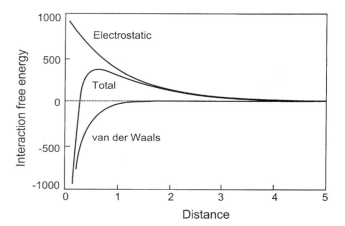

FIGURE 9.3   Schematic illustration of a typical interaction curve versus interparticle separation within the DLVO framework. Shown is the attractive van der Waals interaction and the repulsive electrostatic interaction contributions, as well as the combination of these two contributions.

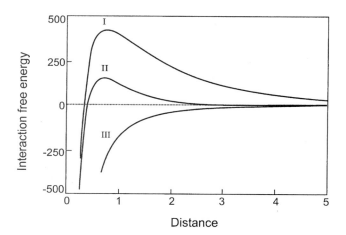

FIGURE 9.4   Schematic illustration of the effect of salt concentration on the magnitude of the secondary repulsive barrier between two colloidal particles. The series I → II → III represent an increasing salt concentration.

Valence of counterion	Negative colloids			Positive colloids		Theory
	As_2S_2	Au	AgI	Fe_2O_3	Al_2O_3	
1	(5.5×10^{-2})	(2.4×10^{-2})	(1.42×10^{-1})	(1.18×10^{-2})	(5.2×10^{-2})	
	1	1	1	1	1	1
2	(6.9×10^{-4})	(3.8×10^{-4})	(2.43×10^{-3})	(2.1×10^{-4})	(6.3×10^{-4})	
	1.3×10^{-2}	1.6×10^{-2}	1.7×10^{-2}	1.8×10^{-2}	1.2×10^{-2}	1.56×10^{-2}
3	(9.1×10^{-5})	(6.0×10^{-6})	(6.8×10^{-5})	-	(8×10^{-5})	
	1.7×10^{-3}	0.3×10^{-3}	0.5×10^{-3}	-	1.5×10^{-3}	1.37×10^{-3}
4	(9.0×10^{-5})	(9.0×10^{-7})	(1.3×10^{-5})	-	(5.3×10^{-5})	
	17×10^{-4}	0.4×10^{-4}	1×10^{-4}	-	10×10^{-4}	2.44×10^{-4}

FIGURE 9.5 Critical salt concentration (in molar units) required to flocculate different dispersions (ccc). Values in parentheses are absolute concentrations, while nonparenthesis values are normalized with the ccc for monovalent counterions. (From Overbeek, in Kruyt, ed., Colloid Science, Elsevier, 1952.)

colloidal systems at high electrolyte or particles concentrations. One such possibility is provided by so-called steric stabilization due to adsorbed or grafted polymer layers. Contrary to electrostatically stabilized systems, little or no destabilization is observed on salt addition. However, polymers can both stabilize and destabilize colloidal dispersions, depending on a number of factors. For a controlled use of polymers in colloidal systems, a basic understanding of factors controlling the stabilization and destabilization is therefore required.

Of major importance for the effect of polymers on the stability of colloidal systems is whether or not the polymers adsorb at the particle surface. If the polymer does not adsorb, it is actually depleted from the interfacial region. This, in turn, results in a surface energy increase, which in turn causes destabilization and flocculation. This is usually referred to as depletion flocculation. Somewhat simplistically, one can see the flocculation as a means for the system to reduce the surface area, and therefore also the volume not accessible for the polymer (Figure 9.6). The depletion attraction depends on both the concentration gradient

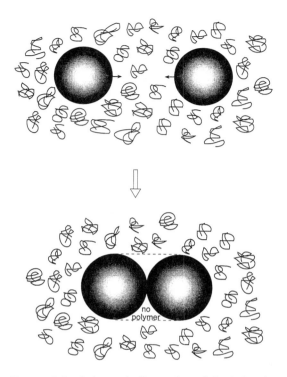

FIGURE 9.6   Schematic illustration of depletion flocculation.

and the width of the depletion zone, the latter governed by, e.g., the polymer molecular weight. Of particular importance is that in order to reach a sufficient driving force for depletion flocculation, the concentration gradient between the bulk and the proximity to the surface must be high, and therefore a quite high polymer concentration (roughly of the order a few percent and above) is required. Thus, only at such concentrations is depletion flocculation observed. Furthermore, it follows that depletion flocculation can generally be reversed simply by diluting the system.

For adsorbing polymers, either colloidal stabilization or destabilization may occur depending on a number of factors. One clear division line can be drawn based on the surface coverage of the adsorbing polymer. Thus, for adsorbing polymers at less than full coverage, one polymer chain may adsorb simultaneously at two or more colloidal particles, thus yielding an attractive interaction (Figure 9.7). The latter causes flocculation, and is usually referred to as bridging

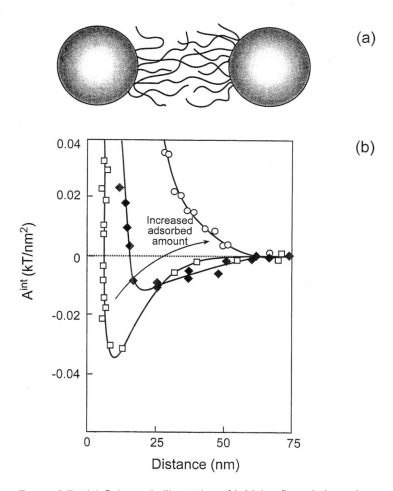

FIGURE 9.7 (a) Schematic illustration of bridging flocculation, where some of the polymer chains adsorb at two or more particles at the same time. (b) Interaction A_{int} between two polymer-coated surfaces as a function of coverage. (Redrawn from Fleer et al., Polymers at Interfaces, Chapman & Hall, 1993.)

flocculation. As an illustration of this, Figure 9.7 shows the interaction between two surfaces coated with an adsorbing polymer at a few different surface coverages. As can be seen, the interaction is monotonically repulsive at high (full) coverage, whereas an attraction is found at partial coverage. Thus, if destabilization is the goal partial coverage is desired, whereas if stabilization is the goal,

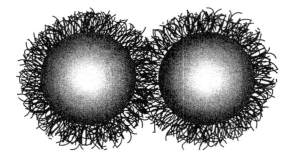

FIGURE 9.8 Schematic illustration of steric stabilization of polymer-coated particles.

one should make sure to be on full coverage, i.e., at the plateau in the adsorption isotherm for the polymer at the particles. It is therefore essential to determine the adsorption isotherm for the system in order to facilitate a controlled stability.

Also for adsorbing polymers at full coverage, either stabilization or destabilization of colloidal systems may occur, depending on the conditions. The key issue in this respect is the role of solvency. As discussed previously in Chapter 8, the free energy of mixing is favored by the mixing entropy, but generally opposed by the enthalpy of mixing. The latter is determined by how good or poor the solvent is, which is usually referred to in terms of solvency. At good solvency conditions, the polymer-solvent interaction is relatively good (or at least not very poor), and a one-phase system is generally formed. With deteriorating solvency, on the other hand, phase separation eventually occurs.

In analogy to this, every process which results in an increased polymer concentration (i.e., demixing) is favorable at poor solvency conditions, but unfavorable at good solvency conditions. When two polymer-coated surfaces (particles) approach each other, there is an overlap between the adsorbed layers. This, in turn, causes the polymer concentration to increase locally in the region between the particles (Figure 9.8). Since this is analogous to a demixing process, the interaction between such surfaces (particles) is attractive at poor solvency conditions and repulsive at good solvency conditions (Figure 9.9).

Therefore, there is generally a good agreement between the critical flocculation point (induced by temperature, solvent composition, pH, cosolute addition, or some other parameter), on one hand, and the onset of phase separation in the polymer solution, on the other. This also means that the critical flocculation point is generally largely independent of the polymer molecular weight and the colloid particle size, chemical nature, and concentration.

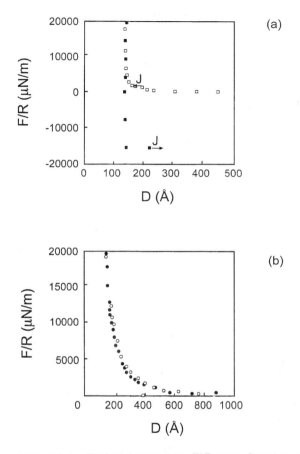

FIGURE 9.9 Typical interaction F/R as a function of distance D between two polymer-coated surfaces at poor (a) and good (b) solvency conditions. Note the attractive interaction (negative F/R) at poor solvency conditions and repulsion (monotonically increasing positive F/R) at good solvency conditions. Open and filled symbols represent forces on approach and separation, respectively. (Redrawn from Malmsten et al., Langmuir 1990, 6, 1572.)

9.2 INTERACTION BETWEEN PARTICLES AND SURFACES

The interaction between particles and macroscopic surfaces follows the same trends as particle-particle interactions, with the exception that the van der Waals interaction is stronger in this geometry. Thus, for similarly charged particle-surface pairs the particle deposition at the surface increases with increasing elec-

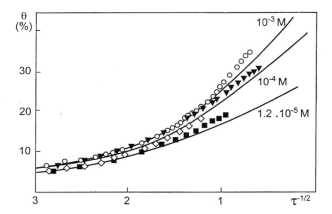

FIGURE 9.10   Effect of ionic strength on the deposition rate $\theta(\tau)$ of latex particles at a surface of a similar charge sign. (Redrawn from Adamczyk et al., Adv. Colloid Interface Sci. 1994, 48, 151.)

trostatic screening or decreased particle and surface charge density (Figure 9.10 and 9.11).

For particle and surfaces of opposite charge, an attractive electrostatic contribution strongly increases the particle deposition rate at the surface, an effect which is opposed on addition of salt. As will be discussed below, this can be used for preparing bioadhesive drug formulations.

In a similar way that particle-particle interactions can be controlled by polymer coatings, the deposition of particles at macroscopic surfaces may be controlled by coating either the particles or the surface or both with polymers. In the present context, polymer coating of particles offers some opportunities to control particle deposition at interfaces, as will be discussed below in relation to bioadhesive drug formulations.

9.3   METHODS FOR STUDYING POLYMER PARTICLE SYSTEMS

For disperse systems in general, the most important parameter to determine is whether or not the system is stable under the conditions of interest. Once this is known, primary information of interest concerns the particle size and size distribution, and possibly also the particle shape and shape distribution. In particular, particle size analysis methods allow simultaneous analysis of whether the system is stable or not, and analysis of particle size and size distribution. Such methods are therefore generally the most important ones for investigations of disperse

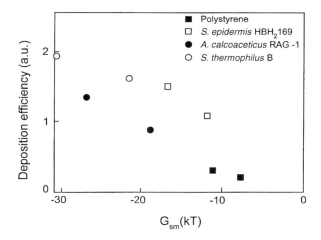

FIGURE 9.11 Effect of particle-surface charge contrast, expressed as the magnitude of the secondary minimum, on the deposition efficiency of polystyrene particles and bacteria with different (negative) surface charge at glass and PMMA. The less negative the particle-surface interaction free energy minimum G_{sm}, the more important the repulsive electrostatic interaction preventing deposition. (Redrawn from Meinders et al., J. Colloid Interface Sci. 1995, 176, 329.)

particle systems. There are many different methods for this, and a few commonly employed techniques and principles will be briefly outlined below.

9.3.1 Dynamic Light Scattering

Dynamic light scattering, or photon correlation spectroscopy (PCS) as it is also frequently called, is a widely used method which is particularly useful for determining the size of small dispersed particles (≤ 500 nm). It is based on the temporal development of light scattering from a particle dispersion. Due to diffusion of the particles, the interference between light scattered from individual particles results in intensity fluctuations. PCS is based on monitoring these time variations in the intensity of light scattered from a dilute dispersion of particles. Since the fluctuations in scattering intensity result from diffusion-dependent local concentration variations, the decay of the scattering intensity autocorrelation function may be used to determine the particle diffusion coefficient (Figure 9.12). This, in turn, may be translated into a particle radius R_h through

$$R_h = \frac{kT}{6\pi\eta D} \tag{9.1}$$

where k, T, η, and D refer to the Boltzmann constant, temperature, the viscosity

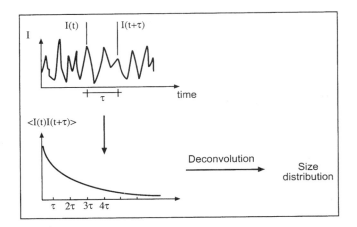

FIGURE 9.12   Schematic illustration of PCS. The intensity *I* is recorded over time *t*, and the time correlation of the intensity fluctuations analyzed. From the correlation function $\langle I(t)\,I(t + \tau)\rangle$, the diffusion coefficient and particle size may be determined.

of the solution surrounding the particles, and the particle diffusion constant, respectively.

For polydisperse particle dispersions size distributions may in principle be obtained by fitting of different mathematical models to the autocorrelation function. Unfortunately, however, these mathematical deconvolution methods are rather ill conditioned, which means that for broad distributions, it is difficult to obtain a unique fit to the autocorrelation function decay. For particle dispersions with narrow fraction sizes, on the other hand, the deconvolution processes may yield valuable information.

Apart from the uncertainty in the extracted particle size distribution for particle dispersions with a wide size distribution, one problem with PCS is that large particles are not straightforwardly analyzed. This means that the occurrence of dilute but large aggregates in a dispersion with a low average size may be difficult to identify and analyze. This may cause significant problems in pharmaceutical formulation development, e.g., in relation to intravenous drug delivery, since even very dilute particle aggregates may cause considerable physiological problems after administration, e.g., related to emboli formation. Care should therefore be employed with PCS in these contexts.

9.3.2   Light Diffraction

Another commonly used optical technique for particle size analysis is light diffraction, which is a potent analysis technique for particles larger than about 0.1

μm. As with dynamic light scattering it requires working with dilute particle samples. The technique is based on measuring the light scattering as a function of the scattering angle, and then applying appropriate optical theories in order to extract the particle size and size distribution. In principle, the method is absolute and does not require calibration, but it is also rather sensitive to input data, e.g., relation to the optical properties of the dispersed particles. Particularly for heterogenous particles (e.g., liposomes or porous polymer particles), such data may be difficult to obtain which may in turn result in uncertainties in the particle size.

9.3.3 Coulter Counter

Contrary to both dynamic light scattering and light diffraction, Coulter counting is not an optical technique. Therefore, Coulter counting does not require strong dilutions in the same manner as these optical techniques, which is advantageous for characterization of more concentrated disperse systems. Instead, Coulter counting is based on the change in resistance resulting from low-conducting particles passing over a thin gap over which a current is flowing (Figure 9.13). This generates voltage pulses when particles pass over the gap, the size of which is proportional to the particle volume, and which therefore may be used for particle size analysis.

Since Coulter counting is based on ''counting'' all particles passing the gap, and since the size of these is monitored, the size distribution is readily obtained with the technique. One limitation with the technique, on the other hand, is that particle size analysis is largely limited to large particles (≥ 1 μm).

9.3.4 Microscopy

The most direct way to obtain information about the size of particles, but also about their shape, and distributions in size and shape, is to use direct visualization by microscopic techniques. Many such techniques are available, e.g., electron microscopies, fluorescence microscopy, light microscopy, different scanning probe microscopies (e.g., AFM), etc. Which of these techniques are best suited for analysis of a particular system largely depends on the system, and in particular the particle size. For example, for particles much smaller than 1 μm, light microscopies provide insufficient resolution, and other methods, e.g., electron microscopy or scanning probe microscopies, must be employed, while for soft systems, e.g., microgel dispersions, scanning probe microscopies may be difficult for mechanical reasons.

A general feature of microscopy techniques is that information about the size and shape of the particles is obtained directly. In suitable cases this allows advanced structural information to be obtained, not only about the particles them-

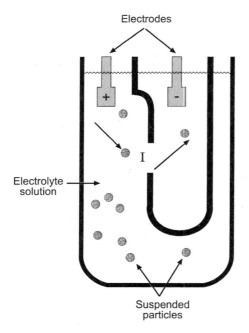

Electrodes

Electrolyte
solution

Suspended
particles

FIGURE 9.13 Schematic illustration of the principle of Coulter counting. A small opening between the electrodes *I* constitutes the sensory zone through which suspended particles pass. In the sensing zone, each particle displaces its own volume of electrolyte. This volume is measured as a voltage pulse. From the volume the particle size is determined.

selves, but also on the structure of aggregates formed by the particles (Figure 9.14 and 9.15).

Since particle size analysis by microscopies is based on probing the structure of a small number of particles, statistics is generally a problem with polydisperse particle systems. In fact, a very large number of microscopy images must be taken in order to secure even rather poor statistical significance. This makes quantitative microscopy techniques very time consuming. Furthermore, since microscopy images are two-dimensional while the systems of interest in drug delivery generally are three-dimensional, there is a risk that the microscopy pictures are flawed by projection artefacts. For example, two particles lying partly on top on each other but not in contact, may appear as being in actual contact in the microscopy images. Care must therefore be taken to identify such effects, unless three-dimensional reconstructions are performed with confocal microscopy. For particle deposition at interfaces, on the other hand, such projection effects are

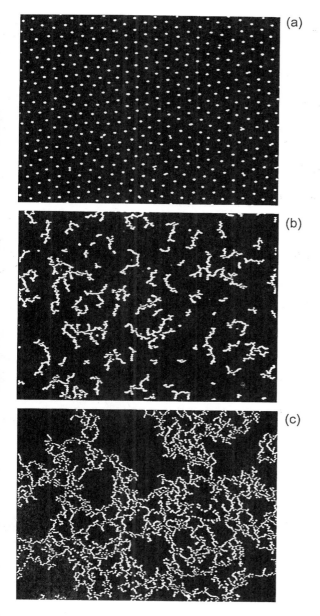

FIGURE 9.14 Microscopic images of shear-induced flocculation of colloidal particles at an interface. Images were taken after 4 (a), 90 (b), and 400 (c) min of shearing. (Redrawn from Hansen et al., J. Colloid Interface Sci. 1999, 218, 77.)

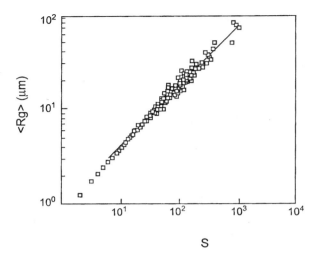

FIGURE 9.15 Data obtained from the pictures in Figure 9.14 presented in the form of a double-logarithmic plot of the radius of gyration R_g vs. the number of particles in the cluster s. The solid line is a fit to a model showing that the system forms a size-invariant structure, with a fractal dimension of 1.57 ± 0.04. (Redrawn from Hansen et al., J. Colloid Interface Sci. 1999, 218, 77.)

less significant, and here microscopy offers real opportunities, e.g., in relation to bioadhesion of colloidal drug carriers.

Apart from the particle size and size distribution, and the particle shape, it is often of significant interest to determine the charge of the particles. As discussed above, this is of importance both for the stability of disperse systems and for the deposition of particles at interfaces. Although a number of methods are currently available for this, particularly those based on electrokinetic phenomena have been applied in pharmaceutical research and development work.

9.3.5 Electrokinetic Methods

When a charged particle is placed in an electric field it will migrate towards the electrode of opposite charge. The speed of this migration, the so-called electrophoretic mobility, may be used to characterize the charge of the particles (Figure 9.16). More precisely, the information obtained from such measurements is the magnitude of the electrostatic potential at the plane of shear, which is usually referred to as the ζ-potential. Alternatively, charge information may be obtained from applying an electric field over an electrolyte solution in contact with a macroscopic surface, and following the induced electroosmotic flow, or by applying

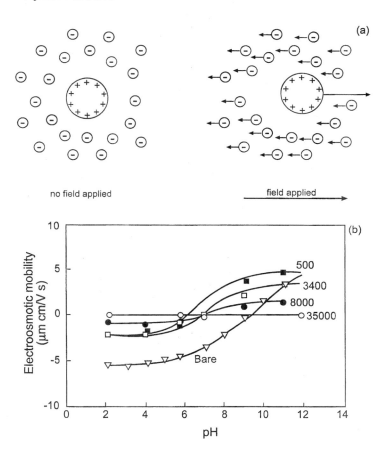

FIGURE 9.16 (a) Schematic illustration of electrophoretic mobility. (b) Effect of pH on the charging of amine-functionalized quartz, and of coating the quartz with uncharged PEO of different molecular weight. Note that the surface modification with high molecular weight PEO in particular results in the charges of the amine-functional surface being effectively masked. (Redrawn from Burns et al., Langmuir 1995, 11, 2768.)

a pressure and following the streaming potential generated from the flow. Irrespective of how the electrokinetic information is obtained, however, it is efficient for following the charging of particles and surfaces, and the effects of surface modifications.

Electrophoresis in particular relies on using dilute systems of nonsettling particles (i.e., not significantly affected by gravity), the movement of which in the

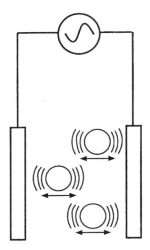

FIGURE 9.17 Schematic illustration of the basis of acoustic size measurements. When an oscillating field is generated, the movement of the suspended particles and the electrolyte solution is different. From the coupling of this relative movement, information can be obtained about both the particle size and charge.

electric field is largely determined by electrophoresis. For such systems, on the other hand, valuable information can be obtained regarding particle coatings, the nature of charged groups on the particle surface, etc.

9.3.6 Acoustic Methods

Another nonoptical method for particle analysis is acoustic measurements. The basis for such methods is the electrophoretic mobility of charged particles in an electric field. By applying an alternating electric field, charged particles can be made to oscillate in space. These oscillations, in turn, couple to the movement of the ambient solution, and generate an ultrasonic signal, which can be analyzed in order to obtain information about both the particle ζ-potential and the particle size (Figure 9.17).

The sensitivity of the method is strongly dependent on the density difference between the dispersed particles and the ambient, and the denser the particles, the better the analysis. At least a 10% difference in density is required to obtain reliable data. Due to the technique being based on an acoustic response, another limitation is that the investigation of highly compressible systems, such as emulsions, liposomes, or dispersed gas bubbles, is precluded.

9.4 POLYMER PARTICLES IN DRUG DELIVERY

Polymer particles used in pharmaceutical applications are mainly those formed by biodegradable polymers, notably polysaccharides, poly(lactide) and poly(glycolide) and their copolymers, the degradation products of which are essentially nontoxic and readily resorbable. As discussed more extensively below, dispersed particles prepared from such polymers are interesting, e.g., for oral delivery of drugs not stable in the stomach, for oral vaccination, and for formulations where bioadhesion is desirable.

9.4.1 Loading of Polymer Particles

Polymer particles for drug delivery can be loaded by drugs in a few different ways:

1. Adsorption of the drug at the particle surface
2. Swelling of the particles in a solvent containing the drug and passive diffusion into the particles
3. Pressure-enhanced incorporation in preformed particles
4. Incorporation of the drug through its presence during the polymerization process
5. Mixing the drug in a polymer melt or a polymer solution, followed by spray cooling or spray drying.

Depending on the system, different loading strategies are preferred. For example, if only low dosages are required and a fast release desired, simple adsorption at the particle surface may be sufficient. In most cases, however, incorporation into the particle interior is desired. For drugs which are readily soluble in a solvent which swells the particles or which can dissolve non-cross-linked polymers, the solvent-based methods may be suitable. Frequently, however, the methods of choice are based on the presence of the drug during the particle formation, e.g., through spray cooling or emulsion polymerization. This often allows a higher drug level to be incorporated, at the same time as a more homogenous distribution of the drug throughout the particles is obtained, the latter advantageous for achieving a sustained drug release.

9.4.2 Release from Polymer Particles

Since polymer particles used in drug delivery are generally designed to be readily biodegradable, it is natural that the drug release rate is addressed mainly by controlling the degradation rate. Often there is a close correlation between the degradation and the drug release rate. This is illustrated in Figure 10.9, showing correlation between the degradation of poly(carbophenoxyvaleric acid) and the release of incorporated p-nitroaniline. The identical behavior regarding degradation and

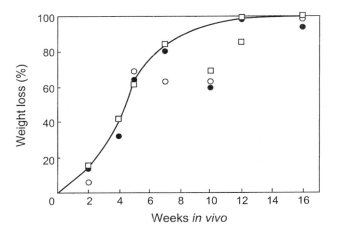

FIGURE 9.18 Weight loss of cross-linked copolymers of ε-caprolactone and δ-valerolactone implanted in rabbit. Results from different experiments are shown. Note that the degradation occurs over more than ten weeks for this polymer. (Redrawn from Pitt et al., in Bruck, ed., Controlled Drug Delivery, CRC Press, 1983.)

release in this case demonstrates that the release occurs as a consequence of the degradation.

As will be discussed in detail in Chapter 10, the degradation rate of polymer particles may be controlled over orders of magnitude through the choice of copolymer composition, and therefore the drug release rate may be widely controlled with some accuracy. Furthermore, a drug release sustained over extremely long times may be reached using this approach (Figure 9.18).

However, the drug release from biodegradable polymer particles is affected also by other factors, notably the drug physicochemical properties. For example, similar to the release of drugs solubilized in micellar, liquid crystalline, liposome, microemulsion and emulsion systems, the drug release from polymer particles depends on the drug hydrophobicity. This is illustrated in Figure 9.19 for a series of nalbuphine prodrugs and polylactide-polyglycolide copolymers of different composition. As can be seen, the drug release rate decreases with an increasing drug hydrophobicity, indicating that the drug partitioning is important to the release rate.

In fact, the relation between degradation, drug partitioning, and drug release may be even more complex than this, since the drug may also affect the degradation rate. For example, basic drugs may behave as base catalysts, which may enhance the degradation rate and hence also the release rate. On the other hand, basic drugs may also neutralize the polymer terminal carboxyl residues of polyes-

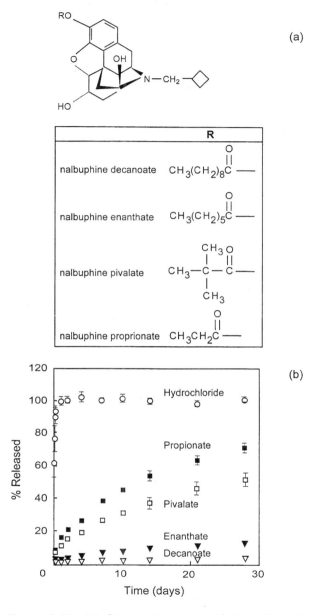

(a)

(b)

FIGURE 9.19 (a) Chemical structure of the nalbuphine prodrugs investigated. (b) Relationship between the release rate and the aqueous solubility of various nalbuphine prodrugs. (Redrawn from Sung et al., Int. J. Pharm. 1998, 172, 17.)

ters, thereby reducing the autocatalysis due to the acidic end groups, and therefore also the degradation rate and the release rate.

9.4.3 Oral Administration of Particles

Both oral and parenteral uptake of colloidal carrier systems have been found to depend on the nature of the carrier as such. For parenteral administration, the uptake of colloidal drug carriers by the reticuloendothelial system depends on a number of factors, notably carrier surface properties, such as hydrophobicity, charge, and chemical functionality. As is discussed in Chapter 4, this is related to the adsorption of certain serum proteins (opsonins) at the carrier surface, initiating various biological responses. By reducing the adsorption of the opsonins at the carrier surface, e.g., by surface modification through PEO derivatives, a very low serum protein adsorption can be reached, thereby prolonging the bloodstream circulation time and obtaining a more uniform tissue distribution.

However, while the factors governing the uptake of intravenously administered colloidal drug carriers are by now rather well known, the oral uptake of such systems is considerably less well known and understood. The oral uptake of such carriers has been found to occur by several different mechanisms and through different parts of the gastrointestinal tract, and also to depend on a number of factors (Tables 9.1. and 9.2).

Some of these factors cannot readily be controlled, and yet others are outside the scope of the formulation as such. Nevertheless, the oral uptake of particles depends strongly on the feeding/fasting state in a similar way as for oral administration of emulsions, i.e., the uptake increases after feeding (Figure 9.20).

As indicated in Figure 9.21, the preferential particle size for uptake depends on the uptake mechanism and the tissue involved. Of particular importance for oral drug delivery of particles, however, is the uptake in Peyer's patches. It is

TABLE 9.1   Mechanisms Involved in the Uptake of Particles

Site/mechanism	Particle size
Villius tips—persorption	5–150 μm
Intestinal macrophages—phagocytosis	1 μm
Enterocytes—endocytosis	<200 nm
Peyer's patches—transparacellular	<10 μm

Source: From O'Hagan et al., J. Anat. 1996, 189, 477.

TABLE 9.2   Factors Affecting the Extent
of Uptake of Particles

Particle size
Particle surface (e.g., hydrophobicity and charge)
Dose of particles administered
Administration vehicle
Use of targeted delivery to M cells
Fed state
Age
Species under investigation
Method used to quantify uptake

therefore interesting to note that the uptake by this mechanism increases with decreasing particle size (Figure 9.21).

Also, the surface properties of the particles play an important role for the oral uptake of particles. As will be discussed below, coating polymer particles by cationic polymers is a way to increase the electrostatic interaction between the particles and negatively charged mucosa or lipid membranes, which promotes bioadhesion and results in an enhanced uptake. Also, the particle surface hydrophobicity has a significant influence on the particle uptake. More precisely, the more hydrophobic the particles, the more pronounced the particle uptake. There-

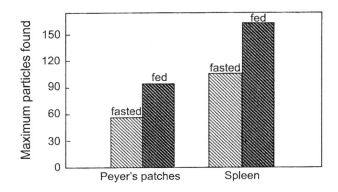

FIGURE 9.20   The effect of fed state on the maximum number of polystyrene particles found in Peyer's patches and spleen. Mice were dosed 10^8 2.65 μm particles by a single oral gavage, and fasting began 12 h prior to dosing. Fed mice were allowed to feed ad libitum. (Redrawn from Ebel, Pharm. Res. 1990, 7, 848.)

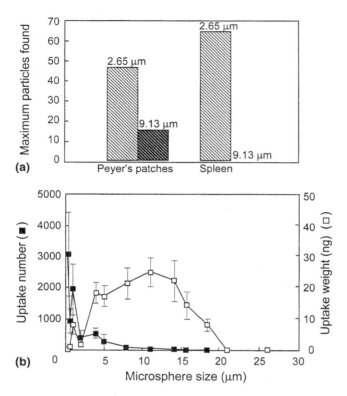

FIGURE 9.21 (a) Size dependence of the maximum number of polystyrene particles found in Peyer's patches and spleen. Mice were dosed 10^8 2.65 μm or 9.13 μm particles by a single oral gavage. No 9.13 μm particles were found in the spleen. (b) Influence of the microsphere size on the uptake in Peyer's patches of polymer particles following oral administration. (Redrawn from Ebel, Pharm. Res. 1990, 7, 848 (a), and Tabata et al., Vaccine 1996, 14, 1677.)

fore, polymer particles may be modified, e.g., through adsorption of water-soluble polymers in order to reduce their intestinal uptake (Figure 9.22).

9.5 BIOADHESION

An issue of some importance in relation to oral drug delivery of particulate drug carriers is that of bioadhesion, by which one usually means the adhesion/adsorption at mucosal surfaces. Since mucins, the main constituent in mucosa, are negatively charged and contain hydrophobic domains (Figure 9.23), it is possible to use a number of approaches for reaching an efficient bioadhesion, including posi-

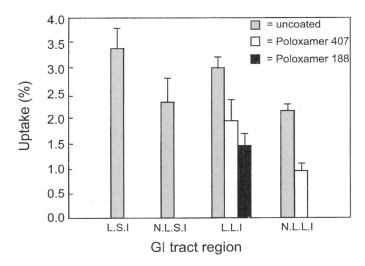

FIGURE 9.22 Uptake of coated and uncoated polystyrene particles in gastrointestinal tract samples. Data are shown for uncoated polystyrene particles, polystyrene particles coated with Poloxamer 407, and polystyrene particles coated with Poloxamer 188. (N)LSI and (N)LLI refer to (non-) lymphoid small intestine and (non-) lymphoid large intestine, respectively. (Redrawn from Florence et al., J. Drug Targeting 1995, 3, 65.)

tively charged carriers, small hydrophobic carriers or carriers containing some hydrophobic parts, or carriers not stable but rather aggregating and depositing at the conditions present at the administration site. By the use of bioadhesive formulations, the residence time at the mucosa can be prolonged, which tends to improve the drug uptake.

Note, however, that bioadhesive formulations are useful not only for oral administration but also for other administration routes, and also for other types of drug carriers than polymeric particles. Nevertheless, the use of mucoadhesive polymers has indeed been found to result in beneficial results in oral administration. Using, e.g., the positively charged polyelectrolyte chitosan has been found to result in a significantly improved bioavailability of particle-based drug delivery systems, which most likely is an effect of an electrostatically driven bioadhesion of the formulation. Furthermore, chitosan particles have been investigated in relation to their clearance characteristics in nasal drug delivery, and found to display a long residence time through bioadhesion (Figure 9.24).

In analogy to this, chitosan-coated alginate beads have been found to adhere more extensively to pig stomach tissue than the corresponding uncoated alginate beads (Figure 9.25).

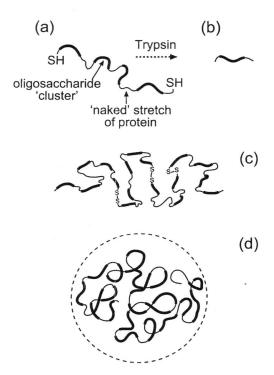

FIGURE 9.23 Schematic illustration of the structure of mucus glycoproteins (mucins). (a) Mucin subunits contain a number (usually 3–5) of (negatively charged) oligosaccharide clusters flanked by (hydrophobic) "naked" stretches of the protein core. (b) Trypsin digestion yields fragments (*T*-domains) corresponding to the oligosaccharide clusters. (c) Mucins are formed by subunits joined end to end. (d) Mucins behave as random coils in dilute solutions. (Redrawn from Carlstedt et al., Ciba Foundation Symposium 1984, 109, 157.)

In a similar way that targeting of liposomes or block copolymer micelles can be used for administration to a selected tissue or cell type, site-specific adherence of orally administered particle formulations may be reached through surface modification of the carrier with entities, e.g., lectins or antibodies, binding to a selected site in the gastrointestinal tract. As an example of this approach, Table 9.3 shows results on how the uptake of polystyrene microparticles into Peyer's patches can be enhanced through incorporation of a monoclonal antibody with specificity to *M* cells.

Similarly, the oral uptake of polystyrene latex particles has been found to be positively affected by modification of the polymer particle surface with specific ligands, e.g., tomato lectin molecules.

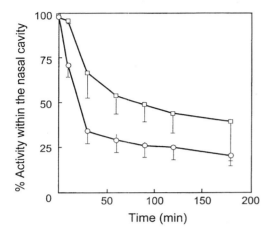

FIGURE 9.24   The clearance of 99m-Tc-sodium pertechnetate and 99m-Tc-diethyl-enetriaminepentaacetic acid, respectively, from the nasal cavity following administration of a chitosan particulate formulation (squares) and the control without such carrier (circles). (Redrawn from Soane et al., Int. J. Pharm. 1999, 178, 55.)

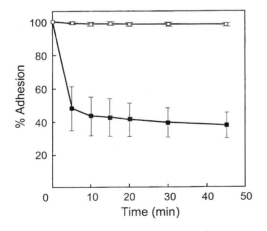

FIGURE 9.25   The adhesion to pig stomach tissue of homogenous alginate beads uncoated (filled squares) and coated (open squares) with chitosan. (Redrawn from Gåserød et al., Int. J. Pharm. 1998, 175, 237.)

TABLE 9.3 Antibody-Dependent Localization of Green or Red Fluorescent Polystyrene Particles in Peyer's Patches. Red and Green Particles Labeled with an anti-M-cell Monoclonal Antibody (5B11) or an Irrelevant Antibody (TEPC183) were Administered Simultaneously, and the Uptake of the Two Particle Types Monitored

Paired combination	Particle count*	Ratio green/red
5B11-green	468 ± 56	3.01 ± 0.28
TEPC 183-red	160 ± 22	
TEPC 183-green	160 ± 38	0.35 ± 0.05
5B11-red	364 ± 77	
5B11-green	363 ± 36	3.46 ± 0.34
-red	105 ± 14	
-green	120 ± 17	0.99 ± 0.11
-red	125 ± 18	

* Mean number of particles ± standard error of the mean of 15 lymphoepithelial domes.
Source: From Pappo et al., Immunology 1991, 73, 277.

Note, however, that also other mechanisms for obtaining bioadhesion than those based on hydrophobic, electrostatic, or specific interactions may be used. In particular, those based on poor solvency of a carrier polymer have been used successfully. For example, polymers displaying reversed temperature-dependent gelation, i.e., gelation on heating, have been investigated in relation to nasal adsorption of insulin in rats. In particular, ethyl(hydroxyethyl)cellulose (EHEC) and poly(N-isopropyl acrylamide), displaying a lower consolute temperature of 30–32°C and 32–34°C, respectively, undergo a transition from relatively low-viscous solutions to relatively rigid gels after administration. Both systems were able to enhance the reduction of the blood glucose level compared to the reference due to gelation-induced bioadhesion of these formulations.

9.6 ORAL VACCINES

An area where biodegradable polymeric drug carriers have been found promising is in the development of oral vaccines. Because most infectious species enter the body through mucosal surfaces, immunization involving these surfaces is an efficient approach for vaccination. Mainly, the gastrointestinal tract has been investigated in this context, although also other mucosal surfaces, e.g., the pulmonary, nasopharyngeal, and genitourinary surfaces are all coated with mucus containing immunoglobulins, notably IgA, and could therefore be of interest in this respect.

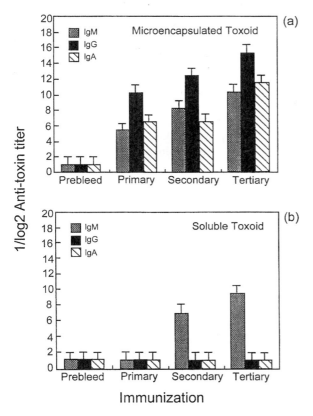

FIGURE 9.26 Plasma antitoxin antibody levels of the IgM, IgG, and IgA isotypes induced following oral immunizations with staphylococcal enterotoxin B vaccine either encapsulated (a) or free (b). (Redrawn from Eldridge et al., J. Controlled Release 1990, 11, 205.)

From a delivery point of view, particle encapsulation is a promising route for successful vaccination through the oral route. There are several reasons for this:

1. The harsh conditions in the stomach cause rapid degradation of the material used for immunization, e.g., peptides, proteins, cells, and viruses. By encapsulation in polymer particles, degradation of the species provoking the immune response may be reduced or eliminated.
2. In analogy to parenteral immunization, particles may be beneficial for immunization also by acting as adjuvants.

3. Since orally administered particles are typically taken up by Peyer's patches, which constitute one of the main immune systems in the gastrointestinal tract, a beneficial localization effect may also occur. In fact, considering the key role played by Peyer's patches, the successful use of particles in oral vaccines seems to depend extensively on the uptake of the latter in these patches.

The most frequently used polymer particle carrier systems for oral vaccination are those consisting of biodegradable poly(lactide), poly(glycolide) or their copolymers. These are interesting in this context since:

1. They are taken up efficiently by Peyer's patches.
2. They are readily biodegradable.
3. The resulting degradation products are essentially non-toxic and readily resorbable.

Much work has been directed over the last decade in particular to investigate the use of this type of particles in oral vaccination, and stimulation of both mucosal (sIgA antibodies) and systemic (IgG antibodies) has been observed. As an illustration of this, Figure 9.26 shows results for *Staphylococcal enterotoxin B* encapsulated in poly(DL-lactide-co-glycolide) particles. As can be seen, immunization based on such particles in the size range $1-10$ μm is efficient. In contrast, the soluble antigen is relatively ineffective.

The use of polymeric microparticles in oral vaccination has been found to be of interest in a range of indications, including, e.g., vaccination against *hepatitis B*, vaccination for fertility control, and vaccination against viruses, including parainfluenza virus and influenza virus.

BIBLIOGRAPHY

Adamczyk, Z., B. Siwek, M. Zembala, P. Belouschek, Kinetics of localized adsorption of colloid particles, Adv. Colloid Interface Sci. 48:151–280 (1994).

Barth, H. G., Modern Methods of Particle Size Analysis, Chemical Analysis, vol. 73, Wiley, New York, 1984.

Eldridge, J. H., R. M. Gilley, J. K. Staas, Z. Moldoveanu, J. A. Meulbroek, T. R. Tice, Biodegradable microspheres: vaccine delivery system for oral immunization, Curr. Topics Microbiol. Immunol. 146:59–66 (1989).

Evans, D. F., H. Wennerström, The Colloidal Domain, Wiley, New York, 1999.

Fleer, G. J., M. A. Cohen Stuart, J.M.H.M. Scheutjens, T. Cosgrove, B. Vincent, Polymers at Interfaces, Chapman & Hall, London, 1993.

Hiemenz, P. C., Principles of Colloid and Surface Chemistry, Marcel Dekker, New York, 1986.

Hunter, R. J., Zeta Potential in Colloid Science, Academic Press, London, 1981.

Israelachvili, J., Intermolecular and Surface Forces, Academic Press, London, 1992.

Jönsson, B., B. Lindman, K. Holmberg, B. Kronberg, Surfactants and Polymers in Aqueous Solution, Wiley, New York, 1998.

Lavelle, E. C., S. Sharif, N. W. Thomas, J. Holland, S. S. Davis, The importance of gastrointestinal uptake of particles in the design of oral delivery systems, Adv. Drug Delivery Rev. 18:5–22 (1995).

Napper, D. H., Polymeric Stabilization of Colloidal Dispersions, Academic Press, London, 1983.

Nielloud, F., G. Marti-Mestres, eds., Pharmaceutical Emulsions and Suspensions, Drugs and the Pharmaceutical Sciences, Marcel Dekker, 2000.

O'Hagan, D. T., in D.T. O'Hagan, ed., Novel Delivery Systems: Oral Vaccines, CRC Press, Boca Raton, 1994.

Porter, C. J. H., Drug delivery to the lymphatic system, Crit. Rev. Ther. Drug Carrier Syst. 14:333–393 (1997).

10

Degradation of Surfactants and Polymers in Drug Delivery

Biodegradable systems are interesting in drug delivery for a number of reasons. In particular, the degradation can be used in order to control the release rate of a drug, but it may also be valuable in order to decrease the risk for accumulation-related diseases, and to control the biological response to the active drug. By the use of biodegradable chemical links, it is possible to make particles, gels, surface coatings, and self-assembled structures, which degrade with orders of magnitude different half-lifes.

10.1 BIODEGRADATION OF POLYMERS

A number of polymers used in pharmaceutical applications are biodegradable, either by chemical or enzymatic action, or both (Figure 10.1). Different polymers are characterized by different stability toward degradation. While some, e.g., polyanhydrides, are very labile and degrading over a time scale of minutes, others are much more stable (Table 10.1).

For polymers to be relevant for pharmaceutical applications for their biodegradation, they should typically degrade, at physiological conditions, over a time scale from minutes to weeks, depending on the application. If the polymers are less stable than this, their controlled preparation and storage may be difficult, while more stable polymers are effectively not biodegradable in the context of

1. Polypeptides

$$\left[N - \underset{\underset{R}{|}}{\overset{\overset{H}{|}}{C}} - \overset{\overset{O}{\|}}{C} \right]$$

2. Poly(lactic acid)

$$\left[O - \underset{\underset{CH_3}{|}}{\overset{\overset{H}{|}}{C}} - \overset{\overset{O}{\|}}{C} \right]$$

3. Poly(glycolic acid)

$$\left[O - \underset{\underset{H}{|}}{\overset{\overset{H}{|}}{C}} - \overset{\overset{O}{\|}}{C} \right]$$

4. Poly(ε-caprolactone)

$$\left[O - (CH_2)_5 - \overset{\overset{O}{\|}}{C} \right]$$

5. Poly(β-hydroxybutyrate)

$$\left[O - \underset{\underset{CH_3}{|}}{\overset{\overset{H}{|}}{C}} - CH_2 - \overset{\overset{O}{\|}}{C} \right]$$

6. Poly(β-hydroxyvalerate)

$$\left[O - \underset{\underset{C_2H_5}{|}}{\overset{\overset{H}{|}}{C}} - CH_2 - \overset{\overset{O}{\|}}{C} \right]$$

7. Polydioxanone

$$\left[O - CH_2 - CH_2 - O - \overset{\overset{O}{\|}}{C} \right]$$

8. Poly(ethylene terephthalate)

$$\left[O - CH_2 - CH_2 - O - \overset{\overset{O}{\|}}{C} - \bigcirc - \overset{\overset{O}{\|}}{C} \right]$$

9. Poly(malic acid)

$$\left[O - \underset{\underset{COOH}{|}}{\overset{\overset{H}{|}}{C}} - CH_2 - \overset{\overset{O}{\|}}{C} \right]$$

10. Poly(tartronic acid)

$$\left[O - \underset{\underset{COOH}{|}}{\overset{\overset{H}{|}}{C}} - \overset{\overset{O}{\|}}{C} \right]$$

11. Poly(ortho esters)

$$R = -(CH_2)_6 - \quad or \quad -CH_2 - \bigcirc - CH_2 -$$

12. Polyanhydrides

$$\left[R - \overset{\overset{O}{\|}}{C} - O - \overset{\overset{O}{\|}}{C} \right]$$

13. Polyacyanoacrylate

$$\left[CH_2 - \underset{\underset{COOR}{|}}{\overset{\overset{CN}{|}}{C}} \right]$$

14. Poly(phosphoesters)

$$\left[O - R - O - \underset{\underset{R'}{|}}{\overset{\overset{O}{\|}}{C}} - O \right]$$

15. Polyphosphazenes

$$\left[N - \underset{\underset{R'}{|}}{\overset{\overset{R}{|}}{P}} \right]$$

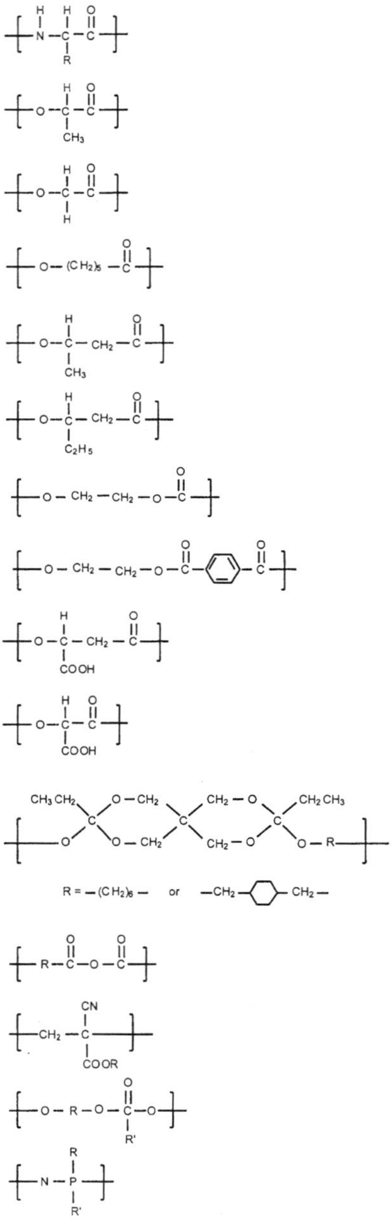

FIGURE 10.1 Chemical structure of some biodegradable polymers.

TABLE 10.1 Typical Hydrolysis Rates
for Some Different Types of Polymers

Class	Hydrolysis rate*
Polyanhydride	0.1 hours
Polyketal	3 hours
Polyorthoester	4 hours
Polyacetal	0.8 years
Polyester	3.3 years
Polyurea	33 years
Polycarbonate	42,000 years
Polyurethane	42,000 years
Polyamide	83,000 years

* Time required for 50% hydrolysis at pH 7 and
25°C.
Source: From Pierre et al., J. Bioact. Compatible
Polym. 1986, 1, 467.

drug delivery. In particular, polyesters have received considerable attention as
biodegradable polymers for drug delivery. Such polymer undergo hydrolysis in
aqueous environment. The rate of the degradation can be controlled straightforwardly, e.g., by controlling the monomer structure or monomer mixture composition. As an illustration, Figure 10.2 shows the effect of composition on the degra-

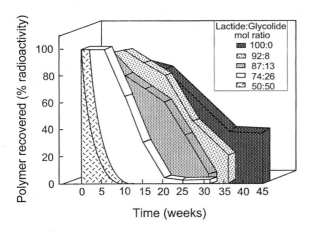

FIGURE 10.2 Effect of the composition on the hydrolytic degradation rate of poly
(lactide)-poly(glycolide) copolymers. (Redrawn from Asano et al., J. Controlled Release 1989, 9, 111.)

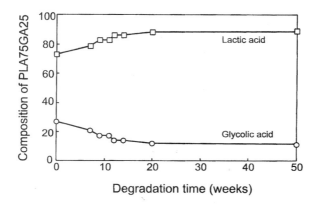

Figure 10.3   Chemical composition of a poly(lactide)-poly(glycolide) (75/25) block copolymer during degradation. (Data from Li et al., J. Mater. Sci. Mater. Med. 1990, 1, 131.)

dation rate of poly(lactide)-poly(glycolide) copolymers (Figure 10.1). Since poly(glycolide) undergoes hydrolytic degradation faster than poly(lactide), increasing the copolymer poly(lactide) content results in a prolonged degradation process (Figure 10.2).

As a result of the faster degradation of one of its components, the composition of biodegradable copolymers generally changes during the degradation process. Thus, due to the preferential degradation of poly(glycolide) blocks, poly(lactide)-poly(glycolide) block copolymers become enriched in poly(lactide) during the degradation process (Figure 10.3).

If the two copolymer components have different tendency for crystallization, degradation may result in a change also in the state of polymer crystallinity. For poly(lactide)-poly(glycolide) copolymers, the preferential degradation of poly(glycolide) has been found to result in a degradation-induced crystallization (Figure 10.4).

In analogy to the protective effect toward hydrolytic degradation of drugs through incorporation in micelles or other drug carriers, the hydrolytic degradation of polymers may be controlled by the accessibility of water to the labile bonds. In particular, by incorporating hydrophobic groups a water-soluble polymer can be made to collapse (Chapter 8), thereby reducing the contact between the hydrolytically labile groups and the aqueous environment, hence also reducing the hydrolysis rate (Figure 10.5).

The hydrolytic degradation rate depends not only on the polymer composition but also on other factors, such as:

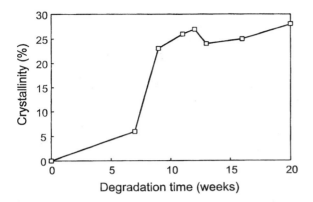

FIGURE 10.4   Crystallinity evolution during degradation of poly(lactide)-poly(glyco-lide) (75/25) block copolymer. (Data from Li et al., J. Mater. Sci. Mater. Med. 1990, 1, 131.)

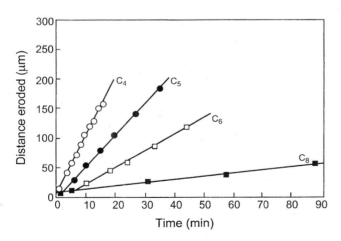

FIGURE 10.5   Effect of polymer substituent (size of ester group in half esters) on the hydrolytic degradation rate. (Redrawn from Heller et al., J. Appl. Polym. Sci. 1978, 22, 1991.)

1. Polymer architecture and crystallinity. (Generally, the degradation increases with decreasing crystallinity.)
2. Polymer architecture and structure formation. (Structures and architectures precluding contact between the labile group and water generally display slower hydrolysis.)
3. Temperature. (Generally, the degradation increases with increasing temperature.)
4. pH. (Generally, the hydrolysis rate increases at low and at high pH.)
5. Presence of a drug. (May both promote and preclude polymer hydrolysis.)

The issue of the effects of polymer self-assembly on the hydrolytic degradation rate is relevant in relation to the use of surface active polymers for drug delivery. An example of this is given by PEO-poly(lactide) ($E_m L_n$) block copolymers, which form micelles with the poly(lactide) residues constituting the hydrophobic micellar core if the poly(lactide) chains are sufficiently long. If the latter are short, on the other hand, they are unable to induce micelle formation (in analogy to other hydrophobic groups). When in the micellar core, the ester groups in the poly(lactide) residues are shielded from contact with water, and hence at least partly protected from hydrolysis. One would therefore expect PEO-poly(lactide) copolymers forming micelles to be characterized by a slower hydrolytic degradation of the poly(lactide) residue than that of block copolymers not forming micelles. Indeed, Figure 10.6 shows that the hydrolysis of $E_{39} L_5$ (which does not form micelles) is considerably faster than that of $E_{39} L_{20}$ (which form micelles). Thus, for $E_{39} L_5$, the ester bonds are constantly exposed to the aqueous environment, and hydrolysis proceeds relatively rapidly. For $E_{39} L_{20}$, on the other hand, the labile bonds are partially protected from hydrolysis and the degradation is slower.

Apart from the polymer structure and composition, the most interesting parameter for varying the hydrolysis of biodegradable polyesters in drug delivery is probably pH. This is due to pH gradients in the gastrointestinal tract (Figure 10.7 and Table 10.2), which may be used together with biodegradable polymers for a directed delivery to a specific region in the gastrointestinal tract.

As with low molecular weight esters, polyester hydrolysis is catalyzed by both acid and base, which means that degradation and degradation-induced drug release is enhanced at high and at low pH, whereas the hydrolytic degradation at neutral pH is generally limited (Figure 10.8). This pH-dependent degradation may allow efficient encapsulation of a drug at storage conditions (often dry or at close to neutral pH), partial or complete acid-catalyzed polymer degradation in the stomach or the small intestine, and drug release either in the stomach or in the intestine, depending on the polymer degradation stability and the drug physicochemical properties.

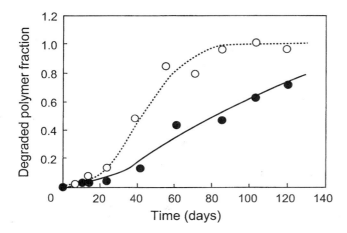

FIGURE 10.6 Hydrolytic degradation of $E_{39}L_5$ (open symbols) and $E_{39}L_{20}$ (filled symbols) at 37°C and unadjusted pH. (Redrawn from Muller et al., J. Colloid Interface Sci. 2001, 236, 116.)

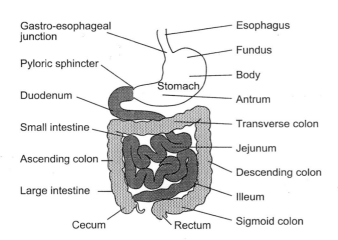

FIGURE 10.7 Schematic illustration of the different regions of the gastrointestinal tract. (Redrawn from Hwang et al., Crit. Rev. Ther. Drug Carrier Syst. 1998, 15, 243.)

TABLE 10.2   Average pH in Healthy Humans in
the Fasted and Fed State at Various Sites in the
Gastrointestinal Tract

Location	pH (fasted)	pH (fed)
Stomach	1.3	4.9
Duodenum (mid-distal)	6.5	5.4
Jujenum	6.6	5.2–6.0
Ileum	7.4	7.5

Source: From Hörter et al., Adv. Drug Del. Syst. 1997,
25, 3.

Besides chemical degradation, polymers may undergo enzyme-catalyzed degradation. While naturally occuring polymers such as polypeptides and polysaccharides are most susceptible to this also numerous synthetic polymers undergo enzymatic degradation (Table 10.3). Indeed, also seemingly inert polymers, such as nylon, poly(ether urethane), poly(terephthalate), poly(hydroxybutyrate), poly(ester-urea), poly(ε-caprolactone), and poly(glycolic acid), are degraded by enzymes.

The enzymatic degradation of polymers depends on a number of factors apart from those related to the polymer chemical structure, including the following and many other, frequently system-specific, parameters.

1.   Temperature
2.   pH
3.   Electrolyte concentration
4.   Presence of enzyme inhibitors
5.   Presence of surfactants, other organic compounds (e.g., urea), cations (certain systems), and other cosolutes
6.   Presence of hydrophobic interfaces (lipases)

As a rule of thumb, enzymes are most efficient at or close to the conditions (e.g., salt concentration, pH, and cation concentration) where they perform their biological function. Departing from these conditions, on the other hand, often results in a decreased enzymatic activity, and therefore also in a decreased enzymatic degradation rate of polymers.

In particular, biodegradable polymer systems are used in drug delivery since they allow a way to control the drug release rate. In many cases, there is a close correlation between the polymer matrix degradation on the one hand, and the drug release rate, on the other (Figure 10.9). Since the degradation rate may be controlled over orders of magnitude through the choice of copolymer composi-

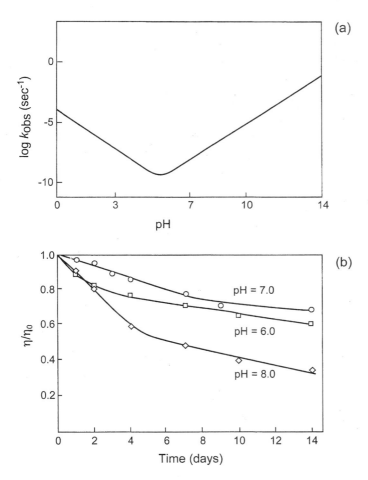

FIGURE 10.8 (a) Effect of pH on the hydrolysis rate constant k_{obs} for ethyl acetate. (b) Influence of pH on the degradation rate, as monitored by a relative viscosity η/η_0 decrease, of a random multiblock polyester-amide. (Redrawn from Bamford et al., eds., Chemical Kinetics, vol. 10, Elsevier, 1972 (a), and de Simone et al., J. Appl. Polym. Sci. 1992, 46, 1813 (b).)

tion and structure and through a number of external parameters, the drug release rate may be widely controlled with some accuracy. Furthermore, a drug release sustained over extremely long times may be reached using this approach. The latter is interesting, e.g., in relation to sustained release of drugs from drug-loaded implants.

TABLE 10.3   Examples of Enzymatic Degradation
of Polymers

Poly(ε-caprolactone)	Chymotrypsin
	Trypsin
	Papain
Poly(dioxane)	Esterase
Poly(ester-urea)	Chymotrypsin
	Elastase
	Subtilisin
Poly(ether urethane)	Cathepsin
	Leucine aminopeptidase
	Papain
	Urease
	Trypsin
Poly(ethylene terephthalate)	Esterase
	Papain
	Leucine aminopeptidase
Poly(glycolic acid)	Esterase
	Ficin
	Carboxypeptidase A
	Clostridiopeptidase A
	Bromleain
	Esterase
	Leucine aminopeptidase
Poly(hydroxybutyrate)	Esterase
Poly(lactic acid)	Pronase
	Proteinase K
	Bromelain
	Lipase
Poly(lysine)	Trypsine
	Chymotrypsin
	Carboxypeptidase B
	Elastase
	Papain
	Ficin

Source: From Park et al., 'Biodegradable Hydrogels for Drug Delivery,' Technomic, 1993.

However, the drug release from biodegradable polymer systems may be determined also by other factors than the polymer degradation rate. An example of this is the drug hydrophobicity, where frequently a slower release is observed for the same polymer system with increasing drug hydrophobicity. Furthermore, basic drugs may behave as catalysts, which may enhance the degradation rate

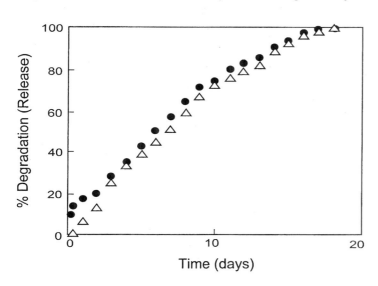

FIGURE 10.9 In vitro release of *p*-nitroaniline (circles) from a poly(carbophenoxy-valeric acid) matrix, as well as the fractional degradation of the matrix (triangles). (Redrawn from Dombs et al., Makromol. Chem. Macromol. Symp. 1988, 19, 189.)

and hence also the release rate. On the other hand, basic drugs may also neutralize the polymer terminal carboxyl residues of polyesters, thereby reducing the auto-catalysis due to the acidic end groups, and therefore also the degradation rate and the release rate.

The degradation of polymers may have also a range of other effects, e.g., relating to gel strength, bioadhesion, responsiveness, etc. For example, when bio-degradable polymers are used as steric stabilizers for colloidal drug carriers, such as liposomes, emulsions, or polymer particles, the colloidal stability of such systems at physiological conditions may depend on the state of degradation. As an illustration of this, Figure 10.10 shows the stability toward salt-induced flocculation of polystyrene particles coated by PEO-poly(lactide) copolymers. In an aqueous solution, these copolymers adsorb at the hydrophobic polystyrene particles with the hydrophobic poly(lactide) block as the anchor. At sufficiently high copolymer concentration, saturation adsorption is achieved, and an efficient steric stabilization of the polystyrene dispersion is obtained also at high salt concentration (Chapter 9).

As degradation of the anchoring poly(lactide) block progresses, the anchoring of the copolymer at the polystyrene particle surface deteriorates. This, in turn, results in a weaker adsorption, and in a decreased amount copolymer adsorbed, which causes the steric protective capacity by the copolymer layer to decrease,

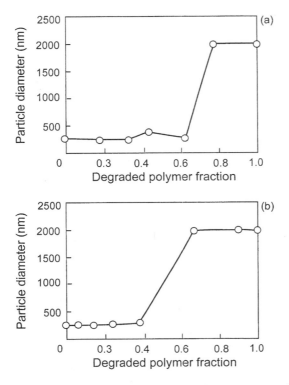

FIGURE 10.10   The aggregate size in polystyrene dispersions stabilized by block copolymers in 10 mM sodium sulfate as a function of degradation of the anchoring poly(lactide) block for $E_{39}L_{20}$ (a) and $E_{39}L_5$ (b). (Redrawn from Muller et al., J. Colloid Interface Sci. 2001, 236, 116.)

and eventually the polystyrene particles to flocculate. The longer the anchoring poly(lactide) block, the more extensive degradation is required in order to weaken and reduce the copolymer adsorption sufficiently to induce flocculation.

In some cases, such a degradation-induced destabilization of colloidal drug carriers may be advantageous. For example, when a good storage stability of a colloidal drug carrier system is required and release to either the stomach or the intestine desired, degradation-induced flocculation through acid-catalyzed hydrolysis (stomach) or enzymatic action (intestine) may be used to localize the colloidal drug carriers at the site of action, thereby improving the drug bioavailability. On the other hand, if colloidal drug carriers stabilized by such polymers are administered intravenously, the degradation-induced flocculation may cause serious side effects relating to emboli formation. In the latter case, therefore, care must be taken to avoid such effects.

As discussed in relation to liposomes (Chapter 4), sterically stabilized and particularly PEO-modified colloidal drug carriers are quite interesting due to prolonged bloodstream circulation time, a comparably even tissue distribution, reduced toxicity effects, etc. The origin of the advantageous effects of PEO-containing coatings of colloidal drug carriers in intravenous drug delivery is the low serum protein adsorption caused by the PEO chains. On biodegradation of the anchoring block of a PEO-containing copolymer, on the other hand, the PEO chains are released and the serum proteins can adsorb. For the PEO-poly(lactide) block copolymers discussed above, the polymer is strongly anchored at hydrophobic particle surfaces when the poly(lactide) moiety is intact, which efficiently prevents serum proteins from adsorbing. On degradation of the poly(lactide) block, however, the polymer does no longer adsorb as extensively and strongly at the surface, and hence is not capable of reducing the protein adsorption (Figure 10.11). Hence, opsonization and RES uptake of colloidal drug carriers stabilized by such polymers will result from this degradation.

Since the circulation time of intravenously administered colloidal drug carriers is rather critically dependent on PEO-chains present on the surface, triggering colloidal drug carriers with such detachable polymer coatings may be

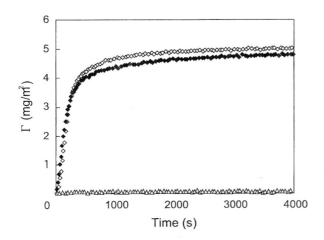

FIGURE 10.11   Adsorption Γ of fibrinogen at a hydrophobic surface from phosphate buffer at 25°C without copolymer (open diamonds), and with adsorbed intact (triangles) or extensively degraded (filled diamonds) $E_{39}L_5$. (Redrawn from Muller et al., J. Colloid Interface Sci. 2000, 228, 326.)

obtained also by other methods, e.g., through incorporation of a disulfide-linked PEO-phospholipid conjugate in liposomes. Such systems offer advantages compared to degradable polymer coatings in that the triggering from stability/circulation to destabilization can be tailored rather straightforwardly by different stability of the linker group between the PEO chain and the hydrophobic domain. In particular, this is interesting from the perspective of a pH-dependent coating, which will allow long circulation in the bloodstream, but which will come off, e.g., on passage through a cancer tissue, where the pH is frequently slightly lower, thereby offering a targeting mechanism. Similarly, pH-dependent detachment of stabilizing PEO chains may offer a mechanism for pH-dependent DNA release in gene therapy (cf. Chapter 4).

As discussed in Chapter 2, block copolymer micelles offer opportunities in intravenous drug delivery, e.g., in the treatment of tumors, or in targeting to selected tissues or cell types. Also here, biodegradable polymers may be used in order to obtain a degradation-induced transition, e.g., from long-circulating micelles containing solubilized drugs to a disintegrated system, thereby resulting in a localized burst release of the drug at low pH, or some other suitable condition. Note, however, that also for such systems, emboli formation may be a real risk. As an illustration of this, Figure 10.12 shows the particle size for a micellar solution of $E_{39}L_{20}$ as a function of the state of degradation of the poly(lactide)

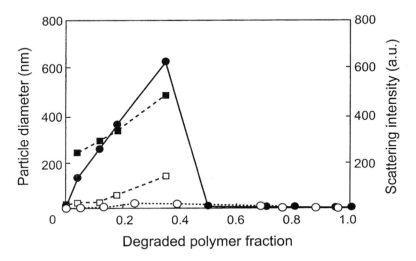

FIGURE 10.12   Particle size (squares) and scattering intensity (circles) of solutions of $E_{39}L_5$ (open) and $E_{39}L_{20}$ (filled) as a function of the degree of degradation of the poly(lactide) block. (Redrawn from Muller et al., J. Colloid Interface Sci. 2001, 236, 116.)

block. For the intact copolymer, small micelles are formed, while for extensively degraded copolymers, only the PEO homopolymer and lactic acid residues are present. At intermediate degradation of the poly(lactide) block, on the other hand, large particles are formed by long blocks of poorly soluble poly(lactide). In comparison, the $E_{39}L_5$ copolymer does not generate as long insoluble poly(lactide) blocks on degradation, and hence less such particle formation occurs. Again, care should be employed when using biodegradable polymers in intravenous drug delivery.

Biodegradable polymer gels are useful, e.g., for oral, buccal, topical, ocular, nasal, and vaginal drug delivery. Gel systems are frequently preferred in these applications due to suitable rheological properties and bioadhesion. Biodegradation of such systems, in turn, offers advantages related to ease of removal or lack of need of removal, and sustained release. Considering the advantageous properties of PEO and PEO-containing copolymers in many drug delivery applications, as well as the general advantages with biodegradable systems, biodegradable gels from functional PEOs offer particularly interesting possibilities (Figure 10.13).

By varying both the nature of the labile link and the architecture of the PEO, different gel dissolution times may be obtained (Table 10.4).

An area where biodegradable gels, and notably biodegradable polysaccharide gels, are useful is colon drug delivery. The main reason for this is that the fermentation of polysaccharide carriers caused by microbial enzymes in the large intestine may be used to obtain efficient controlled release formulations. Examples where such formulations are of interest include, e.g., the treatment of Crohn's

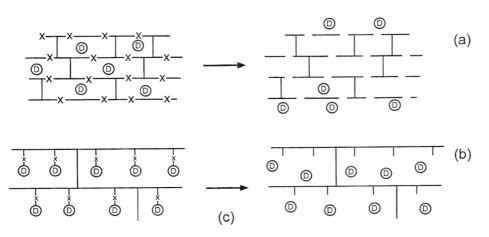

FIGURE 10.13 Schematic illustration of degradation of a gel containing physically entrapped (a) and covalently bound (b) drugs *D*.

TABLE 10.4 Degradation of PEO-Ester-Based Gels at pH 7 and 37°C

	$t_{1/2}$(days)	Dissolution time	
		4-arm PEO	8-arm PEO
Proprionic acid ester	43	20–30	60–70
Carboxymethylated ester	4	2–3	5–7

Source: Data from Zao et al., in Harris et al., eds., Poly(ethylene glycol)—Chemistry and Biological Applications, ACS Symp. Ser. 680, 1998.

disease, ulcerative colitis, spastic colon, constipation, and colon cancer. Moreover, colon administration is also promising for systemic absorption of, e.g., peptides and proteins, which are extensively degraded in the gastrointestinal tract (Table 10.5).

A number of polymer systems are relevant in this context, e.g., coatings by amylose, cyclodextrins, galactomannan or pectin, as well as matrices formed by, e.g., chondroitin sulfate, dextran, pectin, or galactomannan. Just to provide one example, Figure 10.14 shows results on degradation of dextran and degradation-induced drug release for this system.

Another way to control the enzymatic degradation rate and drug release rate is addition of an enzyme inhibitor to the drug formulation. In particular, an approach here is to chemically modify the polymer with an inhibitor, and to control the degradation rate by the concentration and type of inhibitor on the polymer chain (Figure 10.15).

TABLE 10.5 Drugs of Interest in Colon-Specific Drug Delivery

Indication	Drug
Colonic diseases	
Crohn's	Anti-inflammatory agents
Ulcerative colitis	Anti-inflammatory agents
Spastic colon	Anticholinergics
Colorectal diseases	
Constipation	Laxatives
Cancer	Chemotherapeutic agents
Systemic absorption	Peptides, proteins, oligonucleotides
Immunization	Vaccines

Source: From Hovgaard et al., Crit. Rev. Ther. Drug Carrier Syst. 1996, 13, 185.

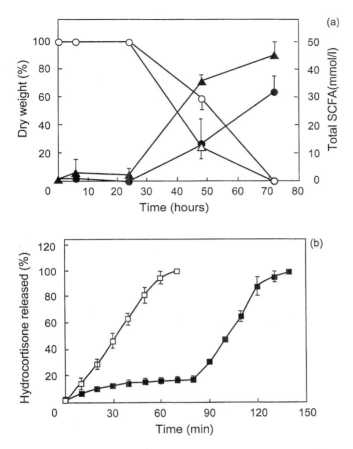

FIGURE 10.14   (a) Degradation, as indicated by loss in dry weight, of dextran hydrogels in a human colonic fermentation model. Results are shown in the form of remaining dry weight (open symbols) and the production of short chain fatty acids (SCFA) (filled symbols) at a dextran gel cross-linking concentration of 4.0% (triangles) and 5.9% (circles). (b) Enzyme-triggered release of hydrocortisone from swollen dextran hydrogels at pH 5.4 and 37°C after addition of enzyme at 80 min (filled symbols) compared with the release in the presence of enzyme at 0 min (open symbols). (Redrawn from Simonsen et al., Eur. J. Pharm. Sci. 1995, 3, 329 (a), and Brønsted et al., STP Pharma Sci. 1995, 5, 65 (b).)

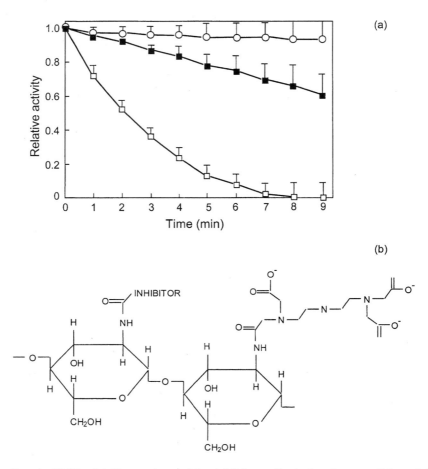

FIGURE 10.15 (a) Comparison of the inhibitory effect of carboxypeptidase A for EDTA-modified chitosan (circles), DTPA-modified chitosan (filled squares), and in the absence of inhibitor-modified chitosan (open squares). (b) Structure of the chitosan-inhibitor conjugate. (Redrawn from Bernkop-Schnürch, Int. J. Pharm. 2000, 194, 1.)

As discussed in Chapter 8, analogous effects were obtained on the release of indomethacin from a calcium pectate gel in the absence and presence pectinolytic enzyme known to be present in the colonic region (Figure 8.42). Together, these examples illustrate that drug release to the colon may be controlled by the stability of the matrix to enzymatic degradation, and that a specific targeting to the colon or large intestine can be obtained by this approach.

As discussed in Chapter 9, biodegradable particles have been found to be promising as drug delivery vehicles, not the least in relation to oral drug delivery. Particular focus in this context has been paid to oral vaccines. From a delivery point of view, particle encapsulation facilitates a successful vaccination through the oral route, since it allows a way to circumvent exposure of the material used for immunization, e.g., peptides, proteins, cells, and viruses, to the harsh conditions in the stomach, thereby reducing their degradation. The polymer particles may also be beneficial for immunization by acting as adjuvants, and by being taken up by Peyer's patches, thereby obtaining a beneficial localization effect.

Although a number of different particle systems may be used for oral vaccination, particularly biodegradable poly(lactide), poly(glycolide) or their copolymers are interesting in this context since they are taken up sufficiently efficient by Peyer's patches, since they are readily biodegradable, and since the resulting degradation products are essentially nontoxic and readily resorbable. Analogous to other forms of biodegradable polymers, the degradation of polymer particles depends on a range of parameters. In particular, the polymer structure and composition are prime parameters for controlling the degradation rate and drug release. However, the particle size and size distribution also affect the degradation rate. In particular, the degradation rate, and consequent drug release, has been found to increase with a decreasing particle size. This is expected, since smaller particles is equivalent to a larger surface area, which favours hydrolytic degradation (Figure 10.16).

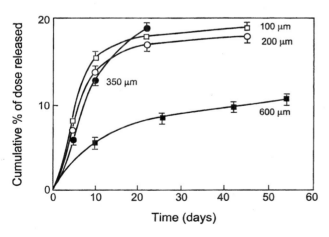

FIGURE 10.16   Release of naltrexone from biodegradable polymer particles of different size. (Redrawn from Yolles et al., in Juliano, ed., Drug Delivery Systems—Characteristics and Biomedical Applications, Oxford University Press, 1980.)

Biodegradable polymers for drug delivery are generally chosen such that the degradation products are essentially harmless, and ideally naturally occuring in the human metabolism. Sometimes, however, biodegradation may result also in negative effects. One such example is the oxidative cleavage which may occur for PEO in the presence of light and oxygen. Although carboxyl groups tend to be the end product after oxidative cleavage, sometimes aldehydes are generated, which may have irritating or even toxic side effects. In pharmaceutical development work, this must be considered by following the metabolic fate of both the drug and the drug carrier.

10.2 BIODEGRADATION OF PHOSPHOLIPIDS

From the perspective of drug delivery, biodegradation of lipids, either chemically or enzymatically, is important since this affects the structure and stability of emulsions, microemulsions, liquid crystalline phases, and dispersed lipid particles. This, in turn, may have implications for the drug release rate and other drug delivery aspects for such systems. Of particular importance in this context is the enzymatic degradation of glycerides or phospholipids through the action of lipases and phospholipases.

The enzymatic degradation rate in lipid and phospholipid systems depends on a range of factors, including the nature of the lipid, the nature of the enzyme, the enzyme concentration, but also on temperature, pH, salt concentration, and many other factors. Here, only a few of these aspects will be discussed in brief.

The effect of lipase addition on the leakage of an encapsulated substance from phosphatidylcholine liposomes is illustrated in Figure 10.17. In these experiments, carboxyfluorescein was incorporated in the aqueous compartment of the liposomes, and its release followed by monitoring the release-related decrease in self-quenching (Chapter 4). As can be seen, addition of lipoprotein lipase causes the encapsulated substance to be released to an extent which depends on the enzyme concentration. The higher the lipoprotein lipase concentration, the faster the phospholipid degradation, and the faster the occurrence of packing defects resulting from the degradation. Therefore, the higher the enzyme concentration, the faster the release of the encapsulated substance.

A central parameter for the rate of enzymatic degradation of phospholipids and glycerides in relation to drug delivery is the length and saturation of the hydrocarbon chains. In general, the degradation rate increases with a decreasing length and an increasing degree of unsaturation of the hydrocarbon chains (Figure 10.18). This is probably due to a combination of packing effects, phospholipid layer cohesion and fluidity. Since the longer and saturated lipids pack more effectively, display larger cohesion, and a decreased fluidity compared to the shorter and unsaturated ones, the lipase action is precluded, hence resulting in a decreased degradation rate.

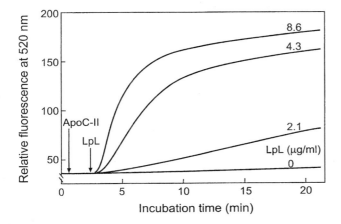

FIGURE 10.17   Effect of lipoprotein lipase (LpL) concentration on the fluorescence from 6-carboxyfluorescein due to its release from phosphatidylcholine liposomes. The lipoprotein lipase concentrations used (μg/ml) are indicated. (Redrawn from Fugman et al., Biochim. Biophys. Acta 1984, 795, 191.)

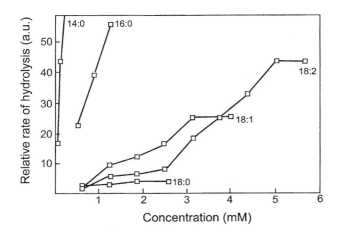

FIGURE 10.18   Relative rate of hydrolysis of sonicated diacyl phosphatidylcholine of different chain length and saturation by phospholipase A_2. (Redrawn from Le-Kim et al., Adv. Prostagland. Thromb. Res. 1978, 3, 31.)

The presence of cholesterol in phospholipid layers reduces the enzyme-catalyzed hydrolysis of gel phase phospholipids. With an increasing concentration of cholesterol, the degradation rate is successively reduced, and at high cholesterol concentrations it is virtually absent (Figure 10.19). The origin of this effect is unclear at present, but may be related to a reduced adsorption capacity of the lipase at the lipid surface in analogy to the decreased adsorption observed for serum lipoproteins (Figure 4.8).

The effects of pH on the enzymatic degradation of lipids and phospholipids is a somewhat complicated issue, notably depending rather strongly on the nature of the enzyme system. All enzymes display a pH-dependent activity, however, and at very high and very low pH, the activity is generally low due to destruction of the protein native conformation and other factors. As an illustration of this, Figure 10.20 shows the pH-dependent hydrolysis of phosphatidylcholine vesicles by phospholipase D.

Phospholipids also display a pH-dependent chemical hydrolysis. In particular, phospholipids display a similar pH-dependent hydrolysis as many esters, i.e., increased degradation at low and high pH due to acid-and base-catalyzed hydrolysis (Figure 10.21). Also, hydrolysis is enhanced at elevated temperature.

Although the examples on the effects of hydrolysis of lipids and phospholipids in the present discussion have been taken from liposome systems, analogous effects occur also in liquid crystalline phases, lipid nanoparticles, and other lipid/phospholipid structures, causing system-dependent effects, e.g., re-

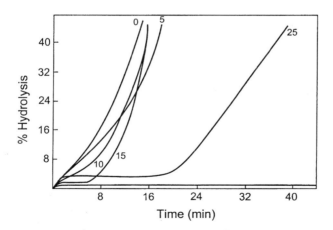

FIGURE 10.19 Effect of cholesterol on the hydrolysis of DPPC-cholesterol mixtures by phospholipase A_2. The mol% of cholesterol is indicated in each curve. (Redrawn from Tinker et al., Can. J. Biochem. 1978, 56, 552.)

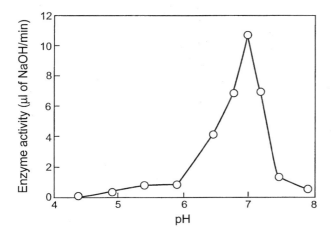

FIGURE 10.20   Effect of pH on the activity of phospholipase D on phosphatidylcholine large unilamellar vesicles. (Redrawn from Kim et al., Bull. Korean Chem. Soc. 1992, 13, 381.)

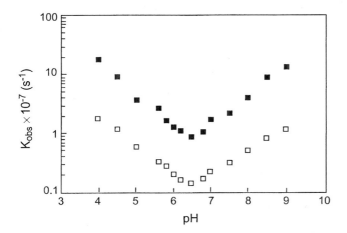

FIGURE 10.21   Effect of pH on the hydrolysis rate K_{obs} of phosphatidylcholine liposomes at 40°C (open symbols) and 70°C (filled symbols). (Redrawn from Grit et al., J. Pharm. Sci. 1993, 82, 362.)

TABLE 10.6   Effect of Degradation Time on the Liquid
Crystalline Phases Formed by the Monoolein/Water/
Sodium Oleate System (50.7/42.2/7.1 wt%) After
Lipase Addition

Time (h)	Space group
0	Ia3d (bicontinuous cubic)
1	Ia3d (bicontinuous cubic)
4	Reversed-hexagonal
13	Reversed-hexagonal
16	Reversed-hexagonal
20	Hexagonal + Fd3m (reversed micellar cubic)
54	Fd3m (reversed micellar cubic)

Source: From Caboi et al., Langmuir, in press.

lating to structure, stability, and drug release. As an illustration of the latter, Table 10.6 shows results on the effect of lipase action on a liquid crystalline phase formed by monoolein/sodium oleate/water. As can be seen, lipase-mediated hydrolysis of monoolein results in a progression of the liquid crystalline phases formed in the order bicontinuous cubic → reversed hexagonal → reversed micellar cubic. This could be expected from simple packing considerations, since an increased degradation results in an increasing amount of sodium oleate (and glycerol), and a decreasing amount of monoolein. An analogous progression can be observed simply by increasing the sodium oleate concentration in monoolein samples.

BIBLIOGRAPHY

Bruch, S. D., Controlled Drug Delivery, CRC Press, Boca Raton, 1983.

Eldridge, J. H., R. M. Gilley, J. K. Staas, Z. Moldoveanu, J. A. Meulbroek, T. R. Tice, Biodegradable microspheres: vaccine delivery system for oral immunization, Curr. Topics Microbiol. Immunol. 146:59–66 (1989).

Hovgaard, L., H. Brøndsted, Current applications of polysaccharides in colon targeting, Crit. Rev. Ther. Drug Carrier Syst. 13:185–223 (1996).

Hwang, S.-J., H. Park, K. Park, Gastric retentive drug-delivery systems, Crit. Rev. Ther. Drug Carrier Syst. 15:243–284 (1998).

Juliano, R. L., ed., Drug Delivery Systems: Characteristics and Biomedical Applications, Oxford University Press, 1980.

O'Hagan, D. T., in D. T. O'Hagan, ed., Novel Delivery Systems: Oral Vaccines, CRC Press, Boca Raton, 1994.

Park, K., W. S. W. Shalaby, Biodegradable Hydrogels for Drug Delivery, Technomic, 1993.

Rubinstein, A., A. Sintov, Biodegradable polymeric matrices with potential specificity to the large intestine, in D. R. Friend, ed., Oral Colon-Specific Drug Delivery, CRC Press, Boca Raton, 1992.

Tarcha, P. J., ed., Polymers for Controlled Drug Delivery, CRC Press, Boca Raton, 1991.

11

Drying of Formulations Containing Surfactants and Polymers

There are numerous instances where drug delivery systems have to be further processed in order to obtain the complete drug formulation. In general, dry formulations are preferred when sufficient storage stability with liquid formulations is difficult or impossible to reach from a chemical and/or physicochemical perspective. For example, this is the case with essentially all protein and peptide drugs, which are generally not sufficiently stable when stored in an aqueous solution. In other cases, dry formulations are preferred for practical or patient compliance reasons. The latter is the case, e.g., with many tablet formulations used primarily for oral administration. Irrespective of the reason for the drying ("lyophilization"), however, it is important to note and control the effects of the lyophilization on the properties of both the drug and the drug delivery system. In this context, surfactants and other surface active compounds, such as polymers and proteins, offer possibilities which have only recently started to be investigated in a reasonably systematic way. In what follows, a few brief examples will be provided to illustrate the use of surfactants, polymers, and proteins in the context of lyophilization of drug delivery systems. In particular, the relationship between the lyophilization and the properties of these compounds in solution and at interfaces is considered. However, no discussion of solid state properties of these systems, or processes less straightforwardly connected to surface activity and self-assembly (e.g., crystallization and precipitation) is provided, since this is considered to be outside the scope of the present volume.

11.1 SPRAY-DRYING

11.1.1 Spray-Drying of Aqueous Protein Solutions

Spray-drying is a method for providing dry powders, which is based on spraying a liquid into hot air through an atomizer, thereby causing the solvent, generally water, to evaporate, and the dissolved material to form solid particles (Figure 11.1).

While spray-drying has found extensive use in food and biotechnical applications, it is generally less extensively used in pharmaceutical applications, and in particular for protein and peptide drugs. One of the reasons for this is the use of high-temperature drying air (typically 180°C at the inlet), which risks denaturing or degrading these substances. It should be remembered, however, that evaporation prevents the spray-dried sample from reaching this temperature. Instead, as long as evaporation proceeds, a cooling effect is achieved, which prevents the temperature of the drying material to reach above the wet bulb temperature of the drying air. Only in the last stages of the drying, when the water activity is low, can the temperature of the particles rise above this temperature. Also here, however, it will still be significantly lower than the air leaving the spray dryer. In quantitative terms, this means that the powder will typically reach a temperature of maximum 40–45°C, and then only for a very short time (typically milliseconds). Considering this, also biological systems relatively unstable toward ther-

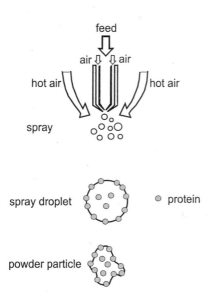

FIGURE 11.1   Schematic illustration of spray-drying of a protein solution.

mal degradation and/or denaturation should be possible to spray-dry with retained biological activity.

Another detrimental factor in spray-drying of proteins and peptides is the presence of a relatively large air-water interface. Due to the surface activity of many proteins and peptides, these will generally adsorb at this surface, and frequently lose biological activity due to surface-induced conformational changes (Figure 11.1). In order to prevent this from happening, surfactants may be added to the drying solution. With the proper choice of surfactant, this can effectively compete with the protein/peptide for the air-water interface, thereby reducing the amount of protein at the surface, and hence also the extent of surface-induced protein/peptide denaturation (Figure 11.2).

The choice of surfactant involves consideration not only of its surface activity and cmc but also of the interaction between the surfactant and the protein. As discussed in Chapter 8, surfactants frequently interact with polymers and proteins, and in some cases cause a denaturation of the latter. Therefore, nonionic surfactants are best suited as surface blocking agents in spray-drying, since they are highly surface active, have a low cmc (and therefore reaching saturation adsorption at low concentrations, requiring only small addition), and do not interact extensively with proteins. Note, however, that if oligo(ethylene oxide)-based surfactants are chosen, they should not have a too low cloud point, since this may cause phase separation in the drying liquid and preclude protein encapsulation in the powder.

11.1.2 Spray-Drying of O/W Emulsions

Encapsulation is relevant for powder processing and manufacturing not only for preserving the biological activity of protein and peptide drugs. It is of interest also for reducing oxidative degradation of hydrophobic drugs, for increasing the powder wettability and dissolution rate, etc. Particular emphasis in relation to this has been placed on o/w emulsions. Through the use of o/w emulsions oil-soluble substances may be encapsulated in a hydrophilic matrix, frequently consisting of carbohydrate (Figure 11.3). In analogy to this, hydrophilic substances can be incorporated in a lipid matrix, which may be of interest, e.g., for lipase-mediated release of protein and peptide drugs, e.g., from a gelatin capsule.

Through the protective properties of the carbohydrate matrix, the emulsion droplets are kept separate from each other, thereby preventing emulsion coalescence, and facilitating emulsion regeneration on redissolution of the powder. As illustrated in Table 11.1 for an o/w emulsion containing griseofulvin some variation in the droplet size of the redissolved emulsions is obtained with both the nature of the carbohydrate and the nature of the oil phase. Also, there is a relatively minor growth in the emulsion droplet size on drying and storage. Overall, however, roughly the same droplet size is obtained after spray-drying and dissolution as before.

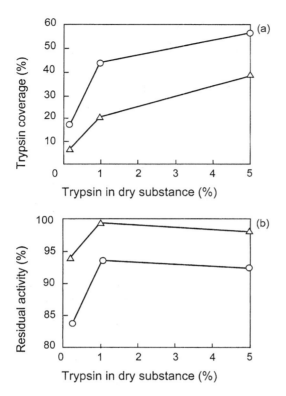

FIGURE 11.2   (a) Surface coverage of trypsin in spray-dried powders composed of lactose and trypsin (lactose/trypsin = 99/1). The overrepresentation of the protein at the powder surface is considerable in the absence of surfactant (circles). Addition of a surfactant (Tween 80) prior to spray-drying reduces the overrepresentation of protein at the surface due to preferential adsorption of the surfactant at the air-water interface of the spray droplets (triangles). (b) Residual activity of trypsin after spray-drying of trypsin/lactose in the presence (triangles) and absence (circles) of surfactant. (Redrawn from Millqvist-Fureby et al., Int. J. Pharm. 1999, 188, 243.)

    In order to reach a successful encapsulation of hydrophobic compounds in powders through the use of o/w emulsions, surface active compounds are added to allow a small droplet size, but also to stabilize the emulsions toward flocculation and coalescence. However, the presence of surface active compounds, e.g., surfactants, surface active polymers or proteins, is beneficial also for the reason that these compounds adsorb at the air-water interface, thereby precluding the adsorption of oil droplets, and contributing to an efficient encapsulation. As be-

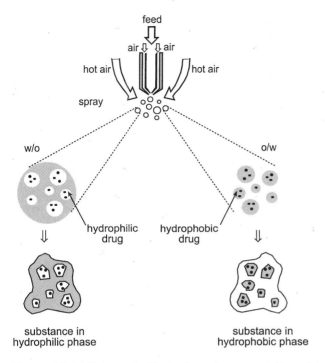

FIGURE 11.3 Schematic illustration of encapsulation of hydrophobic/hydrophilic substance in a powder through spray-drying of o/w and w/o emulsions, respectively.

fore, the surface of the powder particles is dominated by the most surface active compound (Figure 11.4).

In general, spray-drying results in amorphous powder particles. Depending on the matrix carbohydrate, however, recrystallization may occur on storage in humid atmosphere for crystallizing carbohydrates. As a result of this, the oil droplets are expelled from the particle matrix and enriched at the powder particle surface, which can be seen in Figure 11.4 as an increase in the relative oil content at the powder surface. The extent of this oil expulsion depends on the extent and nature of the recrystallization. Since the extent of recrystallization can be controlled by the carbohydrate (mixture) the oil expulsion on humid storage can be reduced by use of a noncrystallizing carbohydrate (mixture).

The encapsulation efficiency of powders based on o/w emulsions affects numerous performance parameters, including oxidative sensitivity of labile drugs, drug evaporation and other types of material loss, and redissolution properties. Regarding the latter, the importance of oil expulsion on humid storage and recrys-

TABLE 11.1   Droplet Size of O/W Emulsions Containing Griseofulvin Before
Spray-Drying and After Reconstitution

	Fat	Carrier	Droplet size
Before drying	Soybean oil	Lactose	0.29 µg
	Coconut oil		0.28 µm
	Rapeseed oil		0.28 µm
	Soybean oil	Lactose + malto-dextrine	0.285 µm
	Coconut oil		0.285 µm
	Rapeseed oil		0.30 µm
Reconstituted after storage (dry atmo-sphere)	Soybean oil	Lactose	0.31 µm
	Coconut oil		0.44 µm
	Rapeseed oil		0.37 µm
	Soybean oil	Lactose + malto-dextrine	0.36 µm
	Coconut oil		0.39 µm
	Rapeseed oil		0.35 µm

* The composition of the dry emulsions were 30% fat (griseofulvin content 4 wt% of the oil phase), 28% sodium caseinate and 42% carbohydrate (42% lactose or 34% lactose + 8% maltodextrine). Hardened coconut oil and rapeseed oil were used.
Source: Data from Pedersen et al., Int. J. Pharm. 1998, 171, 257.

tallization of the carbohydrate matrix is illustrated in Figure 11.5. Thus, on recrystallization and following oil expulsion to the powder surface, the powder particles are less easy to wet and dissolve, resulting in overall much deteriorated dissolution properties. For lyophilized drug delivery systems which should be used after reconstitution, both the safety and efficacy of the therapy depend critically on a complete reconstitution, and therefore it is important to find formulations which allow a fast and complete dissolution (i.e., which do not crystallize extensively on storage).

11.1.3   Spray-Drying of Aqueous Polymeric Two-Phase Systems

Encapsulation in pharmaceutical and other powders can be achieved also through the use of aqueous polymeric two-phase systems. Such systems are frequently formed by solutions containing two uncharged polymers, and in the case of segregative phase separation consists of one phase rich in one of the polymers, and one phase rich in the other (Figure 11.6; see also Chapter 8).

It has been found that some aqueous polymeric two-phase systems, such as those formed by PEO/dextran/water and PVP/dextran/water, may provide efficient partitioning of various biomolecules and other biological entities (Figure

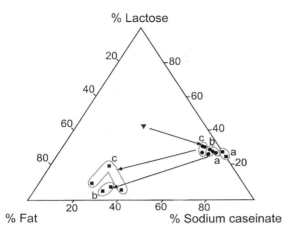

FIGURE 11.4 Surface chemical composition of spray-dried powders determined by ESCA. The composition of the starting material is illustrated by the filled triangle, whereas circles represent the powder surface composition after drying and squares the composition after storage of the powders in a humid atmosphere. (a), (b), and (c) represent samples containing hardened rapeseed oil, soybean oil, and hardened coconut oil, respectively. Note the overrepresentation of the surface active stabilizer (casein) at the powder surface, as well as the surface enrichment of fat after recrystallization of the carbohydrate matrix. (Redrawn from Pedersen et al., Int. J. Pharm. 1998, 171, 257.)

11.6). The partitioning of biomolecules between the two polymer phases depends on a range of parameters, including the nature and molecular weight of the polymers used and the nature of the biomolecule. The important thing for the present discussion, however, is that a strong partitioning toward one of the phases may be obtained, e.g., through the design of the biomolecule, the choice of the two-phase system, or addition of so-called affinity ligands (often surfactantlike compounds), the role of which is to shift the partitioning toward one of the phases (Figure 11.7).

Due to their high water content and the low interfacial tension, aqueous polymeric two-phase systems may be used for mild separation and bioprocessing of proteins, cells, and other types of sensitive biological matter, and also for the separation of sensitive self-assembled structures, such as liposomes.

On stirring of an aqueous two-phase system, one of the water-rich polymer phases will be dispersed in the other, essentially yielding a water-in-water emulsion. By choosing the overall composition of the system, the phase containing the biomolecule may be made to be the dispersed one. This is exemplified in Figure 11.8 for the dextran-PVP system.

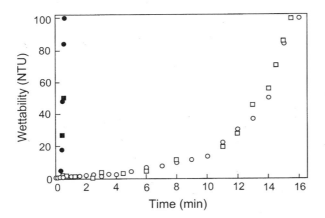

FIGURE 11.5   Wettability as a function of time for spray-dried powders containing an o/w emulsion and lactose. Powders stored dry (i.e., in the absence of recrystallization of lactose) and in 75% relative humidity (i.e., in the presence of recrystallization of lactose) for 3 days are indicated by filled and open symbols, respectively. Duplicate samples are shown. (Redrawn from Fäldt, Thesis, 1995.)

Given the shape of the phase diagram for segregative phase separation, where the tendency for phase separation increases with a decreasing water content, it is clear that polymers which phase separate in a solvent are likely to do so also on successively increasing the polymer concentration through solvent evaporation, e.g., in film casting or spray-drying. Therefore, aqueous polymeric two-phase systems, with one phase containing the substance to be encapsulated dispersed in the other, provide possibilities for encapsulation after spray-drying. The encapsulation, in turn, reduces the exposure of the biomolecules to the spray-droplet surface. Since the air/liquid interface has a high interfacial tension which could cause denaturation, while the interfacial tension between the two aqueous phases is low, this could be expected to be beneficial for the activity retention of also complex and sensitive biological systems (Figure 11.9).

11.2   FREEZE-DRYING

While spray-drying is a relatively simple process from a surface chemical perspective, freeze-drying is considerably more complex. In the latter process, the sample to be lyophilized is frozen, followed by sublimation of the solvent (typically water) under vacuum and a gradually increasing temperature. Without doubt, freeze-drying is the lyophilization process used most extensively in pharmaceutical formulations, and particularly so for protein and peptide drugs.

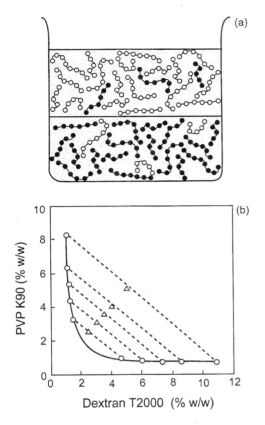

FIGURE 11.6   (a) Schematic illustration of segregative phase separation in a system containing two polymers in a common solvent. (b) Phase diagram for the two-phase system composed of dextran and polyvinylpyrolidone (PVP) in water at room temperature. Triangles and circles represent the overall composition and the composition of the separate phases, respectively. Dashed lines indicate tie lines. (Redrawn from Millqvist-Fureby, J. Colloid Interface Sci. 2000, 225, 54.)

As with spray-drying, lyophilization through freeze-drying risks deactivating protein and peptide drugs through concentration-induced aggregation, deactivation induced through adsorption at various interfaces (notably the ice-water interface), and exposure of the active compound to air through incomplete encapsulation after completed lyophilization. As with spray-drying, various compounds, notably carbohydrates and polyalcohols, are used as "protectants." The role of these protectants is probably manifold, but still not very well known. For

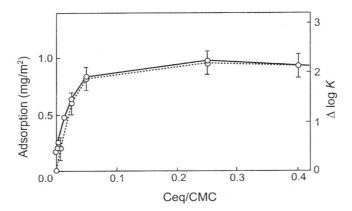

FIGURE 11.7   Adsorption of a PEO-fatty acid ester ($C_{18:2}$-EO_{151}) at phosphatidylcholine surface (solid line) as a function of concentration c_{eq}, and its effects on the partitioning K of the corresponding liposomes in a PEO/dextran/water two-phase system (dashed line). (Redrawn from Van Alstine et al., Langmuir 1997, 13, 4044.)

example, during the freezing process, any solute is concentrated, which may result in an aggregation difficult to reverse on dissolution of the powders. Cryoprotectants may help reducing this effect through effectively "diluting" molecules with a tendency for aggregate formation, e.g., proteins. Cryoprotectants may also help maintaining pH during the freeze-drying process, again reducing aggregation and following deactivation. They may also slow down phase separation during freezing due to their typically high concentration, which results in a substantial

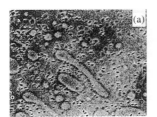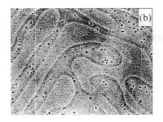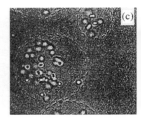

FIGURE 11.8   Phase separation at various PVP/dextran ratios as observed by light microscopy. The dextran-rich phase is identified by the presence of *E. faecium* cells, which partition quantitatively to this phase. Samples were mixed by inversion immediately before taking a small sample for microscopy. (a), (b), and (c) represent a PVP/dextran ratio of 30/70, 40/60, and 70/30 w/w, respectively. Note that sample (a) is dextran-continuous, sample (b) bicontinuous, and sample (c) PVP continuous. (Redrawn from Millqvist-Fureby, J. Colloid Interface Sci. 2000, 225, 54.)

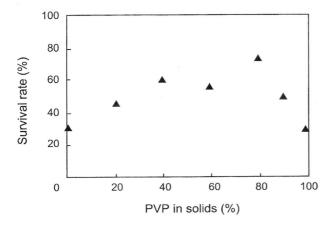

FIGURE 11.9 Survival rate after spray-drying of *E. faecium* in PVP/dextran/water polymeric two-phase systems. Note the increased survival on encapsulating the bacteria in dextran droplets (i.e., on increasing the PVP concentration from 0% to 20–40%). (Redrawn from Millqvist-Fureby et al., J. Colloid Interface Sci. 2000, 225, 54.)

viscosity. Probably the most important role of cryoprotectants in freeze-drying, however, is that they replace hydration water molecules after lyophilization. Since the activity of proteins may depend rather critically on its hydration, complete dehydration of proteins may result in deactivation. Particularly with carbohydrates, however, the solvation water may be replaced and the protein structure and activity retained after lyophilization.

Another interesting aspect in this context is the occurrence of ice-water interfaces during the freeze-drying process. In analogy to other interfaces, such as the air-water interface in spray-drying discussed above, protein adsorption at the ice-water interface may potentially result in surface-induced conformational changes and a consequent activity loss. Unfortunately, adsorption at the ice-water interface is experimentally very difficult to investigate, and not surprisingly, therefore, little is known about the real importance of this effect. However, a clear correlation has been found between freeze-induced and surface-induced denaturation for a series of proteins (Figure 11.10). Although no direct proof of surface-induced protein deactivation at the ice-water interface is provided, this still suggests that the adsorption at the ice-water interface may be detrimental for protein activity in freeze-drying.

Given the above, one would expect that activity preservation of proteins during freeze drying to benefit from formation of an amorphous glass state during lyophilization, thereby precluding material redistribution through adsorption or

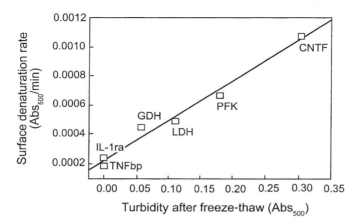

FIGURE 11.10 Correlation between freeze-induced denaturation (inferred from the turbidity of the protein solution after freeze-thaw) and surface-induced denaturation (Teflon) for a series of proteins. (Redrawn from Chang et al., J. Pharm. Sci. 1996, 85, 1325.)

concentration. This, in turn, puts requirements on both the freezing rate, the freezing temperature, and the nature and concentration of the solute.

During freezing of an aqueous solution, the concentration of all solutes will increase as a result of ice formation. If the temperature is sufficiently low, this solute concentration eventually results in a transition from a viscous solution to a glass state. The water content of this glass state depends on temperature, more specifically decreasing with increasing temperature. The maximum temperature where this transition can occur without concentration-induced crystallization is generally referred to as T'_g. Considering this, keeping the temperature below this temperature for as much of the freeze-drying process as possible is expected to be advantageous (Figure 11.11).

The occurrence of material reorganization above T'_g as a result of concentration-induced crystallization or adsorption at the ice-water interface can be investigated by first freezing a sample fast to well below T'_g, and then taking the sample up to a temperature above T'_g but below the ice melting temperature, and keeping it there for a defined time prior to drying, and comparing the powder surface composition to that obtained for samples stored well below T'_g all the time until drying.

As can be seen in Tables 11.2 and 11.3, such "annealing" above T'_g prior to drying results in an increased surface concentration of both BSA and trypsin for a range of carbohydrates, the latter with T'_g values spanning over rather wide temperatures. Quantitatively, the protein concentration at the freeze-dried powder

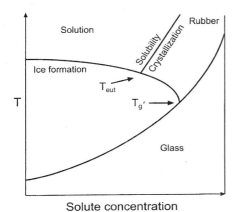

FIGURE 11.11 Schematic phase diagram of an aqueous system showing ice formation, solute crystallization, eutectic point, and glass transition during freezing. (Redrawn from Wang, Int. J. Pharm. 2000, 203, 1.)

surface is much higher than expected from the average composition. This clearly illustrates that above T'_g, significant material redistribution occurs as a consequence of ice crystal formation and growth.

Interestingly, there is little effect of annealing on the degree of crystallinity, except in the case of sucrose, for which an annealing-induced crystallization is observed. In the other cases, the increased surface concentration after annealing

TABLE 11.2 Comparison of Surface Protein Content of Freeze-Dried BSA/Carbohydrate (1/99 W/W) Powders Obtained from ESCA*

Excipient	Processing	BSA coverage (%)
Mannitol	Reference	5
Mannitol	Annealing	5
Lactose	Reference	<2.5
Lactose	Annealing	6
α-Cyclodextrin	Reference	<2.5
α-Cyclodextrin	Annealing	17

* Freeze-dried samples were obtained by rapid freezing to −28°C, followed by annealing at −5°C for 48 hours, and subsequent cooling to −28°C prior to drying. The reference samples were stored at −28°C for 48 hours instead of the annealing period.
Source: Data from Millqvist-Fureby et al., Int. J. Pharm. 1999, 191, 103.

TABLE 11.3   Surface Coverage and Relative Activity of Freeze-Dried
Trypsin/Carbohydrate (1/99 W/W) Powders*

Sample	Trypsin coverage (%)	Relative activity (%)	Crystallinity (%)
Lactose, reference	<2	81	Amorphous
Lactose, annealed	5.0	81	Amorphous
Lactose/Tween 80, reference	2.2	65	Amorphous
Lactose/Tween 80, annealed	5.2	68	Amorphous
Sucrose, reference	2.0	63	42
Sucrose, annealed	6.1	58	63
Dextrin, reference	6.5	74	Amorphous
Dextrin, annealed	7.5	74	Amorphous
Mannitol, reference	10.5	73	63
Mannitol, annealed	16.2	77	65
α-Cyclodextrin, reference	3.3	92	Amorphous
α-Cyclodextrin, annealed	<2	90	Amorphous

* Samples were rapidly frozen at $-28°C$, followed by annealing at $-5°C$ for 48 h, and subsequent cooling to $-28°C$ prior to freeze-drying. Reference samples were stored at $-28°C$ for 48 h instead of annealing treatment.
Source: Data from Millqvist-Fureby et al., Int. J. Pharm. 1999, 191, 103.

therefore results from adsorption at the ice–water interface. Furthermore, in the case of trypsin for these particular excipients, there is little activity loss due to the annealing as such, indicating that the surface accumulation of trypsin does not affect its native conformation. This is suggested also by the lack of a positive effect of Tween 80 in the case of lactose. Crystallization-induced reorganizations as those occurring in the case or sucrose, on the other hand, seem to be detrimental for the trypsin activity.

11.3   DRYING OF SELF-ASSEMBLED STRUCTURES

In a similar way that drying, heating, and freezing induce strains on proteins in spray-drying and freeze-drying, drying of self-assembled structures with these methods may be detrimental for the stability and performance of the latter systems. In particular, disperse systems such as liposomes risk undergoing destabilization on drying and dry storage, such that the particle size after drying and dissolution is larger than that prior to drying.

Also analogous to spray-drying and freeze-drying of protein and peptide drugs, the nature of protectants used for drying of self-assemblied systems is important for the result of the drying process. For freeze-drying, this can be understood in a similar way as freeze-drying of proteins. Thus, effective cryoprotection of liposomes should be favored by rapid freezing to a temperature well below T'_g for as long a period as possible during the drying period in order to reduce freeze concentration and following liposome coalescence and destabilization. Also, different protectants have been found to interact with the polar head group of phospholipids, which should affect the liposome stability in both freeze-drying and spray-drying. For spray-drying, it may be necessary to reduce the accumulation of liposomes at the air-water interface, which can be achieved by introduction of a surface-active compound in the drying dispersion or increasing the viscosity of the drying medium through addition of polymer. The important thing in the present context, however, is that liposome systems may be both freeze-dried and spray-dried in such a way that they do not flocculate or coalesce, but rather keep their overall structure (Table 11.4 and Figure 11.12).

A more difficult issue in relation to drying of self-assembled structures such as liposomes is that of retained encapsulation of solubilized drug also during and after drying. Instead, the stresses caused by the drying processes risk to significantly reduce the degree of encapsulation of drugs by such systems after drying (Figure 11.13).

However, having protective agents such as carbohydrates or polyalcohols on both sides of the membrane, i.e., both on the outside and the inside of the liposome, may significantly increase the amount of drug retained by the liposomes after drying (Table 11.5). Since the concentration of such protectants is generally quite high both in freeze-drying and spray-drying, this is most likely

TABLE 11.4 Effects of Various Saccharides and Polyalcohols on the Size of Liposomes Prepared by Egg Phosphatidylcholine Before and After Freeze-Drying

	D (nm) before	D (nm) after
Disaccharide		
Trehalose	28 ± 7	30 ± 4
Sucrose	26 ± 5	28 ± 4
Maltose	28 ± 4	32 ± 4
Monosaccharide		
Glucose	28 ± 6	29 ± 4
Mannose	28 ± 4	27 ± 6
Galactose	20 ± 4	21 ± 4
Polyalcohol		
Sorbitol	27 ± 5	37 ± 15
Inositol	26 ± 7	1760 ± 350
Mannitol	28 ± 4	1900 ± 441

Source: Data from Tanaka et al., Chem. Pharm. Bull. 1992, 40, 1.

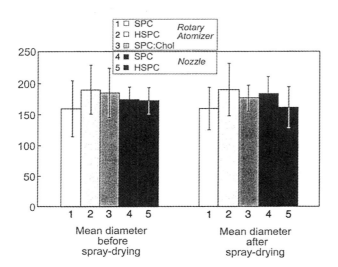

FIGURE 11.12 Effect of spray-drying on the size (in nm) of liposomes containing atropin. Lactose was used as the protectant. SPC, HSPC, and Chol refer to soybean phosphatidylcholine, hydrogenated SPC, and cholesterol, respectively. (Redrawn from Goldbach, et al., Drug Dev. Ind. Pharm. 1993, 19, 2623.)

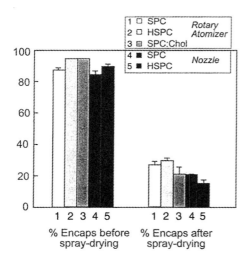

FIGURE 11.13 Encapsulation of atropin in liposomes before and after spray-drying with lactose. (Redrawn from Goldbach et al., Drug Dev. Ind. Pharm. 1993, 19, 2623.)

TABLE 11.5 Effect of Trehalose on Preservation of Vesicle Structure
in the Dry State*

Sample	Drying time (h)	$^{22}Na^+$ retained (%)	Residual water (%)
Trehalose	24	94	5.6
(both sides)	48	84	5.4
	72	84	5.2
Trehalose	24	68	5.4
(outside)	48	49	5.0
	72	17	4.2

* A trehalose concentration of 250 mM was used throughout.
Source: Data from Madden et al., Biochim. Biophys. Acta 1985, 817, 67.

an effect of reducing the osmotic stress over the membrane due to the difference
in protectant concentration on the two sides of the membrane, hence also reducing
leakage over the membrane due to this stress.

BIBLIOGRAPHY

Chang, B. S., B. S. Kendrick, J. F. Carpenter, Surface-induced denaturation of proteins
during freezing and its inhibition by surfactants, J. Pharm. Sci. 85:1325–1330,
1996.

Crowe, J. H., L. M. Crowe, Factors affecting the stability of dry liposomes, Biochim.
Biophys. Acta 939:327–334 (1988).

Giunchedi, P., U. Conte, Spray-drying as a preparation method of microparticulate drug
delivery systems: an overview, STP Pharma Sci. 5:276–290 (1995).

Johnson, K. A., Preparation of peptide and protein powders for inhalation, Adv. Drug
Delivery Rev. 26:3–15 (1997).

Levine, H., L. Slade, Principles of "cryostabilization" technology from structure/property
relationships of carbohydrate/water systems—A review, Cryo-Letts. 9:21–63
(1988).

Maa, Y.-F., C. C. Hsu, Protein denaturation by combined effect of shear and air-liquid
interface, Biotechnol. Bioeng. 54:503–512 (1997).

Maa, Y.-F., P.-A. T. Nguyen, S. W. Hsu, Spray-drying of air-liquid interface sensitive
recombinant human growth hormone, J. Pharm. Sci. 87:152–159 (1988).

Madden, T. H., M. B. Bally, M. J. Hope, P. R. Cullis, H. P. Schieren, A. S. Janoff, Protection of large unilamellar vesicles by trehalose during dehydration: retention of vesicle contents, Biochim. Biophys. Acta 817:67–74 (1985).

Millqvist-Fureby, A., M. Malmsten, B. Bergenståhl, Spray-drying of trypsin—surface
characterisation and activity preservation, Int. J. Pharm. 188:243–253 (1999).

Millqvist-Fureby, A., M. Malmsten, B. Bergenståhl, An aqueous polymer two-phase system as carrier in the spray-drying of biological material, J. Colloid Interface Sci. 225:54–61 (2000).

Millqvist-Fureby, A., M. Malmsten, B. Bergenståhl, Surface characterisation of freeze-dried protein/carbohydrate mixtures, Int. J Pharm. 191, 103–114 (1999).

Nail, S. L., L. A. Gatlin, in K. E. Avis, H. A. Lieberman, and L. Lachman, eds., Pharmaceutical Dosage Forms, vol. 2, Marcel Dekker, New York, 1993.

Pedersen, G. P., P. Fäldt, B. Bergenståhl, H. G. Kristensen, Solid state characterisation of a dry emulsion: a potential drug delivery system, Int. J. Pharm. 171:257–270 (1998).

Wang, W., Lyophilization and development of solid protein pharmaceuticals, Int. J. Pharm. 203:1–60 (2000).

Index